Caries Excavation: Evolution of Treating Cavitated Carious Lesions

Monographs in Oral Science

Vol. 27

Series Editors

A. Lussi Bern
M.A.R. Buzalaf São Paulo

Caries Excavation: Evolution of Treating Cavitated Carious Lesions

Volume Editors

Falk Schwendicke Berlin

Jo Frencken Nijmegen

Nicola Innes Dundee

69 figures, 59 in color, and 19 tables, 2018

KARGER

Basel · Freiburg · Paris · London · New York · Chennai · New Delhi · Bangkok · Beijing · Shanghai · Tokyo · Kuala Lumpur · Singapore · Sydney

Falk Schwendicke
Operative and Preventive Dentistry
Charité – Universitätsmedizin Berlin
Corporate Member of Freie Universität Berlin
Humboldt-Universität zu Berlin
DE–14197Berlin (Germany)

Jo Frencken
Radboud University Medical Centre
Department of Oral Function and Prosthetic Dentistry
NL–6525 AX Nijmegen (The Netherlands)

Nicola Innes
School of Dentistry, University of Dundee
2 Park Place
Dundee DD1 4HR (UK)

Library of Congress Cataloging-in-Publication Data

Names: Schwendicke, Falk, editor. | Frencken, Jo, 1950- editor. | Innes, Nicola, editor.
Title: Caries excavation : evolution of treating cavitated carious lesions / volume editors, Falk Schwendicke, Jo Frencken, Nicola Innes.
Other titles: Monographs in oral science ; v. 27. 0077-0892
Description: Basel ; New York : Karger, 2018. | Series: Monographs in oral science, ISSN 0077-0892 ; vol. 27 | Includes bibliographical references and indexes.
Identifiers: LCCN 2018017608| ISBN 9783318063684 (hbk. : alk. paper) | ISBN 9783318063691 (e-ISBN)
Subjects: | MESH: Dental Caries--therapy | Dental Restoration, Permanent | Pit and Fissure Sealants--therapeutic use
Classification: LCC RK331 | NLM WU 270 | DDC 617.6/7--dc23 LC record available at https://lccn.loc.gov/2018017608

Bibliographic Indices. This publication is listed in bibliographic services, including Current Contents® and Index Medicus.

www.karger.com
Printed on acid-free and non-aging paper (ISO 9706)
ISSN 0077–0892
e-ISSN 1662–3843
ISBN 978–3–318–06368–4
e-ISBN 978–3–318–06369–1

Contents

List of Contributors

Imad About
Aix Marseille University, CNRS
ISM, Institute of Movement Sciences
FR Marseille (France)
E-Mail imad.about@univ-amu.fr

Lars Bjørndal
Section of Cariology and Endodontics
Department of Odontology
Faculty of Health and Medical Sciences
University of Copenhagen
Nørre Allé 20
DK–2200 Copenhagen (Denmark)
E-Mail labj@sund.ku.dk

Uwe Blunck
Charité Centre for Dental Medicine
Department for Operative and Preventive Dentistry
Assmannshauser Strasse 4-6
DE–14197 Berlin (Germany)
E-Mail uwe.blunck@charite.de

Clarissa Bonifacio
Department of Conservative Dentistry
Academic Centre for Dentistry Amsterdam – ACTA
Amsterdam (Netherlands)
E-Mail c.bonifacio@acta.nl

Georg Conrads
Division of Oral Microbiology and Immunology
Department for Operative Dentistry
Periodontology and Preventive Dentistry
RWTH Aachen University Hospital
Pauwelsstrasse 30
DE–52074 Aachen (Germany)
E-Mail gconrads@ukaachen.de

Sophie Doméjean
UFR d'Odontologie
2 rue de Braga
FR–63100 Clermont-Ferrand (France)
E-Mail sophie.domejean@uca.fr

Margherita Fontana
Cariology, Restorative Sciences and Endodontics
School of Dentistry, Room 2393
University of Michigan
1011 N University Avenue
Ann Arbor, MI 48109-1078 (USA)
E-Mail mfontan@umich.edu

Jo Frencken
Philips van Leijdenlaan 25
NL–6525 AX Nijmegen (The Netherlands)
E-Mail jo.frencken@radboudumc.nl

Gerd Göstemeyer
Charité Centre for Dental Medicine
Department for Operative and Preventive Dentistry
Assmannshauser Strasse 4-6
DE–14197 Berlin (Germany)
E-Mail gerd.goestemeyer@charite.de

Brigitte Grosgogeat
Université Lyon 1, UFR Odontologie, Laboratoire des Multimatériaux et Interfaces, UMR CNRS 5615, and Hospices Civils de Lyon, Service de Consultations et de Traitements Dentaires, FR–38670 Lyon (France)
E-Mail brigitte.grosgogeat@recherche.univ-lyon1.fr

Nicola Innes
School of Dentistry, University of Dundee
2 Park Place
Dundee DD1 4HR (UK)
E-Mail n.p.innes@dundee.ac.uk

Thomas Lamont
School of Dentistry, University of Dundee
2 Park Place
Dundee DD1 4HR (UK)
E-Mail t.lamont@dundee.ac.uk

Soraya Leal
Campus Darcy Ribeiro, Faculdade de Ciências da Saúde
Departamento de Odontologia
Universitdade de Brasília
Brasília, DF 70670-410 (Brazil)
E-Mail sorayaodt@yahoo.com

Colin Levey
School of Dentistry, University of Dundee
2 Park Place
Dundee DD1 4HR (UK)
E-Mail c.levey@dundee.ac.uk

Adrian Lussi
Department of Preventive, Restorative and
Pediatric Dentistry
University of Bern
Freiburgstrasse 7
CH–3010 Bern (Switzerland)
E-Mail adrian.lussi@zmk.unibe.ch

Klaus W. Neuhaus
Department of Preventive
Restorative and Pediatric Dentistry
Freiburgstrasse 7
CH–3010 Bern (Switzerland)
E-Mail klaus.neuhaus@zmk.unibe.ch

Daniela Raggio
Department of Orthodontics and Pediatric Dentistry
School of Dentistry, University of São Paulo
São Paulo (Brazil)
E-Mail danielar@usp.br

David Ricketts
School of Dentistry, University of Dundee
2 Park Place
Dundee DD1 4HR (UK)
E-Mail d.n.j.ricketts@dundee.ac.uk

Mark Robertson
School of Dentistry, University of Dundee
2 Park Place
Dundee DD1 4HR (UK)
E-Mail m.robertson@hotmail.co.uk

Ruth M. Santamaría
Department of Preventive and Pediatric Dentistry
Ernst-Moritz-Arndt University of Greifswald
Rotgerbergstrasse 8
DE–17487 Greifswald (Germany)
E-Mail ruth.santamaria@uni-greifswald.de

Falk Schwendicke
Operative and Preventive Dentistry
Charité – Universitätsmedizin Berlin
Corporate Member of Freie Universität Berlin
Humboldt-Universität zu Berlin, and
Berlin Institute of Health
Assmannshauser Strasse 4-6
DE–14197 Berlin (Germany)
E-Mail falk.schwendicke@charite.de

Guus van Strijp
Department of Cariology Endodontology
Pedodontology
Academic Centre for Dentistry (ACTA)
University of Amsterdam and VU University Amsterdam
Gustav Mahlerlaan 3004
NL–1081 LA Amsterdam (The Netherlands)
E-Mail a.vstrijp@acta.nl

Cor van Loveren
Department of Cariology Endodontology
Pedodontology
Academic Centre for Dentistry (ACTA)
University of Amsterdam and VU University Amsterdam
Gustav Mahlerlaan 3004
NL–1081 LA Amsterdam (The Netherlands)
E-Mail c.v.loveren@acta.nl

Foreword

A monograph addresses a single subject and this book is about caries excavation – everyday dentistry for many. How should soft, infected dentine be managed? The authors have studied, discussed, and researched this question and distilled contemporary knowledge for you. Intriguingly, with one notable exception, it may not matter what you do. Brush, seal, or selectively remove, all have their place but with each you must understand what is being attempted and why.

So what is the exception? What must you not do? You must never pick up a sharp excavator or burr and remove soft tissue vigorously because this could damage the tooth and even prejudice its survival. Perversely, this might be precisely what you were taught to do in dental school! This just goes to show how research changes clinical practice and how important it is to keep up to date.

So read and enjoy the book!

Edwina Kidd, London
Em. Professor in Cariology

Preface

There is a reason why medical researchers do their work. They wish to contribute to improving people's health and well-being through eradicating diseases, to improve existing treatments and change disease-causing behaviour, and much more, through the study of these areas.

An astronomically high number of medical publications appear in the literature monthly. The number of oral health-related publications is very high, too high for a dental practitioner to read them all. Some of these have a quality that leaves one wondering how the manuscript passed the review process. Others are of extremely good quality and provide new worthwhile information.

The scientific world is assisting medical professionals by producing systematic reviews and/or meta-analyses on an ever-growing number of topics. A systematic review merely appraises the available evidence on a topic in the literature on the basis of research quality criteria and then draws conclusions. They are not designed to make recommendations on treatment. Therefore, these reviews and/or meta-analyses cannot be left on their own as the impacts of the individual results need to be merged to facilitate change, for example in improving (oral) health or aspects of it. It is like bricks that need cement to build a solid structure. A way of combining newly acquired knowledge into contemporary disease management concepts is to write a book, or in this particular case a monograph. Another way is to develop guidelines.

The current monograph was written by dedicated researchers who are experts in the various subfields of cariology and restorative dentistry. The chapters are built on evidence-based results and take the reader through the development of dental caries, assess the devices for diagnosing it in clinical practice and in an epidemiological setting, and provide new insights in the way a dentine carious cavity can be managed both from a tissue removal and a restoration point of view. Examples of dental tissue-preserving methods are presented and the necessity for sealing a dentine carious cavity with a quality restorative material is highlighted with ample evidence. Also, an update on how to conduct a randomised clinical trial is presented, and a chapter is included on terminology to support better verbal communication and interactions between members of the oral health profession from all corners of the world. The monograph concludes with recommendations and suggestions of areas in dentine carious cavity treatment that are not fully understood yet.

In essence, dental caries is a preventable, behaviour/life-style disease. It implies that members of the public do not need to go through the ordeal of drilling and filling teeth regularly as the generation following the Second World War had to undergo. At that time, oral health research was in its infancy. Over the past decades, oral science has yielded information that benefits the public. It is the duty of the oral health profession to embrace philosophies of managing dental caries, such as the minimal intervention dentistry concept, which aims to keep healthy teeth healthy throughout life by preserving sound and remineralisable tooth tissue. The expectation in many parts of the world as people are getting older is that they wish to enjoy a well-functioning, pain-free oral cavity. Therefore, tissue-saving procedures should be commonplace after caries prevention has failed, in order for the elderly to have a sufficient number of functioning teeth to assist them.

The idea for writing this monograph on the *Evolution of Treating Cavitated Carious Lesions* was born at the memorable congress of the European Organisation of Dental Research (ORCA) in Liverpool in 2014. It became operational first at the 2015 Leuven meeting, where the International Caries Consensus Cooperation (ICCC) was established. The ICCC published 4 papers in 2016 that form the basis of a number of chapters contained in the current monograph.

We wish the reader very many happy moments reading this work. We hope that this monograph finds its way to undergraduates in all dental schools and to postgraduate education courses around the world. The oral health profession has the knowledge and tools, as well as the duty to participate together with people/patients to "prevent restorations" and to "prevent root canal treatment and extraction on the basis of dental caries," and to prolong a healthy dentition into older age. Let's collectively do it.

Falk Schwendicke, Berlin
Jo Frencken, Nijmegen
Nicola Innes, Dundee

Schwendicke F, Frencken J, Innes N (eds): Caries Excavation: Evolution of Treating Cavitated Carious Lesions.
Monogr Oral Sci. Basel, Karger, 2018, vol 27, pp 1–10 (DOI: 10.1159/000487826)

Pathophysiology of Dental Caries

Georg Conrads[a] · Imad About[b]

[a]Division of Oral Microbiology and Immunology, Department for Operative Dentistry, Periodontology and Preventive Dentistry, RWTH Aachen University Hospital, Aachen, Germany; [b]Aix Marseille University, CNRS, ISM, Institute of Movement Sciences, Marseille, France

Abstract

Carious lesion dynamics are dependent predominantly on the availability of fermentable sugars, other environmental conditions, bacteria, and host factors. Our current understanding of the microorganisms involved in the initiation and progression of caries is still rather incomplete. The most relevant acidogenic-aciduric bacterial species known to date are *Streptococcus mutans*, bifidobacteria, and lactobacilli. Whereas mutans streptococci are initiators, bifidobacteria and lactobacilli are more enhancers for progression. Boosters for microbial activity are specific environmental conditions, such as the presence of fermentable dietary sugars and the absence of oxygen. Based on these conditions, the necrotic and/or contaminated zone fulfils all criteria for disease progression and has to be removed. For those deep lesions where the pulp vitality is not affected, a selective removal of the contaminated leathery dentine should take place as this approach lowers the risk of regrowth of the few embedded microbial cells here. In repelling the microbial attack and repairing damage, the host has developed several ingenious strategies. A major resistance to carious lesion progression is mounted by the dentine-pulp tissues. The signalling molecules and growth factors released upon dentine demineralisation upregulate the odontoblast activity and act as sensor cells. After carious stimulation, odontoblasts initiate an inflammatory reaction by producing chemokines and synthesise a protective tertiary dentine. After the destruction of these cells, the pulp still has a high capacity to synthesise this tertiary dentine thanks to the presence of adult stem cells within the pulp. Also, in addition to the systemic regulation, the pulp which is located within the inextensible confines of the dentine walls has a well-developed local regulation of its inflammation, regeneration, and vascularisation. This local regulation is due to the activity of different pulp cell types, mainly the fibroblasts, which secrete soluble molecules that regulate all these processes.

Microbiology of Tooth Decay

Dentistry dates as far back as 5,000 BC when people in India, Egypt, Japan, and China thought dental caries were a result of a "tooth worm." The term "dental caries" first appeared in the literature around 1634 and is derived from the Latin word cariēs for decay and from ancient Irish ara-*chrinn*, it decays. The term was originally used simply to describe holes in the teeth with little knowledge of the aetiology and pathogenesis of the disease [1].

Concepts and beliefs about the cause of dental caries have evolved over many centuries, with the involvement of microorganisms recognised since the late 1800s. Readers interested in the concepts in caries microbiology and their development over time can find comprehensive literature on the topic [2, 3]. Despite thousands of publications, however, the central question of the relative importance of different bacteria in the disease remains unanswered.

With technical advances in our ability to identify, cultivate, and count different microorganisms, our views have evolved regarding the contribution of particular species of plaque bacteria to the caries process [4]. But it might take another 20–50 years, as a rough estimate, before deep-sequencing technologies and the gene databases have reached such a quality that the entire gene repertoire and interactions within a carious tissue can be determined. The limits so far are the length of an ambiguity-free sequence read (which is currently as short as 500 bp applying the leading Illumina sequencing technology) and, as a consequence, the need to select a short but taxon-representative region, usually a variable region, e.g., V1-V3, V3-V4, or V3-V5 of the 16S rDNA (total length 1,545 bp) or – even better – of the 23S rDNA (total length 2,905 bp). For instance, V3-V4 sequence results will leave many saccharolytic *Streptococcus* and *Actinomyces* species as "unclassified." That means our current picture about the microorganisms involved in the initiation and progression of caries or other especially polymicrobial diseases is still rather incomplete. However, the species known to be involved so far and the correlated pathomechanisms of dental caries can be taken as a draft model and are thus discussed below.

In dental caries, we see an ecologic shift within the dental biofilm environment, driven by frequent access to fermentable dietary carbohydrates. This leads to a move from a balanced population of microorganisms of low cariogenicity to a consortium of high cariogenicity and to an increased production – and correlated tolerance – of organic acids promoting dental hard tissue net mineral loss. That is why we call this consortium acidogenic and acidophil (synonym aciduric). Besides the presence of fermentable dietary carbohydrates and selection of acidogenic-aciduric bacterial species, the host susceptibility, which is a rather simplified term for a multifactorial complexity, is the third major player.

The acidogenic-aciduric bacterial species *Streptococcus mutans* is recognised as being eminently involved in cariogenic processes, including early childhood caries, enamel carious lesions, cavitated lesions, or carious dentine. However, over time its attributed role changed from that of a true pathogen (specific plaque hypothesis [5]) to enhancer (active role) and/or indicator (passive role) of a sugar-triggered cariogenic vicious circle (extended caries ecological hypothesis [6, 7]), and the discussion still goes on [8]. As a matter of fact, *S. mutans* is detected in a few caries-free and found absent in several caries-active individuals, impairing its outstanding caries indicatory potential. Furthermore, most relevant acidogenic-aciduric bacterial species are: (i) *S. mutans* relatives (called mutans streptococci or MS) with a similar virulence potential, namely *S. sobrinus*; (ii) bifidobacteria, including *Bifidobacterium dentium* and other closely related oral *Bifidobacterium* spp., but also the more distantly related species *Scardovia wiggsiae*, and (iii) lactobacilli, especially those with pellicle-adhesive potential [9].

A number of epidemiological and in vitro studies suggested that *S. sobrinus* – under circumstances yet to be determined – may be even more cariogenic than *S. mutans* [8–11]. In addition, targeted clinical studies have suggested that preschool and 15-year-old school children harbouring both *S. mutans* and *S. sobrinus* had a higher incidence of dental caries than those with *S. mutans* alone (for a review see Conrads et al. [10]).

Unlike MS, the highly aciduric bifidobacteria, especially *B. dentium*, do not colonise hard surfaces per se, since denture plaque associated with denture stomatitis harboured high levels of MS, lactobacilli, and yeasts, but not *B. dentium*. This indicates that *B. dentium* does not simply colonise intact dental hard surfaces but instead suggests that it is the lesion initiated by other species that facilitate the attachment and proliferation of *B. dentium*. In contrast to MS, the presence of this species might therefore be more a result than the cause of initial lesions. Clearly, *B. dentium* and MS are significant independent indicators [9].

A similar role (more profiteer than initiator) was recently proposed for lactobacilli, with *Lactobacillus fermentum*, *L. rhamnosus*, *L. gasseri*, *L. salivarius*, *L. plantarum*, and the *L. casei-paracasei* group as the most abundant species. According to this concept, precaries lesions become a retentive, low pH niche for lactobacilli accumulation, which take advantage of their proclivity for making and surviving in an increasingly reduced pH environment. In some cases, the lactobacilli can even outcompete and exclude the MS that created the retentive niche, which might explain why caries lesions are sometimes free of MS but not or very rarely free of lactobacilli [9].

Other less investigated but interesting caries-indicator candidates are *Atopobium* spp., *Slackia exigua* and a few others [11, 12]. The entire network of microbial organisms involved, which are not only bacteria but also saccharolytic yeasts (e.g., *Candida albicans*), *Archaea* (enhancer of fermentation processes by consuming end products such as CO_2 and H_2), or bacteriophages (enhancer of lateral gene transfer and thus of evolution), is extremely complex and diverse.

Taken together, every cavity might have its own demineralising consortium of active organisms and genes, but the following simple principles are universal:

1 Presence of acidogenic-aciduric microorganisms and their ability to attach to the pellicle-coated tooth surface, either directly (pioneers such as MS) or indirectly (beneficiaries such as bifidobacteria and lactobacilli; for a review see Conrads et al. [10]).

2 Environmental conditions favouring the multiplication and metabolism of such species: access to low-molecular sugars, especially sucrose, and low redox potential at the same time. High sugar and low oxygen leads to rapid fermentation and acid production.

With these simple principles, it is possible to identify (constitute) what a carious tissue actually is and how much tissue must or should be removed or excavated to stop further decay.

Histology of a Carious Tissue – The Microbiological Perspective

The degree of success in eliminating bacteria during cavity preparation and prior to the insertion of a restoration may increase the longevity of the restoration and therefore the success of the restorative procedure. The complete eradication of bacteria in a caries-affected tooth during cavity preparation is considered a difficult clinical task and – from the perspective of a microbiologist – almost impossible, and also not required anymore, as is discussed in the chapter by Bjørndal [this vol., pp. 68–81]. Attempts to excavate completely extensive carious tissue may affect the vitality of the pulp and weaken the tooth structure. In principal, disinfection of the cavity preparation after caries excavation can aid in the elimination of bacterial remnants, reducing the risk for recurrent caries and failure of the restoration. However, the side effects of chemical disinfectants (e.g., chlorhexidine or benzalkonium chloride) on the restorative treatment, including reduced dentine bond strength, have been a major concern for both dental clinicians and researchers [13], and therefore alternatives still have to be found and their efficacy proven.

As shown in Figure 1, the carious tissue consists of 4 different zones, but only 3 clinically noticeable

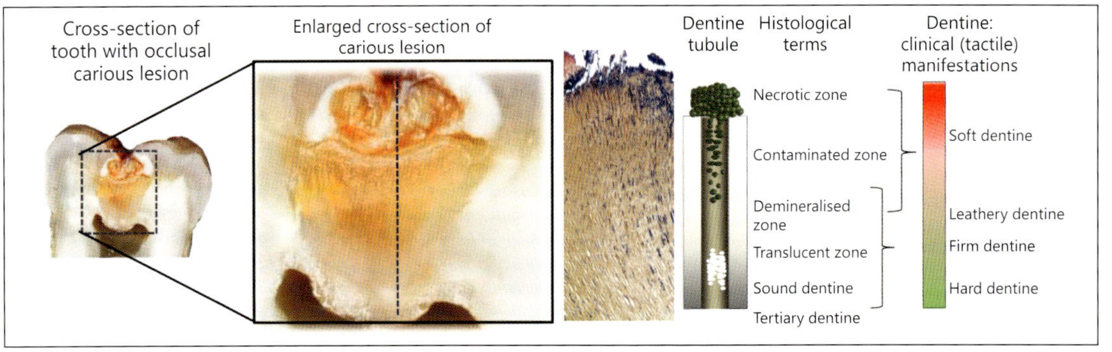

Fig. 1. Histology of carious tissue. Note the correlations between cross-section, ultrastructure zones, and clinical (tactile) manifestations. Modified from Innes et al. [14] and Ogawa et al. [15]. Reprinted by Permission of SAGE Publications, Inc.

layers. The outer layer, clinically the soft dentine, consists of the necrotic zone with the microbial biofilm attached, and the contaminated zone. The soft dentine is characterised by a gradient of microorganisms with cell-numbers between 10^1 and 10^8 per mg (measured from the inside to outside, pulpal to coronal), including aciduric, facultative anaerobic bacteria. Comparing the conditions here with the principles mentioned above, this necrotic and/or contaminated zone fulfils all criteria for disease (demineralisation) progression as it is anaerobic (low redox potential demanding a fast substrate turnover for sufficient energy resourcing) and, at least temporarily, fed by high concentrations of fermentable dietary carbohydrates. This layer has to be removed.

The next layer is the demineralised zone, which correlates clinically with leathery dentine. This zone is characterised by few microorganisms per milligram, very little nutrients (since already consumed by the bacteria and yeasts in the outer layer), and a strictly anaerobic atmosphere. While the latter condition favours demineralisation by acid production, the sheer low number of fermenting bacteria and the very low nutritional source prohibits substantial multiplication and metabolism. It is the consensus that for deep lesions, extending beyond the inner (pulpal) third or quarter of dentine radiographically, selective removal (incomplete excavation to protect the pulp) should be limited to soft dentine, excluding the removal of contaminated leathery dentine [14]. From the microbiological point of view, this approach is tolerable as electron transport within, and acid production by, the few cells is also very low in this zone. However, bacteria have several strategies to overcome harsh conditions and – after preparation, disinfection if applicable, infiltration if applicable, and restoring – might still be alive although in a dormant state [16, 17]. This means the lesion and the bacteria are arrested, but only temporarily. If there is gap formation at the tooth-restoration interface, possibly further supported by the microleakage of fluids and salivary proteins to the gap, this leads to inevitable microbial colonisation from saliva, but also to the possible regrowth of dormant cells and, ultimately, secondary caries formation. Therefore, for less deep lesions, selective removal should take place down to firm dentine, which not only has clinical advantages (more depth for a solid restoration), but also lowers the risk of regrowth of surviving microbial cells.

Finally, pulpally the translucent zone of firm softer dentine is characterised by demineralisation since acids, but not the bacterial cells, penetrate to this depth. Here, the plate-form apatite crystals apparently dissolve and recrystallise into

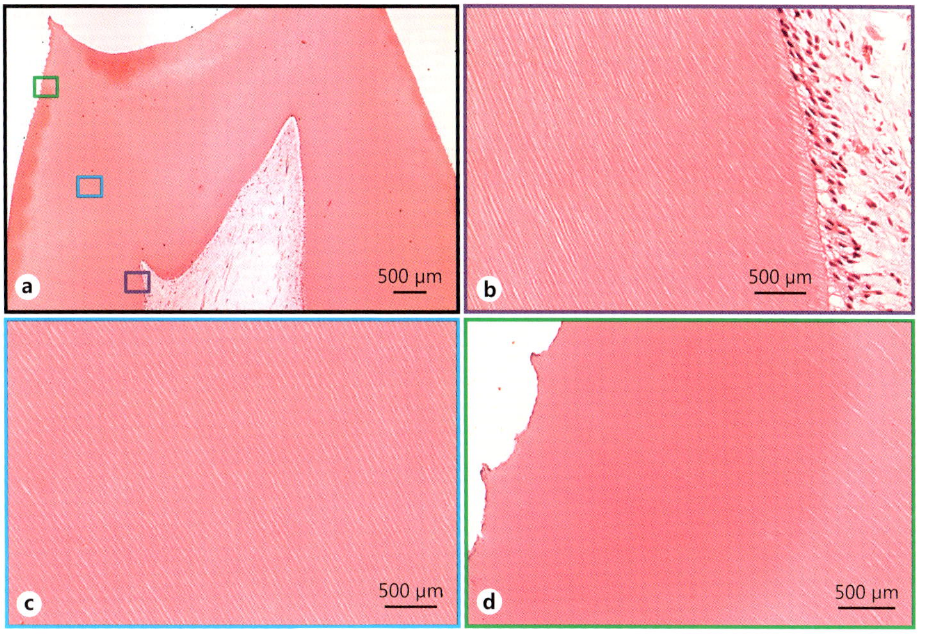

Fig. 2. a Histology of sound dentine in a premolar. **b** Dentine tubules are numerous and wide open on the pulp side. **c** They are less numerous and appear more narrow at mid-distance between the pulp and the dentine-enamel junction. **d** Dentine tubules are very narrow and many of them appear completely obliterated upon approaching the dentine-enamel junction.

a rhomboid form, defined as whitlockite [$Ca_9(MgFe)(PO_4)_6PO_3OH$]. This crystalline form seems to be softer and less resistant to cutting and acids [15]. This layer might not be absolutely sterile, but metabolism of aciduric microorganisms is almost impossible and thus negligible. For repelling and combatting the microbial attack and repairing damages, the host has developed several ingenious strategies.

Pulp Response to Dental Caries

Host pulp response to dental caries is a key element in understanding the carious process and its consequences. In this regard, enamel acts as a physical mineralised barrier preventing bacterial infiltration into the dentine and pulp. Also, the underlying dentine histology, composition, and function provide significant information on how bacteria invasion is hindered by the dentine itself and how this dentine provides signalling molecules to induce dentine regeneration during the carious process. In the case of a deep carious lesion reaching the odontoblasts, the pulp tissue itself has also elaborated efficient strategies to hinder or even arrest the carious lesion progression and the bacterial infiltration into the pulp.

Dentine Histology at the Dentine Enamel Junction Is Different from that of Deep Dentine

Dentine has a unique histological tubular appearance. The tubules close to the dental pulp are numerous and wide open. Their diameter decreases gradually as they get away from the pulp and become very narrow or completely obliterated upon approaching the dentine-enamel junction (Fig. 2).

This suggests that the superficial dentine hinders bacterial infiltration when they reach the dentine surface. On the other hand, when bacteria reach the open dentine tubules they can invade the dental pulp more rapidly through the tubules. This may suggest significant consequences to the underlying pulp only if we consider the bacterial invasion consequences. However, the dental pulp established efficient protective mechanisms against this invasion.

Dentine Matrix Contains Sequestered Signalling Molecules

While the major dentine inorganic component is hydroxyapatite, its organic matrix is mainly composed of collagen I and non-collagenous proteins such as dentine sialoprotein [18] and dentine matrix protein-1 [19]. These are involved in the initiation and the regulation of dentine mineralisation. In addition, different signalling molecules have been reported to be secreted by the odontoblasts and sequestered in the dentine matrix, mainly in an inactive form. Among others, these include transforming growth factor-β_1 (TGF-β_1), basic fibroblast growth factor (FGF-2), vascular endothelial growth factor (VEGF), and platelet derived growth factor (PDGF) [20, 21]. During the carious dissolution of the dentine matrix, these molecules can be released and reach the underlying odontoblasts leading to the upregulation of their synthetic activity.

In addition to the responsiveness to these growth factors, recent data demonstrated that odontoblasts act as sensor cells as they express transient potential channel receptors. These receptors allow the odontoblast to be responsive to the external stimulations, such as noxious heat, noxious cold, as well as chemical and mechanical stimulations [22]. Thus, upon stimulation, odontoblasts synthesise a new tertiary dentine at the pulp periphery facing the stimulation site. This focally secreted dentine can also be deposited within the dentine tubules to decrease their permeability to cariogenic bacteria and their toxins, leading to the protection of the underlying pulp.

Thus, odontoblasts represent the first defence mechanism in case of carious lesion development. Indeed, these cells also express receptors called Toll-like receptors (TLRs) 2 and 4 [23, 24], which recognise specific structures on Gram-positive and Gram-negative bacteria, respectively. These TLRs belong to a big family of pattern recognition receptors that are activated after contact with common molecules on the pathogen surface. In moderate carious injuries, TLRs 2 are highly expressed in the underlying odontoblasts [25]. Upon activation, these TLRs induce the secretion of antimicrobial molecules such as β-defensins and nitric oxide by the odontoblasts which have an antibacterial effect against *S. mutans*, thus limiting cariogenic bacteria progression towards the pulp [26]. Also, upon activation of their receptors, odontoblasts secrete proinflammatory chemokines which lead to dendritic cell recruitment in order to eliminate the pathogenic agents [27].

Overall, in the case of moderate dentine carious lesions, the odontoblasts act as a barrier exerting antimicrobial effects and initiating the secretion of a tertiary dentine to protect the underlying pulp (Fig. 3).

However, in the case of severe and rapidly progressive carious lesions, tertiary dentine focal synthesis may not be enough and bacteria may destroy the newly synthesised tertiary dentine, reach the underlying pulp, and induce an inflammatory reaction (Fig. 4).

The Dental Pulp Defence Strategies

When the odontoblastic barrier is destroyed by the carious lesion and either bacteria or their toxins reach the underlying pulp, a tertiary dentine secretion can still be observed. This dentine, which is secreted after the odontoblast destruction, is synthesised by another cell type originat-

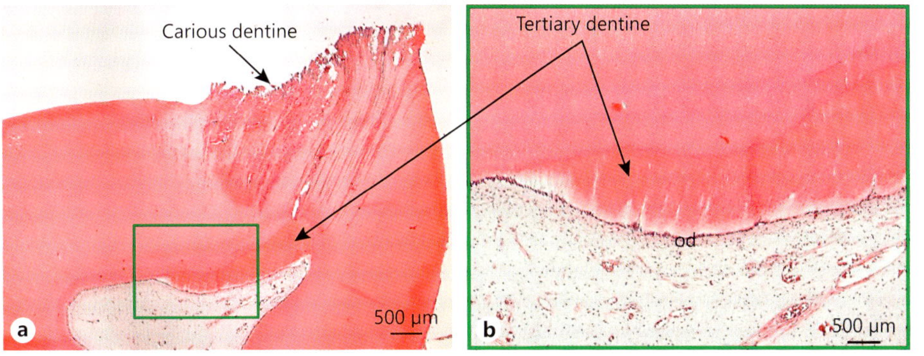

Fig. 3. a Histology of a moderate carious lesion in a molar. It is characterised by a disorganised dentine with a loss of the typical tubular structure at the carious site. **b** Tertiary dentine is secreted locally by the underlying odontoblasts (od). At this stage, bacterial infiltration is arrested at a distance from the pulp, which has a normal aspect.

ing for the differentiation of adult pulp stem cells. This reparative dentine usually contains fewer tubules than the physiological one. This might decrease the bacterial infiltration or their toxins to the underlying pulp. While little was known about the cells secreting this dentine, the discovery of adult stem cells within the dental pulp provided a significant step forward. Indeed, all dental pulps in permanent and primary teeth and at all ages comprise, at least, a population of adult stem cells [28]. This was first demonstrated in a culture system of cells isolated from the pulps of third molars, where pulp cells were able to produce a mineral matrix with molecular and mineral characteristics of dentine [29]. Additionally, when isolated with specific mesenchymal stem cell markers such as STRO-1 and transplanted after mixing with hydroxyapatite/tricalcium phosphate ceramic powder subcutaneously in mice, they generated a dentine/pulp-like tissue [30]. There is converging evidence that one of the niches of these stem cells is located in the perivascular area. After pulp injury, these cells are activated and migrate to the injury site to synthesise the tertiary dentine [31]. It has been reported that TGF-β_1, which can be released after the dissolution of dentine, is involved in the recruitment of these cells and their differentiation into odontoblast-like cells secreting the tertiary dentine [32].

Additionally, recent investigations on dental pulp, which has a terminal circulation, revealed that, in addition to the systemic regulation, it has a local regulation of its vascularisation, inflammation, and regeneration. This allows the dental pulp to resist bacterial invasion by different mechanisms, as explained below.

Dental Pulp Local Regulation

It is well established that carious injury leads to pulp hypoxia. Different pulp cell types, such as fibroblasts, endothelial, and stem cells, have been reported to upregulate the synthesis of hypoxia-inducible factor, which increases the synthesis of angiogenic growth factors such as VEGF, FGF-2, and PDGF. This leads to vasodilation and the increased formation of blood vessels at the carious injury site. Overall, this increases nutrient, blood, and oxygen supply to the injured tissue. This also allows inflammatory cell recruitment to carry out phagocytosis of pathogens. After complete pulp healing, there is a downregulation of angiogenic factor secretion and a return to normoxia with normal pulp vascularisation [33].

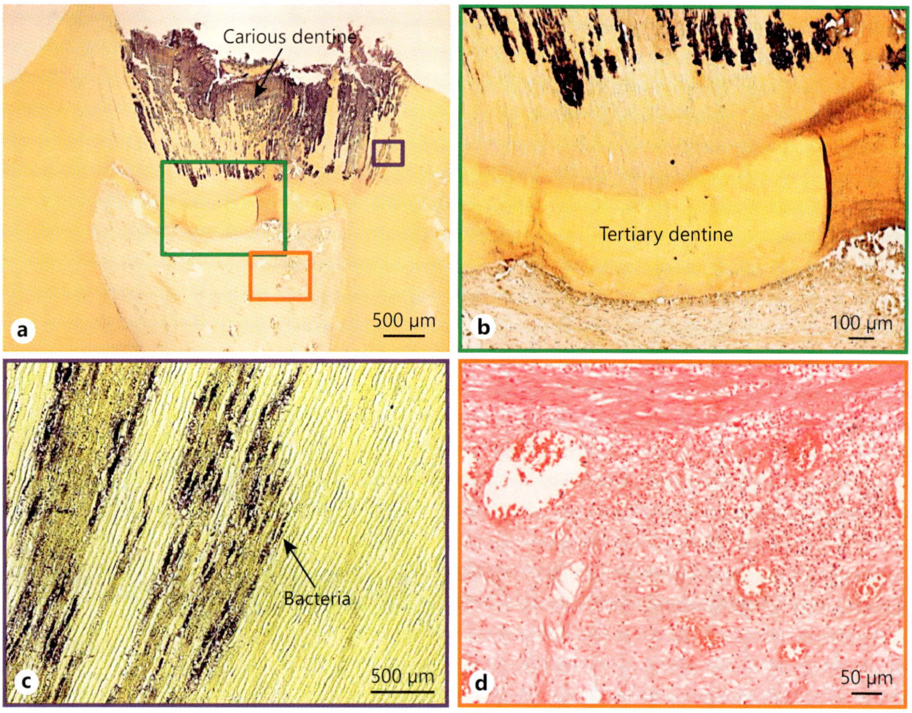

Fig. 4. a Histology of a severe carious lesion in a molar. It is characterised by a disorganised dentine at the carious site. **b** Tertiary dentine is produced in the form of a bridge by the underlying odontoblasts. At this stage, bacteria infiltrated the dentine tubules (**c**) and the pulp, which appears inflamed and infiltrated by numerous inflammatory cells (**d**).

Carious injury also leads to a pulp inflammatory reaction initiated by complement activation. Complement is the name given to about 40 proteins synthesised mainly by the liver and released in the plasma. During the inflammatory process, the complement is activated, leading to the synthesis of biologically active complement fragments. These play a major role in eliminating pathogenic agents. Pulp fibroblasts have been recently reported as the only non-immune cell capable of synthesising all complement proteins [34]. After complement activation, biologically active fragments are released. Recent investigation of these fragments revealed their involvement in the pulp anti-inflammatory and regeneration processes. Indeed, pulp complement can be activated by lipoteichoic acids of Gram-positive bacteria, such as *S. mutans* and *S. sanguinis*. Upon activation, several biologically active molecules are released. Among these, C5a has been shown to be involved in the recruitment of pulp stem cells [35] and in the guidance of nerve growth to the stimulation site [36]. Another fragment, C3a, is involved in the proliferation of both pulp fibroblasts and stem cells and in guiding fibroblast migration to the stimulation site [37]. This clearly illustrates the involvement of complement in the pulp regeneration process facing bacterial infiltration during carious disease. Indeed, reparative dentine is efficient in arresting the carious injury progression (Fig. 3). This may be partially explained by the fact that pulp complement activation also leads to the synthesis of a complex molecular structure called membrane attack complex. This complex structure can be produced by the fibroblasts and has been shown not only to be fixed on *S. mutans* and *S. sanguinis*, but also to kill these cariogenic bacteria [33]. When this complex polymerises on bacteria walls, it creates numerous holes leading to the entry of electrolytes and water, which results in bacteria destruction. Thus, the fibroblasts dampen down, and may even arrest the bacterial invasion to the pulp and provide the adequate signals not only to kill cariogenic bacteria, but also to initiate the regeneration process by recruiting the stem cells and nerve regeneration.

Overall, a carious lesion should be regarded as a dynamic process. Its progression does not only depend on the bacterial infiltration and the local environment, but also on the host pulp response.

References

1 Bowen WH: Dental caries – not just holes in teeth! A perspective. Mol Oral Microbiol 2016;31:228–233.
2 Russell RR: How has genomics altered our view of caries microbiology? Caries Res 2008;42:319–327.
3 Russell RR: Changing concepts in caries microbiology. Am J Dent 2009;22:304–310.
4 Tanner AC, Kressirer CA, Faller LL: Understanding caries from the oral microbiome perspective. J Calif Dent Assoc 2016;44:437–446.
5 Loesche WJ: Chemotherapy of dental plaque infections. Oral Sci Rev 1976;9:65–107.
6 Marsh PD: Microbial ecology of dental plaque and its significance in health and disease. Adv Dent Res 1994;8:263–271.
7 Takahashi N, Nyvad B: Caries ecology revisited: microbial dynamics and the caries process. Caries Res 2008;42:409–418.
8 Rosier BT, De Jager M, Zaura E, Krom BP: Historical and contemporary hypotheses on the development of oral diseases: are we there yet? Front Cell Infect Microbiol 2014;4:92.
9 Henne K, Rheinberg A, Melzer-Krick B, Conrads G: Aciduric microbial taxa including *Scardovia wiggsiae* and *Bifidobacterium* spp. in caries and caries free subjects. Anaerobe 2015;35:60–65.
10 Conrads G, de Soet JJ, Song L, Henne K, Sztajer H, Wagner-Döbler I, Zeng AP: Comparing the cariogenic species *Streptococcus sobrinus* and *S. mutans* on whole genome level. J Oral Microbiol 2014;6:26189.
11 Lif Holgerson P, Ohman C, Ronnlund A, Johansson I: Maturation of oral microbiota in children with or without dental caries. PLoS One 2015;10:e0128534.
12 Tanner AC, Kent RL Jr, Holgerson PL, Hughes CV, Loo CY, Kanasi E, Chalmers NI, Johansson I: Microbiota of severe early childhood caries before and after therapy. J Dent Res 2011;90:1298–1305.
13 Hewlett ER, Cox CF: Clinical considerations in adhesive restorative dentistry – influence of adjunctive procedures. J Calif Dent Assoc 2003;31:477–482.
14 Innes NP, Frencken JE, Bjørndal L, Maltz M, Manton DJ, Ricketts D, van Landuyt K, Banerjee A, Campus G, Domejean S, Fontana M, Leal S, Lo E, Machiulskiene V, Schulte A, Splieth C, Zandona A, Schwendicke F: Managing carious lesions: consensus recommendations on terminology. Adv Dent Res 2016;28:49–57.
15 Ogawa K, Yamashita Y, Ichijo T, Fusayama T: The ultrastructure and hardness of the transparent layer of human carious dentine. J Dent Res 1983;62:7–10.
16 Rheinberg A, Swierzy IJ, Nguyen TD, Horz HP, Conrads G: Cryptic *Streptococcus mutans* 5.6-kb plasmids encode a toxin-antitoxin system for plasmid stabilization. J Oral Microbiol 2013;5:19729.
17 ten Cate JM: Biofilms, a new approach to the microbiology of dental plaque. Odontology 2006;94:1–9.
18 Butler WT, Bhown M, Brunn JC, D'Souza RN, Farach-Carson MC, Happonen R-P, Schrohenloher RE, Seyer JM, Somerman MJ, Foster RA, et al: Isolation, characterization and immunolocalization of a 53-kdal dentine sialoprotein (DSP). Matrix 1992;12:343–351.
19 Butler WT, Ritchie H: The nature and functional significance of dentine extracellular matrix proteins. Int J of Dev Biol 2003;39:169–179.
20 Finkelman RD, Mohan S, Jennings JC, Taylor AK, Jepsen S, Baylink DJ: Quantitation of growth factors Igf-I, SGF/IGF-II, and TGF-β in human dentine. J Bone Miner Res 1990;5:717–723.
21 Roberts-Clark DJ, Smith AJ: Angiogenic growth factors in human dentine matrix. Arch Oral Biol 2000;45:1013–1016.
22 El Karim IA, Linden GJ, Curtis TM, About I, McGahon MK, Irwin CR, Lundy FT: Human odontoblasts express functional thermo-sensitive TRP channels: implications for dentine sensitivity. Pain 2011;152:2211–2223.
23 Jiang H-W, Zhang W, Ren B-P, Zeng J-F, Ling J-Q: Expression of toll like receptor 4 in normal human odontoblasts and dental pulp tissue. J Endod 2006;32:747–751.
24 Veerayutthwilai O, Byers MR, Pham TT, Darveau RP, Dale BA: Differential regulation of immune responses by odontoblasts. Mol Oral Microbiol 2007;22:5–13.
25 Farges J-C, Keller J-F, Carrouel F, Durand SH, Romeas A, Bleicher F, Lebecque S, Staquet M-J: Odontoblasts in the dental pulp immune response. J Exp Zoolog B Mol Dev Evol 2009;312:425–436.

26 Farges JC, Bellanger A, Ducret M, Aubert-Foucher E, Richard B, Alliot-Licht B, Bleicher F, Carrouel F: Human odontoblast-like cells produce nitric oxide with antibacterial activity upon TLR2 activation. Front Physiol 2015;6:185.
27 Keller J-F, Carrouel F, Colomb E, Durand SH, Baudouin C, Msika P, Bleicher F, Vincent C, Staquet M-J, Farges J-C: Toll-like receptor 2 activation by lipoteichoic acid induces differential production of pro-inflammatory cytokines in human odontoblasts, dental pulp fibroblasts and immature dendritic cells. Immunobiology 2010;215:53–59.
28 Huang GTJ: Pulp and dentine tissue engineering and regeneration: current progress. Regen Med 2009;4:697–707.
29 About I, Bottero M-J, de Denato P, Camps J, Franquin J-C, Mitsiadis TA: Human dentine production in vitro. Exp Cell Res 2000;258:33–41.
30 Gronthos S, Brahim J, Li W, Fisher LW, Cherman N, Boyde A, DenBesten P, Robey PG, Shi S: Stem cell properties of human dental pulp stem cells. J Dent Res 2002;81:531–535.
31 About I: Dentine-pulp regeneration: the primordial role of the microenvironment and its modification by traumatic injuries and bioactive materials. Endod Top 2013;28:61–89.
32 Mathieu S, Jeanneau C, Sheibat-Othman N, Kalaji N, Fessi H, About I: Usefulness of controlled release of growth factors in investigating the early events of dentine-pulp regeneration. J Endod 2013;39:228–235.
33 Jeanneau C, Rufas P, Rombouts C, Giraud T, Dejou J, About I: Can pulp fibroblasts kill cariogenic bacteria? Role of complement activation. J Dent Res 2015;94:1765–1772.
34 Chmilewsky F, Jeanneau C, Laurent P, About I: Pulp fibroblasts synthesize functional complement proteins involved in initiating dentine-pulp regeneration. Am J Pathol 2014;184:1991–2000.
35 Chmilewsky F, Jeanneau C, Laurent P, Kirschfink M, About I: Pulp progenitor cell recruitment is selectively guided by a C5a gradient. J Dent Res 2013;92:532–539.
36 Chmilewsky F, About I, Chung SH: Pulp fibroblasts control nerve regeneration through complement activation. J Dent Res 2016;95:913–922.
37 Rufas P, Jeanneau C, Rombouts C, Laurent P, About I: Complement C3a mobilizes dental pulp stem cells and specifically guides pulp fibroblast recruitment. J Endod 2016;42:1377–1384.

For microbiology: Georg Conrads
Division of Oral Microbiology and Immunology, Department for Operative Dentistry, Periodontology and Preventive Dentistry, RWTH Aachen University Hospital
Pauwelsstrasse 30
DE–52074 Aachen (Germany)
E-Mail gconrads@ukaachen.de

For histology: Imad About
Aix Marseille University, CNRS, ISM, Institute of Movement Sciences
FR–13385 Marseille (France)
E-Mail imad.about@univ-amu.fr

Schwendicke F, Frencken J, Innes N (eds): Caries Excavation: Evolution of Treating Cavitated Carious Lesions.
Monogr Oral Sci. Basel, Karger, 2018, vol 27, pp 11–23 (DOI: 10.1159/000487827)

Caries Epidemiology and Its Challenges

Jo Frencken

Department of Oral Function and Prosthetic Dentistry, Radboud University Medical Center, Nijmegen, The Netherlands

Abstract

Despite their limitations, caries epidemiology continues to rely predominantly on visual/tactile indices for detecting and assessing carious lesion-related conditions. Over the last 4 to 5 decades, the prevalence and severity of dental caries in primary and permanent dentitions have been reduced in a number of countries based on the published studies. Despite this achievement, the prevalence and severity of dental caries remains too high at a world level. Pits and fissures in occlusal surfaces of first molars and pits in buccal surfaces of lower first molars are most vulnerable for developing a carious lesion. Dental caries is a preventable, behavioural/life-style disease that is age related and life-long. Preventing dental caries should start at mother-and-child clinics in conjunction with the available educational and health care programmes. Oral health (caries) epidemiological surveys should be held periodically.

Detection and Assessment Devices

In essence, carious lesions can be detected and assessed using visual/tactile and electronic devices. Over the past decades a number of electronic devices have been introduced in response to some of the limitations of traditional methods such as the radiograph and visual/tactile devices. While perhaps suitable for use in the dental clinic, not all electronic devices appear suitable for use in epidemiological surveys. In addition, a number of them have no proven or poor validity and many are not field-proof [1, 2]. Therefore, dental practitioners should not place much reliance on these electronic devices. It means that despite their limitations, caries epidemiology continues to rely predominantly on visual/tactile indices for detecting and assessing carious lesion-related conditions in a field setting [3].

Visual/Tactile Devices Currently in Use

A caries assessment device should fulfil some prerequisites before it can be applied clinically. These include: manageability (be cheap, fast, acceptable, and easy to learn), reproducibility (ability to show the same results when a sample is measured twice or more by the same observer), and accuracy (to be able to detect and determine whether a disease is truly present or not, and whether the codes and descriptions are unambiguously presented) [4]. To what extent commonly applied visual/tactile devices have been tested for the presence of these prerequisites is worth investigating. Validity testing is particularly important and not always performed correctly [5, 6]. The following paragraphs introduce some visual/tactile devices currently in use.

While it is accepted that the explorer should not be used to detect carious lesions, as damage can occur to enamel when pushing the explorer into pits and fissures and in brittle enamel carious lesions, the explorer is part of the assessment of the level of "activity" of the lesion. Activity is assessed by removing biofilm from stagnation areas with the explorer and to "sense" the roughness and hardness of the lesion as the tip of the instrument is drawn gently across the lesion. Nyvad et al. [7] described activity assessment and developed a carious lesion activity assessment system. In addition to assessing various stages of carious lesions in enamel and dentine, this system also includes an evaluation of restorations but not for teeth missing due to dental caries. The Nyvad system appears to have predictive validity on the basis of a single study. However, whether a carious lesion was active or inactive at the start of the intervention that tested the predictive value had no influence on the outcome after 3 years [8].

The International Caries Detection and Assessment System (ICDAS) Collaboration Group developed and promoted the ICDAS 2-digit index as a new classification system in caries epidemiology by emphasising the importance of assessing various stages of enamel carious lesions in reaction to the reduction of dentine carious lesions in a number of western countries [9]. However, many visual/tactile indices that contain enamel carious lesions codes have been introduced since the mid-1950s [10] and provide useful information with respect to the suitability of more than 1 code for the reliable assessment of enamel carious lesions [11]. ICDAS was upgraded to ICDAS II, followed a couple of years later by ICDAS II-PUFA, and most recently by the International Caries Classification and Management System (ICCMS) [12]. The presence of face, content, and construct validity of ICDAS II has been questioned [13]. Researchers who used ICDAS (II) have altered the system over the years because of difficulties encountered when using it in epidemiological surveys in the field [14–16]. Another limitation in using ICDAS relates to reporting results. Initially, the DMFT/S unit was used to report results, followed later by the DMFT/S+PUFA modification, and later again by the DMFT/$S_{ICDAS/LA}$ where "LA" stands for "lesion activity." To be trained and calibrated in 3 differentiating codes for carious lesions in enamel, and then to group these codes together with code 0 to produce a dmf/DMF score seems like a great deal of additional work to end up with a simplified coding system that could have been used all along. After testing 2 codes for recording stages in a carious lesion in enamel, Marthaler [11] concluded that 1 code is sufficient. With the introduction of the ICCMS in 2013 [12], the ICDAS II index became split into a care index (former 1st digit) and a carious lesion index (former 2nd digit), with various options to merge the 7 caries-related codes for reporting results. With many changes in ICDAS over a relatively short period of time, it is difficult to see whether each of these steps, and upgraded steps, have been validated, especially in an epidemiological setting. Therefore, one should think twice before using ICDAS (II) or ICCMS in epidemiological surveys.

Around 2010, the pulp/ulceration/fistulae/abscess (pufa/PUFA) index was introduced [17].

The index assesses the pathological consequences of the caries process only and appears to be a valuable addition to recording caries-related conditions in epidemiology. It does not assess enamel or dentine carious lesions that can be restored, neither does it determine the presence of restorations or teeth lost due to dental caries. A few studies have been published and none have reported the validity of the index.

The index used most frequently in caries epidemiological surveys worldwide is that developed by the World Health Organisation (WHO) [18]. The index basically assesses whether or not a carious lesion is cavitated into dentine. Teeth missing due to dental caries and tooth restorations are also recorded.

The visual/tactile indices described above each have their limitations for use in caries epidemiological surveys. For example, the pufa/PUFA index needs to be complemented by an index that assesses enamel and dentine carious lesions without pulpal involvement; the Nyvad criteria needs the addition of a "missing teeth due to caries" category, the ICDAS II (double digits) needs the pufa/PUFA index, while the WHO index needs to be supplemented with an index that includes enamel carious lesions and the pufa/PUFA index.

The disadvantages of the visual/tactile indices described above are overcome by a newly developed assessment instrument termed the "Caries Assessment Spectrum and Treatment" (CAST) instrument [19]. It was introduced for the assessment of dental caries-related conditions and treatment in epidemiological surveys and designed to overcome the shortcomings of the indices/systems described above. It permits the registration of sound teeth, sealants, restorations, enamel, and dentine carious lesions, advanced stages of carious lesions into the pulp and tooth-surrounding tissues, and teeth lost from dental caries (Table 1). The assessment is performed visually, with the naked eye, and does not use compressed air for drying tooth surfaces. CAST consists of 10 codes that are ordered hierarchically. This implies that a sealant (code 1) is less severe than an enamel carious lesion (code 3), and that a dentine carious lesion that can be restored (code 5) is less severe than a tooth with a carious lesion with pulpal involvement (code 6).

Research showed that the CAST instrument has face, content, construct, and external validity for use in children and adults [20, 21] and has a high level of reproducibility [22]. The CAST codes can be converted to dmf/DMF counts so that dmf/DMF scores can be compared with those obtained from using the WHO index [23]. A restoration (code 2) and a tooth lost due to dental caries (code 8) is considered not diseased. With CAST, a caries-diseased tooth is one that has a dentine carious lesion (codes 4, 5) or has pathology (code 6, 7). This affects the determination of the prevalence of dental caries in a population, as discussed in the next section.

The CAST instrument needs to be tested in populations of different ages and backgrounds than those studied so far. CAST has been used or is in use in epidemiological surveys in Brazil [23], India [24], Pakistan [25], Poland [26], Mozambique, Peru, Russia, Surinam, and Turkey.

Reporting Data from Caries Epidemiological Surveys

The manner in which results are reported is important. Documents that describe epidemiological surveys are not restricted to dental professionals. Policy makers, medical practitioners, politicians, and the public have access to such documents, which requires clear reporting and should be straightforward and supported with easily understandable tables and figures. To make caries epidemiological reports easy to read a few typical dental inherited approaches from the past need to be changed, such as the use of the dmf/DMF index, which dates back to 1938 and contains a number of deficiencies.

Table 1. The validated CAST characteristics, codes and descriptions

Characteristic	Code	Description
Sound	0	No visible evidence of a distinct carious lesion is present
Sealant	1	Pits and/or fissures are at least partially covered with a sealant material
Restoration	2	A cavity is restored with an (in)direct restorative material
Enamel	3	Distinct visual change in enamel only; a clear caries-related discolouration is visible, with or without localised enamel breakdown
Dentine	4	Internal caries-related discolouration in dentine; the discoloured dentine is visible through enamel which may or may not exhibit a visible localised breakdown of enamel
	5	Distinct cavitation into dentine; the pulp chamber is intact
Pulp	6	Involvement of the pulp chamber; distinct cavitation reaching the pulp chamber or only root fragments are present
Abscess/fistula	7	A pus-containing swelling or a pus-releasing sinus tract related to a tooth with pulpal involvement
Lost	8	The tooth has been removed because of dental caries
Other	9	Does not correspond to any of the other descriptions

An inherent deficiency is its use in calculating the prevalence of dental caries. By definition, the presence of carious lesions into dentine, restored dentine lesions, and missing teeth due to dental caries (D_3MFT) make up the prevalence of dental caries. If required, the code for enamel carious lesion(s) can be included in the prevalence calculation, but this has to be clearly stated (D_1MFT or D_2MFT). The present definition covers not only actual disease but also past disease (restored and missing teeth). The advantage of considering teeth restored and teeth lost due to dental caries not diseased anymore is that dental caries prevalence is calculated on the bases of the actual presence of the disease in the individual. This reasoning was one of the cornerstones of the development of CAST. It holds the advantage of depicting the state of the disease and monitoring its changes over time in society more reliably. For example, successful interventions cannot be evidenced by a lower prevalence score [27].

In principle, studies that use CAST do not report the results in dmf/DMF counts but a dmf/DMF count can be calculated using CAST codes [23]. CAST uses frequency distributions per caries code or for maximum CAST code, depending on the aim of the survey (Fig. 1, 2). The severity of caries-related conditions within an individual or group after using CAST is calculated according to a mathematical formula in which the CAST codes have been assigned a weighted coefficient of severity [28]. Those wishing to know more about how to apply CAST and how to report data are referred to the CAST manual [29].

Global Epidemiology of Dental Caries

A recent publication reported on the global epidemiology of dental caries [30]. The paper was based on a systematic review of systematic reviews on the prevalence and incidence of dental caries. As only one systematic review was retrieved covering 1990–2010, and this review had limited background variables [31], the WHO Data Bank at Malmö University Dental School [32] was used to obtain more detailed information. The Data Bank contains dental caries-related data, covers several decades of studies, and is periodically updated. The country dental caries prevalence and the dmf/DMF and d/D-component data from the recommended WHO age groups were used as outcome measures for the period

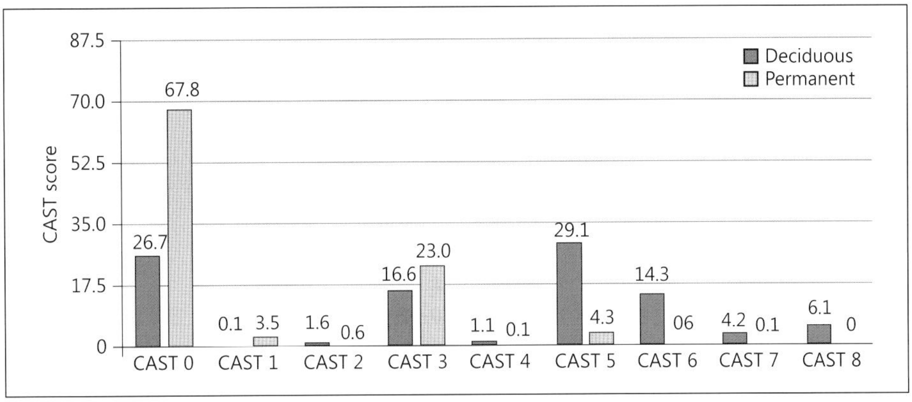

Fig. 1. Maximum CAST score per subject and type of dentition based on hypothetical results. Modified from Leal et al. [57].

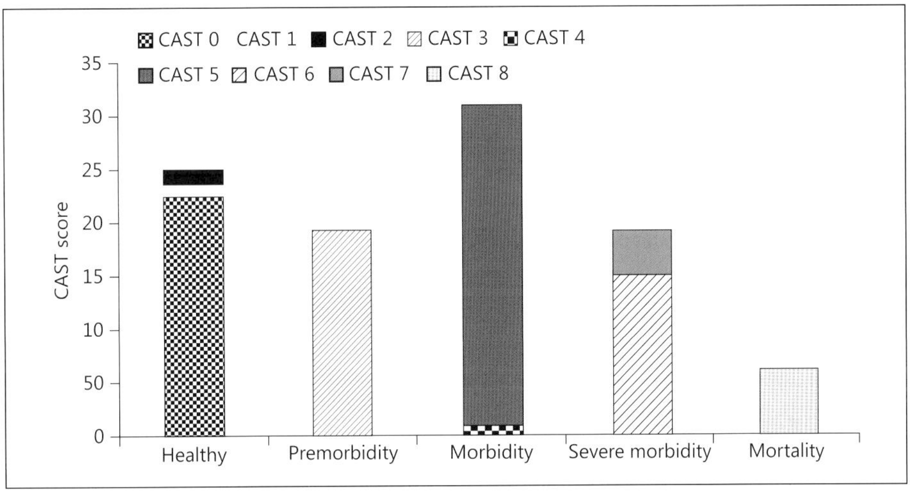

Fig. 2. Severity of dental caries based on the maximum CAST score per subject. Modified from Leal et al. [57].

from 2000 to 2016. These data were related to the countries' gross national income [33], developed by the World Bank, according to high-, upper-middle-, lower-middle-, and low-income countries.

The publication also reported trend studies that had covered a period of at least 20 years, from 1999 to 2016. The caries assessment criterion developed by the WHO (1971) was used most frequently.

Global Burden of Untreated Cavitated Dentine Carious Lesions

The systematic review dealt with the global burden of untreated cavitated dentine carious lesions and covered 187 countries [31]. The age-standardised prevalence of untreated dentine carious lesions in the primary dentition in the global population did not change during the 2 decades and constituted the 10th most prevalent health condi-

Table 2. Median prevalence of cavitated dentine carious lesions in 5- and 6-year-olds, median of mean dmft scores and range interval, and proportion of d-component and range interval by category of country income, using WHO Data Bank data from 2000 to 2015 (data from Frencken et al. [30])

	Country income			
	low	lower-middle	upper-middle	high
Lesion prevalence				
Countries, *n*	3	12	13	33
%	64.4	83.4	76.4	49.0
Range	49.2–93.1	64.0–88.6	53.4–93.2	21.0–93.4
Mean dmft scores				
Countries, *n*	3	16	15	33
Median	4.4	4.1	3.9	2.0
Range	3.0–9.0	1.4–8.0	2.4–6.7	0.3–6.7
D-component				
Countries, *n*	2	9	11	22
%	96.1	96.4	88.0	75.0
Range	93.3–98.9	91.3–100	78.6–97.3	33.3–100

n, number.

tion, affecting 621 million children worldwide. There were no significant differences between boys and girls.

The global age-standardised prevalence of untreated dentine carious lesions in the permanent dentition did not change between 1990 and 2010 and reached a peak at age 25 years, with a second peak at around 70 years of age. There were no significant differences between gender. The authors concluded that untreated cavitated dentine carious lesions in permanent teeth remained the most prevalent health condition across the globe in 2010, affecting 2.4 billion people [31].

Prevalence and Extent of Carious Lesions in Infants and Young Children

It is technically and behaviourally possible to keep healthy primary teeth healthy. Unfortunately, this is not the reality in many world communities. Frencken [34] reported that "(severe) early childhood caries ([S-]ECC) is prevalent in many countries with large populations in deprivation. Epidemiological surveys from Brazil, Canada, Vietnam, China, Switzerland, and Thailand show alarming results. High prevalence figures for S-ECC for 38% (Canada) and 44.1% (Thailand) of 3-year olds have been reported while the prevalence of ECC was 24.8% in Switzerland and 74.4% in Vietnam among 1- to 6-year olds. The mean dmft-score for 1- to 6-year olds was 3.6 in China and 3.9 in Canada" [31]. The heterogeneity of data collection methods between these studies notwithstanding, these figures show that something is drastically wrong in many world communities despite some improvements achieved over the last 3 decades in other countries and communities [27].

One of the risk indicators for developing dental caries is the level of deprivation. The major driver of deprivation is the availability of funds/income. Therefore, a country's caries-related data from the WHO database have been linked to their gross national income. Table 2 shows that cavitated dentine carious lesions in 5- and 6-year-old children are prevalent in all countries but that there was a difference in the severity of cavitated dentine carious lesions across the groups of income countries. The lowest median dmft count was found in the high-income group (2.0) compared to 3.9 and 4.1 in the upper-middle- and lower-middle-income groups, respectively. The percentage of the d-component was high in all income groups in each country [30]. These findings confirm the outcome of the study by Kassebaum et al. [31] and paint a poor picture of the dental caries situation in youngsters in world communities.

Fortunately, good news can also be reported. Although considered poor, the current dental caries situation may not be as bad as 40 years ago. Table 3 shows trends in the prevalence of cavitated dentine carious lesions and the mean dmft scores in 5 countries. In all countries, the prevalence and mean dmft scores decreased remarkably over time. The highest reduction rate in the prevalence of cavitated dentine carious lesions was reported for the UK and Sweden: 46 and 45%, respectively, over 40 years [30]. Dentine carious lesions are now concentrated in a minority of children in these and perhaps more countries. Trend studies show the importance of monitoring the disease situation in a country/community regularly.

Table 3. Trends in the prevalence of cavitated dentine carious lesions and in mean dmft scores in 4-, 5-, and 5- to 6-year-olds over decades in a number of countries (data from Frencken et al. [30])

Country/period	Age, years	Prevalence, %	dmft mean
South Africa [48]	5–6		
1947		88	6.7
2002		57	3.1
Sweden [49]	4		
1967		83	4.0
2007		38	3.4
UK [35]	5		
1973		72	4.0 (dft)
2013		26	0.7
China [50]	5		
1987–1994		80	–
2010–2013		56	–
Czech Republic [51]	5		
1994		76	3.5
2006		58	2.7

Prevalence and Extent of Carious Lesions in Children

On the basis of the data from the WHO database and compared to the other 3 income groups, the median prevalence of cavitated dentine carious lesions and median mean DMFT score of 12-year-old children in the upper-middle-income group were high, at 69.4% and 2.1%, respectively (Table 4). The median percentage of the D-component was high in the low-income (100%), lower-middle-income (80%), and upper-middle-income groups (79%) compared to the high-income group (45.5%), which varied between 0.0 and 92.9% [30].

Similar to the dental caries situation in young adults, the situation in children was worse a couple of decades ago than now. Trend studies have shown a large reduction in the prevalence of cavitated dentine carious lesions and in mean DMFT scores in some countries irrespective of the continent they are conducted in (Table 5) [30]. The reduction in Poland is less pronounced in numbers compared to the other countries and the prevalence of cavitated dentine carious lesions and severity scores in adolescents in 2012 are high in comparison to comparable results in the other countries. The number of sound teeth in 15-year-old adolescents in the UK was 10 higher than among 16- to 24-year olds 45 years earlier [35].

The decline in the prevalence and severity of dental caries has not affected children of different socioeconomic status (SES) equally. Particularly in affluent societies, children from low-SES are worse off than their peers with a high SES. Reasons for this difference are related not only to income, but also to culture, ethnicity, and parental education and dental attender [36, 37]. Overall, inequality in life is a major risk factor for developing carious lesions in children.

Table 4. Median prevalence of cavitated dentine carious lesions in 12-year-olds, median of mean DMFT scores and range interval, and median proportion of D-component and range interval by category of country income, using WHO Data Bank data from 2000 to 2015 (data from Frencken et al. [30])

	Country income			
	low	lower-middle	upper-middle	high
Lesion prevalence				
Countries, *n*	5	15	20	36
%	42.2	41.9	69.4	46.6
Range	19.1–97.3	22.4–75.7	37.0–87.0	22.3–84.0
Mean DMFT scores				
Countries, *n*	9	21	27	44
Median	0.9	1.4	2.1	1.3
Range	0.3–5.5	0.4–4.5	1.1–4.9	0.4–4.8
D-component				
Countries, *n*	3	13	16	27
%	100.0	80.0	79.0	45.5
Range	–	66.6–100	36.4–94.1	0.0–92.9

n, number.

Which Are the Most Carious Lesion-Susceptible Permanent Teeth and Surfaces in Child Populations?

This question was discussed by Frencken [34] in the following manner. "The fluoride studies from the 1950s to the 1980s showed that the largest reduction in the extent and severity of carious lesions in children took place in smooth surfaces, followed by approximal surfaces. Fluoride was less effective in occlusal surfaces." Other researchers have also reported this hierarchy in carious lesion susceptibility [11, 38, 39]. On the basis of data from 20,000 schoolchildren aged 5–16 years in the USA, it was established that the predominant susceptible tooth sites in low dentine carious lesion individuals (DMFS <5) were pits and fissures (95%). The proportion of approximal surfaces and smooth surfaces increased with an increase in mean DMFS score in this age group. In high-dentine carious lesion individuals (DMFS >25), the proportion of dentine carious lesions was about 20% for smooth surfaces, 30% for approximal surfaces, and 50% for pits and fissures [39].

Is there also a hierarchy in dentine carious lesions by tooth type? On the basis of the findings of the same US study, it could be concluded that occlusal surfaces of first molars and buccal pits of lower first molars were the most carious lesion-susceptible type of tooth and tooth surface. If all the first molars are affected, then a high probability exists that the second molars will be affected. The occlusal surfaces of the second molars and the buccal surfaces of the lower second molars are the second most susceptible sites for dentine carious lesion development in children with a low DMFS count. Smooth surfaces on the lower anterior region are least susceptible. A New Zealand birth-cohort study confirmed that the first followed by second permanent molars are most affected by dental caries over a period of 38 years [40].

All in all, pits and fissures in occlusal and pits in buccal tooth surfaces appear to be the most vulnerable sites for dentine carious lesions in the permanent teeth of children and adolescents. In children at high-caries risk these sites may need extra protection to keep them healthy.

Table 5. Trends in the prevalence of cavitated dentine carious lesions and in mean DMFT scores in adolescents, young adults, and 35- to 44-year-olds, and number of sound teeth over decades in a number of countries (data from Frencken et al. [30])

Country/period	Prevalence, %	Mean DMFT	Mean DMFS	Sound teeth, *n*
South Africa [48]				
11- to 13-year olds (urban)				
1977	70	4.4		
2002	37	1.5		
14- to 17-year olds (urban)				
1977	95	7.5		
2002	50	2.0		
Brazil [52]				
12- to-13-year olds				
1971	98	9.2		
2011	37	0.7		
Norway [53]				
12-year olds				
1985	81	3.4		
2004	60	1.7		
UK [35]				
15-year olds				
1968				16.3[a]
1973	97	8.4		
2013	42	1.2		26.6[b]
Poland [54]				
12-year olds				
1978	98	6.3		25.0[c]
2012	84	3.5		17.0[c]
The Netherlands [55]				
Low SES				
9-year olds				
1990	28		3.0	
2009	23		2.5	
14-year olds				
1990	67		6.3	
2009	51		4.1	
20-year olds				
1990	94		14.7	
2009	74		7.7	
High SES				
9-year olds				
1990	26		2.9	
2009	15		1.8	
14-year olds				
1990	75		3.1	
2009	38		3.5	
20-year olds				
1990	94		9.4	
2009	70		6.7	

Table 5. (continued)

Country/period	Prevalence, %	Mean DMFT	Mean DMFS	Sound teeth, *n*
Americas [56][d]				
12-year olds				
North				
1970s		4.4 (2.6–5.3)		
1990s		1.6 (1.4–1.8)		
Central/Caribbean				
1970s		5.1 (4.8–5.6)		
1990s		2.9 (1.1–4.9)		
South[e]				
1970s		5.8 (1.2–8.6)		
1990s		3.1 (1.3–4.7)		

SES, socioeconomic status.
[a] 16- to 24-year-olds.
[b] 15-year-olds.
[c] Mean DMFT score in 35- to 44-year-olds.
[d] Data for the Americas are presented as the median mean DMFT (range).
[e] 12-year olds.

Table 6. Median mean DMFT scores and range interval among 35- to 44-year-olds, proportion of D-component and range interval by category of country income, using WHO Data Bank data from 2000 to 2015 (data from Frencken et al. [30])

	Country income			
	low	lower-middle	upper-middle	high
Mean DMFT scores				
Countries, *n*	3	6	8	20
Median	3.1	7.5	11.4	13.5
Range	2.9–4.7	2.6–14.6	6.0–14.8	6.8–20.0
D-component				
Countries, *n*	2	5	7	16
%	53.6	39.7	17.9	9.6
Range	45.1–62.0	24.0–54.0	13.3–52.6	3.4–27.9

n, number.

Prevalence and Extent of Carious Lesions in Adults and the Elderly

Using the data of the WHO database, the median mean DMFT score among 35- to 44-year-old adults was high in the high-income group (13.5) and low in the low-income group (3.1; Table 6). Unfortunately, only a small number of countries was included in the low-income group. The mean percentage of the D-component was low (9.6%) in the high-income group and high (53.6%) in the low-income group.

Although there have been few trend studies, they show a clear picture. The mean number of teeth present among 50-, 60-, and 70-year olds from Sweden increased from 21.5 to 26.1 among 50-year olds and from 13.3 to 20.7 among 70-year olds between 1973 and 2003 [41]. Among 50-year-old Swedish women, the mean number of teeth increased from 14.6 in 1968/69 to 27.3 in 2004/05. The percentage of edentulous women decreased from 18.2 to 0.3 between 1968/69 and 2004/05 [42]. This pattern has also been reported in the UK, Canada, and Australia [43].

The prevalence of root carious lesions in subjects aged over 60 years in Japan was 39% in 2006, with poor oral hygiene and a low salivary flow rate being potential risk factors [40]. More recently, in southern Brazil, approximately 36% of dentate individuals had carious lesions and/or restorations that affected, on average, 5.0 teeth [41]. In an older age group of over 80-year-old Swedish elders, untreated coronal dentine carious lesions were present for between 36 and 56% of the subjects, while between 54 and 75% had untreated root carious lesions [42]. A review on this topic is available from Tonetti et al. [44].

The fact that people are getting older with more natural teeth than in previous times increases the risk for carious lesion development, both in crown and root surfaces, because of an increase in the number of teeth and improvement in living conditions. This risk implies that adequate care needs to be organised on the basis of realistic treatment options that include the possibility to deliver care at home and in institutions where many elderly people remain for longer. This implies that the care, including restorative treatments, needs to be mobile. An example of such an approach is atraumatic restorative treatment (ART) [45, 46].

Challenges

Dental caries is a behavioural/life-style disease which is preventable in nature through diet (sugar-free consumption) control and daily plaque removal with a toothbrush and fluoride toothpaste. Despite being preventable, dental caries is widespread and untreated dentine carious lesions in permanent and primary dentitions are ranked number 1 and 10, respectively, on the list of most prevalent medical diseases and conditions [47].

Pits and fissures in occlusal first molars and pits in buccal mandible first molars are the tooth types and sites that are the most susceptible for developing dentine carious lesions. In children at high risk for carious lesion development, these tooth types and sites need to be monitored well.

Progress has been made in oral health over the last 3–4 decades, but the extent to which the reduction in prevalence and severity of dental caries is applicable to countries around the world is unknown as many countries do not carry out epidemiological surveys or do not publish the results in the English-language dental literature. However, monitoring and comparing trends in caries prevalence and severity requires studies to have the same outcome measures and use the same assessment instruments.

Considering the need and importance for monitoring dental caries over time, only validated carious lesion assessment indices/systems should be used. Not all currently used indices/systems have sufficient validation. The CAST instrument is an exception, but it requires further testing for its applicability in different age groups.

Generally speaking, dental caries is an age-related and a life-long disease. Despite progress made in improving oral health, the fact that people are living longer and that more teeth remain at risk at old age than before does not reduce the burden of dental caries in society. This conclusion calls for the introduction of a massive behavioural/preventive programme that targets parents and dental/medical professionals, and should start at mother and child health care centres and continue throughout the primary educational system. Dental practitioners should leave their comfort zone of the dental surgery and make themselves available for providing care at the community level, while oral health care financial systems should allow for a gradual shift from predominantly rewarding curative care (damage repair) to preventive and promotional oral healthcare.

References

1 Twetman S, Axelsson S, Dahlén G, Espelid I, Mejàre I, Norlund A, Tranæus S: Adjunct methods for caries detection: a systematic review of literature. Acta Odontol Scand 2013;71:388–397.
2 Tassery H, Manton DJ: Detection and diagnosis of carious lesions; in Eden E (ed): Evidence-Based Caries Prevention. Cham, Springer International, 2016.
3 Gimenez T, Piovesan C, Braga MM, Raggio DP, Deery C, Ricketts DN, Ekstrand KR, Mendes FM: Visual Inspection for caries detection: a systematic review and meta-analysis. J Dent Res 2015;94:895–904.
4 Sturmans F: Epidemiologie: Theorie, Methoden en Toepassing, ed 3. Nijmegen, Dekker & van de Vegt, 1986, p 46.
5 Ismail AI, Sohn W, Tellez M, Amaya A, Sen A, Hasson H, Pitts NB: The International Caries Detection and Assessment system (ICDAS): an integrated system for measuring dental caries. Community Dent Oral Epidemiol 2007;35:170–178.
6 Jablonski-Momeni A, Stachniss V, Ricketts DN, Heinzel-Gutenbrunner M, Pieper K: Reproducibility and accuracy of the ICDAS-II for detection of occlusal caries in vitro. Caries Res 2008;42:79–87.
7 Nyvad B, Machiulskiene V, Baelum V: Reliability of a new caries diagnostic system differentiating between active and inactive caries lesions. Caries Res 1999;33:252–260.
8 Nyvad B, Machiulskiene V, Baelum V: Construct and predictive validity of clinical caries diagnostic criteria assessing lesion activity. J Dent 2003;82:117–122.
9 Pitts N: "ICDAS" – an international system for caries detection and assessment being developed to facilitate caries epidemiology, research and appropriate clinical management. Community Dent Health 2004;21:193–198.
10 Ismail AI: Visual and visuo-tactile detection of dental caries. J Dent Res 2004; 83:C56–C66.
11 Marthaler TM: A standardized system of recording dental conditions. Helv Odontol Acta 1966;10:1–18.
12 Ismail AI, Pitts NB, Tellez M: The International Caries Classification and Management system (ICCMS): an example of a caries management pathway. BMC Oral Health 2015;15(suppl 1):S9.
13 de Souza Hilgert AL: Caries Assessment Spectrum and Treatment (CAST): A new epidemiological instrument; PhD thesis, Radboud University, Nijmegen, 2015, pp 134–137.
14 Agustsdottir H, Gudmundsdottir H, Eggertsson H, Jonsson SH, Gudlaugsson JO, Saemundsson SR, Eliasson ST, Arnadottir IB, Holbrook WP: Caries prevalence of permanent teeth: national survey of children in Iceland using ICDAS. Community Dent Oral Epidemiol 2010; 38:299–309.
15 Cadavid AS, Lince CMA, Jaramillo MC: Dental caries in the primary dentition of a Colombian population according to the ICDAS criteria. Braz Oral Res 2010; 24:211–216.
16 Almerich-Silla JM, Boronat-Ferrer T, Montiel-Company JM, Iranzo-Cortés JE: Caries prevalence in children from Valencia (Spain) using ICDAS II criteria, 2010. Med Oral Patol Oral Cir Bucal 2014;19:e574–e580.
17 Monse B, Heinrich-Weltzien R, Benzian H, Holmgren C, van Palenstein Helderman W: PUFA – an index of clinical consequences of untreated dental caries. Dent Oral Epidemiol 2010;38:77–82.
18 World Health Organization: Oral Health Surveys: Basic Methods, ed 1. Geneva, WHO, 1971.
19 Frencken JE, de Amorim RG, Faber L, Leal SC: The Caries Assessment Spectrum and Treatment (CAST) index: rational and development. Int Dent J 2011; 61:117–123.
20 de Souza AL, van der Sanden WJM, Leal SC, Frencken JE: The Caries Assessment Spectrum and Treatment: face and content validation. Int Dent J 2012;62:270–276.
21 de Souza AL, Leal SC, Chaves SB, Bronkhorst EM, Frencken JE, Creugers NHJ: The Caries Assessment Spectrum and Treatment (CAST) instrument: construct validation. Eur J Oral Sci 2014; 122:149–153.
22 de Souza AL, Bronkhorst EM, Creugers NHJ, Leal SC, Frencken JE: The Caries Assessment Spectrum and Treatment (CAST) instrument: its reproducibility in clinical studies. Int Dent J 2014;64: 187–194.
23 de Souza A, Leal S, Bronkhorst E, Frencken JE: Assessing caries status according to the CAST instrument and WHO criterion in epidemiological studies. BMC Oral Health 2014;14:119.
24 Reddy ER, Rani ST, Manjula M, Kumar LV, Mohan TA, Radhika E: Assessment of caries status among schoolchildren according to decayed-missing-filled teeth/decayed-extract-filled teeth index, International Caries Detection and Assessment System, and Caries Assessment Spectrum and Treatment criteria. Indian J Dent Res 2017;28:487–492.
25 Malik A, Shaukat MS, Qureshi A: Prevalence of dental caries using novel Caries Assessment Index: CAST. J Dow Uni Health Sci 2014;8:7–10.
26 Baginska J, Rodakowska E, Wilczko M, et al: Caries Assessment Spectrum and Treatment (CAST) index in the primary molars of 6- to 7-year-old Polish children. Oral Health Prev Dent 2016;14: 85–92.
27 Baelum V, Fejerskov O: How big is the problem? Epidemiological features of dental caries; in Fejerskov O, Nyvad B, Kidd (eds): Dental Caries: The Disease and Its Clinical Management, ed 3. Oxford, Wiley Blackwell, 2015.
28 Ribeiro APD, Maciel IP, de Souza Hilgert AL, Bronkhorst EM Frencken JE, Leal SC: Caries Assessment Spectrum Treatment (CAST): the severity score. Int Dent J 2018;68:84–90.
29 Frencken JE, de Souza Hilgert AL, Bronkhorst EM, Leal SC: CAST: Caries Assessment Spectrum and Treatment: Manual. Enschede, Ipskamp Drukkers, 2015.
30 Frencken JE, Sharma P, Stenhouse L, Green D, Laverty D, Dietrich T: Global epidemiology of dental caries and severe periodontitis – a comprehensive review. J Clin Periodontol 2017;44:S94–S105.
31 Kassebaum NJ, Bernabé E, Dahiya M, Bhandari B, Murray CJ, Marcenes W: Global burden of untreated caries: a systematic review and metaregression. J Dent Res 2015;94:650–658.
32 Oral Health Care System and Services. Malmö University. https://www.mah.se/CAPP/Country-Oral.../Oral-Health-Care-System-and-Services (accessed July 15, 2016).

33 Gross National Income (GNI; Atlas Method) Per Capita, 2014. https://en.wikipedia.org/wiki/List_of_countries_by_GNI (accessed July 17, 2016).
34 Frencken JE: Dental caries and caries epidemiology; in Eden E (ed): Evidence-Based Caries Prevention. Cham, Springer, 2016.
35 Murray JJ, Vernazza CR, Holmes RD: Forty years of national surveys: an overview of children's dental health from 1973–2013. Br Dent J 2015;219:281–285.
36 André Kramer AC, Petzold M, Hakeberg M, Östberg AL: Multiple socioeconomic factors and dental caries in Swedish children and adolescents. Caries Res 2017;52:42–50.
37 Lambert MJ, Vanobbergen JSN, Martens LC, De Visschere LMJ: Socioeconomic inequalities in caries experience, care level and dental attendance in primary school children in Belgium: a cross-sectional survey. BMJ Open 2017; 7:e015042.
38 Batchelor PA, Sheiham A: Grouping of tooth surfaces by susceptibility to caries: a study in 5–16 year-old children. BMC Oral Health 2004;4:2.
39 Sheiham A, Sabbah W: Using universal patterns of caries for planning and evaluating dental care. Caries Res 2010;44: 141–150.
40 Broadbent JM, Foster Page LA, Thomson WM, Poulton R: Permanent dentition caries through the first half of life. Br Dent J 2013;215:E12.
41 Hugoson A, Koch G, Göthberg C, Helkimo AN, Lundin SA, Norderyd O, Sjödin B, Sondell K: Oral health of individuals aged 3–80 years in Jönköping, Sweden, during 30 years (1973–2003). II. Review of clinical and radiographic findings. Swed Dent J 2005;29:139–155.
42 Wennström A, Ahlqwist M, Stenman U, Björkelund C, Hakeberg M: Trends in tooth loss in relation to socio-economic status among Swedish women, aged 38 and 50 years: repeated cross-sectional surveys 1968–2004. BMC Oral Health 2013;13:63.
43 MacEntee MI, Bryant SR, Keller H, Nguyen CT, Yao CS: Caries control for frail elders; in Fejerskov O, Nyvad B, Kidd E (eds): Dental Caries: The Disease and Its Clinical Management, ed 3. Oxford, Wiley Blackwell, 2015.
44 Tonetti MS, Bottenberg P, Conrads G, Eickholz P, Heasman P, Huysmans MC, López R, Madianos P, Müller F, Needleman I, Nyvad B, Preshaw PM, Pretty I, Renvert S, Schwendicke F, Trombelli L, van der Putten GJ, Vanobbergen J, West N, Young A, Paris S: Dental caries and periodontal diseases in the ageing population: call to action to protect and enhance oral health and well-being as an essential component of healthy ageing – consensus report of group 4 of the joint EFP/ORCA workshop on the boundaries between caries and periodontal diseases. J Clin Periodontol 2017;44(suppl 18):S135–S144.
45 Amer RS, Kolker JL: Restoration of root surface caries in vulnerable elderly patients: a review of the literature. Spec Care Dentist 2013;33:141–149.
46 da Mata C, Allen PF, McKenna G, Cronin M, O'Mahony D, Woods N: Two-year survival of ART restorations placed in elderly patients: a randomised controlled clinical trial. J Dent 2015;43:405–411.
47 Marcenes W, Kassebaum NJ, Bernabé E, Flaxman A, Naghavi M, Lopez A, Murray CJ: Global burden of oral conditions in 1990–2010: a systematic analysis. J Dent Res 2013;92:592–597.
48 Cleaton-Jones P, Fatti P: Dental caries in children in South Africa and Swaziland: a systematic review 1919–2007. Int Dent J 2009;59:363–368.
49 Stecksén-Blicks C, Kieri C, Nyman JE, Pilebro C, Borssén E: Caries prevalence and background factors in Swedish 4-year-old children – a 40-year perspective. Int J Paediatr Dent 2008;18:317–324.
50 Zhang X, Yang S, Liao Z, Xu L, Li C, Zeng H, Song J, Zhang L: Prevalence and care index of early childhood caries in mainland China: evidence from epidemiological surveys during 1987–2013. Sci Rep 2016;6:18897.
51 Lenčová E, Pikhart H, Broukal Z: Early childhood caries trends and surveillance shortcomings in the Czech Republic. BMC Public Health 2012;12:547.
52 Constante HM, Souza ML, Bastos JL, Peres MA: Trends in dental caries among Brazilian schoolchildren: 40 years of monitoring (1971–2011). Int Dent J 2014;64:181–186.
53 Haugejorden O, Birkeland JM: Ecological time-trend analysis of caries experience at 12-years of age and caries incidence from age 12 to 18 years: Norway 1985–2004. Acta Odontolog Scand 2006; 64:368–375.
54 Gaszyńska E, Wierzbicka M, Marczak M, Szatko F: Thirty years of evolution of oral health behaviours and dental caries in urban and rural areas in Poland. Ann Agric Environ Med 2014;21:557–561.
55 Schuller AA, van Dommelen P, Poorterman JH: Trends in oral health in young people in the Netherlands over the past 20 years: a study in a changing context. Community Dent Oral Epidemiol 2014; 42:178–184.
56 Beltrán-Aguilar ED, Estupiñán-Day S, Báez R: Analysis of prevalence and trends of dental caries in the Americas between the 1970s and 1990s. Int Dent J 1999;49:322–329.
57 Leal SC, Ribeiro APD, Frencken JE: Caries Assessment Spectrum and Treatment (CAST): a novel epidemiological instrument. Caries Res 2017;51:500–506.

Jo Frencken
Philips van Leijdenlaan 25
NL–6525 AX Nijmegen (The Netherlands)
E-Mail jo.frencken@radboudumc.nl

Schwendicke F, Frencken J, Innes N (eds): Caries Excavation: Evolution of Treating Cavitated Carious Lesions.
Monogr Oral Sci. Basel, Karger, 2018, vol 27, pp 24–31 (DOI: 10.1159/000487828)

Carious Lesion Diagnosis: Methods, Problems, Thresholds

Klaus W. Neuhaus · Adrian Lussi

Department of Preventive, Restorative and Pediatric Dentistry, Bern, Switzerland

Abstract

The difference between carious lesion diagnosis and carious lesion detection is discussed here. Concerning carious lesions, 3 diagnostic requirements should be fulfilled: to detect lesions, to assess surface integrity, and to assess lesion activity to support clinical decision making. The first and most important diagnostic method is meticulous visual-tactile inspection. This is the only method that potentially contributes to all 3 diagnostic requirements. All other methods that are presented in this chapter, i.e., bitewing radiography, fluorescence-based technologies, and transillumination methods, are limited to assessing lesion depth in surfaces that are not visible to the eye and thus contribute to lesion detection only. At the end of the chapter, recent developments in objective lesion activity assessment are presented.

Detection versus Diagnosis of Caries

In general, most dental practitioners' use the term "caries diagnosis" synonymously with "caries detection" [1]. This might derive from the fact that the therapeutic step is indirectly linked to the diagnostic step [2, 3]. Because therapy is remunerated, and operative intervention more so than non-operative intervention, a dichotomous "caries yes/no thinking" is often employed in daily practice – although this is not sufficient. However, it is worthwhile considering the distinct differences between these two terms.

"Caries detection" means the discrimination between a healthy tooth surface and a tooth surface affected by a carious lesion to a certain degree. To a great extent the different methods of caries detection aim at staging the caries process in order to facilitate treatment decision making: initial stages of caries usually require different treatment options than further progressed stages. In this respect, caries detection also and most importantly involves the assessment of surface integrity of a tooth. Once a frank cavitation occurs on a tooth surface, removal of the biofilm in that place is hampered. Thus, non-operative intervention is usually not recommended anymore, and the dental practitioner treats the lesion by cleaning, restoring, and sealing the cavity in order to facilitate plaque removal at the restored tooth surface [4].

Detecting a carious lesion does not say anything about whether the lesion is in a progressing or in a stagnating stage [5]. The lesion's specific behaviour over time is referred to as "lesion activity" [6]. Lesion activity assessment is a crucial factor because its outcome contributes to clinical decision making [7]. Furthermore, in a broader perspective "caries diagnosis" also considers the local environment in which the respective tooth is embedded. Several patient-specific factors (location/position of the tooth or the lesion, saliva, microbiota, fluoride availability, cleaning habits, diet) that contribute to individual caries risk also play a significant role in the decision-making process of caries diagnosis. However, this chapter deals with the first two aspects, caries detection and lesion activity assessment.

Caries Detection Methods

Visual-Tactile Inspection

The first and most important method to detect and to diagnose caries is visual-tactile inspection [8]. The eyes are able to discriminate by colour matching all clinically relevant caries stages from sound tooth surfaces to dental restorations. The eyes are also capable of seeing surface discontinuities, ranging from microcavities to large cavities. Further advantages include clinical visual inspection being fast, inexpensive, radiation-free, and helping to establish doctor-patient contact. As a prerequisite, the eyes should be functioning perfectly [9]. It is known that after the age of about 40 years the eyes have lower accommodation capabilities, the reflection glare increases, and the visual acuity decreases [10, 11]. Therefore, the use of moderately high magnification loupes (about ×2.5) [12] is recommended to compensate for reduced vision at increased age [13]. It has been shown that magnification greater than ×2.5 significantly decreased specificity, irrespective of the duration of clinical experience [13]. Additional illumination is helpful, but if too intense (>20,000 lx) it might actually reduce the accuracy of caries detection [14]. Lastly, a visual caries detection system should be used that takes into account the different stages of carious lesion development, and not only those that have reached a stage of cavitation. Several main caries detection and notation systems are available (Nyvad system [6], The International Caries Detection and Assessment System (ICDAS) [15], and the Caries Assessment Spectrum and Treatment (CAST) [16]). CAST covers the total spectrum of dental caries and has been designed for epidemiological purposes, whereas ICDAS and the so-called Nyvad criteria can be used also in the private office. For epidemiological data acquisition, ICDAS and Nyvad criteria have their limitations [see the chapter by Frencken; this vol., pp. 11–23]. It has been shown that proper training is needed to use either system to increase reliability, validity, and accuracy. The outcome of visual caries detection trials is dependent on the circumstances under which clinical visual inspection takes place, on the caries prevalence of the respective patients/subjects or, in laboratory experiments, on caries levels [17], and caries detection thresholds [18, 19]. Thus, in a recent review, a moderate to high degree of heterogeneity was found in visual caries detection studies [20]. In visual caries detection studies assessing initial and more advanced caries lesions, pooled sensitivities and specificities were reported to be 0.27–0.81 and 0.73–0.99, respectively, with a tendency towards lower sensitivity and higher specificity in clinical settings [20].

Visual-tactile inspection works well on visible surfaces, but the detection of carious lesions in the approximal surface is more difficult, and therefore more biased [20]. Furthermore, dentine carious lesions in occlusal surfaces with seemingly intact fissures (so-called "hidden caries") is usually detected at a relatively late stage when discolouration of dentine shines through the enamel [21]. Approximal surfaces and occlusal grooves and fissures are the sites where most carious lesions are found. On approximal surfaces, a small hook-like probe might add information on a present cavitation, but this test is reliable only when the cavitation itself or the area beneath the contact zone of two adjacent teeth are large enough for the probe to enter. A sharp-ended probe should only be used to gently touch the surface of the tooth to assess lesion roughness, but this test seems to be not reliable [22]. Firm pressing of a sharp probe in order to test the "stickiness" of a fissure should be refrained from because irreversible damage occurs that results in more invasive treatment [23]. The use of a periodontal probe is recommended to scan the surface for irregularities, such as microcavities [24].

Theoretically, visual inspection can be performed on approximal surfaces when the patient receives orthodontic separating rubber bands for 2 to 3 days to create space between the teeth [examples of this are shown in Fig. 3 in Schwendicke, Lamont and Innes, this vol., p. 36 and Fig. 3 in Fontana and Innes, this vol., p. 107]. This method works well for single approximal spaces and has been used as a gold standard in several clinical trials [25, 26]. For multiple approximal spaces, however, the effect would be less pronounced. This method also has the disadvantages of discomfort for the patient and requiring several appointments. Whilst in other medical disciplines several appointments for several tests to derive a complex diagnosis are usually accepted by patients, in dentistry there seems to be a need for immediate findings and treatment decisions [2].

Cleaning of teeth is necessary to inspect the tooth surfaces [27, 28]. Having defined approximal surfaces and occlusal fissures and grooves as high-risk caries sites, these sites are often covered by plaque or even food remnants that render a meticulous visual inspection impossible without prior cleaning. It is essential that plaque present be identified by means of a probe, because the position of the plaque may be an indicator for the presence of "active" enamel carious lesion(s) [6]. Clinically, the patient can be asked to brush the teeth in the usual way before inspection. This facilitates the identification of chronically neglected sites easier. Depending on the cleaning habits of the patients, chronically swollen and bleeding papillae hamper visual inspection of the interdental areas, and an initial periodontal therapy might be necessary before assessing the surface for the presence of a carious lesion.

Regarding occlusal caries diagnostics, some authors recommend the use of air abrasion because the small particles are able to clean the fissures better than pumice and brush or rubber cup [29]. Dental practitioners should be aware of the powder they use, because alumina air abrasion changes the surface morphology, especially of brittle enamel in carious fissures [30]. Sodium bicarbonate powder will cause bleeding when targeting the gums [31], so for cleaning prior to visual inspection air-abrasion with atraumatic glycine or erythritol powders should always be used [32].

Radiography

In order to enhance the detection of approximal carious lesions on bitewing, radiography is usually recommended. This technique allows the visualisation of the demineralisation depth both in enamel and in dentine. For dental practitioners, bitewing radiography is the primary means of supplementing findings obtained by visual inspection. Bitewing radiography shows mineral loss by change of radiolucency. It should be kept in mind that the change of radiolucency is a mere estimate for the degree of demineralisation. It does not show if active biofilm is present and thus if the lesion is progressing or is in a stagnating phase. Only the comparison with previous or future radiographs allows for lesion activity judgement. It is not possible to see on a bitewing radiograph whether the surface is cavitated or not [33]. There is too much overlap of dental hard tissue both in occlusal and approximal surfaces that does not allow the determination of whether cavitation has already occurred in the outermost surface. In a recent meta-analysis, sensitivity and specificity for carious lesion detection in approximal surfaces have been reported to be 0.36 and 0.94, respectively, at the dentine level [34]. When enamel carious lesions are included, sensitivities and specificities changed to 0.24 and 0.97 [34].

Because dental radiography consists of ionising radiation, its use should be justified [35]. Practically all dental scientific societies have published regulations on the frequency for bitewing radiographs, depending on the individual caries risk and on the age of the patient [35–38].

Depending on the detection threshold, bitewing radiography can be both helpful and misleading. It has been shown that if enamel carious lesions are included in the detection threshold level, more enamel lesions can be detected visually than radiographically [19, 20]. This might be because the crowns should be free from overlapping structures on the radiograph for superficial enamel carious lesion detection. Crowding of teeth, height of the palate, compliance of the patient and positioning of the intraoral film can reduce the quality of the radiographs, resulting in less diagnostic information for the dentist. When the caries prevalence is low, the possible risk of false-positive diagnoses outweighs the risk of overlooked carious lesions [3].

Several clinical studies have been carried out to assess the state of the surface in relation to depth of radiolucency in bitewing radiographs (for a review see Wenzel [33]). If dentinal carious lesions are visible in approximal surfaces, the surface has been found to be broken in earlier studies in more than 70% of cases [33].

If occlusal dentinal carious lesions are visible radiographically on otherwise clinically inconspicuous occlusal surfaces, the clinician should be aware of ongoing demineralisation, and a minimally invasive restoration should be applied [22]. However, it is not possible to see occlusal carious lesions restricted to enamel in bitewing radiographs.

As a more recent development, cone beam computerised tomography (CBCT) has been advocated by some authors who reported that a higher sensitivity with unchanged specificity might be achieved in vitro [39–41]. Under optimum circumstances, with high resolution, crowns without restorations can be viewed with CBCT almost as well as with microcomputed tomography, and it might be possible to even detect a cavitation in the transverse plane. However, since most devices have a limited field of view, one CBCT scan would be necessary for each side. Taking this into account and the fact that CBCT images are compromised by radiation artefacts from existing fillings or even from thick enamel [42], the much higher radiation dose, costs, and, last but not least, the necessity to interpret all radiologic findings for legal reasons [43], CBCT cannot be regarded as a recommended means for caries lesion detection. It is safe to stipulate that for caries detection, CBCTs absolutely cannot be justified.

Fluorescence-Based Technologies

The interaction of light with matter may lead to several specific phenomena: light can be reflected, or scattered (back-scattering or diffuse transmission), there can be transmission of the light, absorption with heat production or absorption with fluorescence [44]. Under the impact of suitable wavelengths, bacteria, or rather their porphyrins, can have a characteristic red fluorescence [45]. Fluorescence is thus an indirect measure of the degree of tooth demineralisation [46–48]. It is applicable on occlusal surfaces, smooth surfaces, and some devices also measure carious lesions in approximal surfaces [49].

There are pen-type devices that measure the red fluorescence locally in small areas and camera-based systems that can visualise the fluorescence for one or more tooth surfaces at once. One of the most popular pen-type fluorescence devices operates on a wavelength of about 650 nm and has a numeric output between 0 and 99 (DIAGNOdent pen, KaVo, Biberach, Germany). This device measures the fluorescence and allows for monitoring over time. In numerous studies a greater reliability was found for the pen-type fluorescence device compared to visual caries detection [49–51]. Among the camera-based systems, there are devices that visualise fluorescence qualitatively (e.g., Sopro, Acteon, La Ciotat, France), and other devices that have a quantitative output (e.g., Vistacam iX, Dürr, Bietigheim-Bissingen, Germany). There is a heterogeneous body of evidence derived from clinical studies [52]. While certain authors found that use of fluorescence devices increased the diagnostic accuracy [53–58], others found that it did not add to clinical decision making compared to visual inspection and radiography [59, 60], at least not in primary teeth [61].

Like radiography, fluorescence-based methods cannot detect surface cavitation, but they may add to the information on lesion depth. This might be helpful especially when radiography cannot be applied (repeatedly in children or pregnant women, anxious patients etc.) and visually dubious or conspicuous sites are present. One problem with fluorescence is the sensitivity to false positive results because of the inherent autofluorescence of biofilm, calculus, some prophylaxis pastes [62] or some filling materials [63, 64]. Fluorescence-based methods therefore require professional tooth cleaning before application, and – within the limits outlined above – they are most notably suitable for adjunct primary caries detection. Although thresholds have been published indicating the presence of enamel caries or dentine caries, the use of fluorescence-based methods is usually advocated as a "second opinion" device [46, 47], and treatment decisions should not be based on fluorescence measurements alone.

Transillumination

Especially for anterior teeth, fibre optic transillumination (FOTI) is an easy, inexpensive, and fast method to improve the visualisation of the depth of approximal decay. A bright light source is necessary to transilluminate the teeth. Light is applied to the side of the tooth and its transmission observed from either the opposing side or occlusally in the case of molars and premolars. Because light is scattered more in carious dental tissue than in sound dental tissue, caries appears darker against the healthy surrounding tissues. Thus, FOTI can assist the judgement as to whether the lesion is confined to enamel or if it has already extended to dentine because it enhances the contrast between sound and carious tissue. However, it is not possible to see cavitation or lesion activity with transillumination. Temporary tooth separation with a spatula or gentle flossing can add valuable information on surface continuity [25]. For premolars and molars, the digitised FOTI (DIFOTI), where a charge-coupled device sensor replaces the human eye, has produced heterogenous results with limited evidence [52]. Compared to radiographs, for detecting enamel carious lesions, a better agreement with the reference standard was reported for DIFOTI, while the detection of dentinal carious lesions was similar [65]. However, differences between reported studies might be attributable to inadequate light source or insufficient calibration [66].

Recently, a device with advanced near-infrared light transillumination (NILT) technology has been marketed and validated in clinical studies (DIAGNOcam, KaVo). This device consists of an intraoral camera with a wide-angle objective. The light source operates on a near-infrared wavelength of about 760 nm. Two branches illuminate the apical region from the oral and buccal aspect; the light enters the tooth via the roots, and the illuminated tooth is viewed from the occlusal aspect. This method is primarily suitable for approximal caries detection. Sound enamel looks shiny and transparent because light is transmitted in an unhampered way, while approximal enamel lesions are depicted as grey shadows. Because lesion depth in dentine is visible only in very deep dentine lesions for diagnostic purposes, the geometry of the approximal enamel lesion as viewed from the occlusal aspect is linked to lesion depth [67]. It has been found that an enamel shadow in broader contact with the enamel-dentine junction is indicative of a dentinal carious lesion, and in a clinical trial with 127 lesions in 85 patients the agreement between NILT and bitewing radiography for dentine carious lesion detection was reported to be almost 100% [68]. However, approximal lesions restricted to enamel were less likely to be reliably detected with interexaminer reliability of 0.51 (weighted kappa) [69].

Unfortunately, with NILT it is neither possible to detect surface cavitation nor to visualise approximal cervical secondary lesions, because the restauration hampers light transmission. For occlusal surfaces, no validated lesion detection criteria have been described so far.

Lesion Activity Assessment

Active enamel carious lesions are more likely to turn into cavitated lesions than inactive enamel lesions [6, 7]. Using visual-tactile criteria, active enamel carious lesions look whitish, matte, and opaque, they feel rough on gently running a probe across the surface and are often covered by "tacky" plaque before professional tooth cleaning [6]. By contrast, inactive enamel carious lesions look shiny and they feel smooth on running a probe over the surface. In a 2-year survey, it was found that these criteria are more predictive for occlusal sites than for smooth surfaces [70]. This is probably due to the fact that, as with carious lesion detection, lesion activity assessment in approximal surfaces is hampered by the neighbouring teeth and by the gingival papilla and/or gingival bleeding. Therefore, and because lesion activity assessment despite calibration can result in less than perfect agreement [71], objective methods using reflection intensity [72] or chemiluminescence [73] have been described. However, these have only a limited body of evidence to support their use. Attempts have been carried out to use fluorescence to measure lesion activity by measuring a suspected area after air drying with compressed air [74], but the positive predictive value was reported to be 0.5, meaning one could achieve the same chance of being correct by the flip of a coin.

Visual-tactile inspection, correctly performed, has been and remains the method of choice for carious lesion diagnosis. If indicated, the diagnostic process may be supported by methods that contribute to lesion detection and to the assessment of lesion depth, especially for surfaces that are concealed to direct vision.

References

1 Nyvad B: Diagnosis versus detection of caries. Caries Res 2004;38:192–198.
2 Bader JD, Shugars DA: What do we know about how dentists make caries-related treatment decisions? Community Dent Oral Epidemiol 1997;25:97–103.
3 Baelum V: What is an appropriate caries diagnosis? Acta Odontol Scand 2010;68: 65–79.
4 Ekstrand KR, Ricketts DN, Kidd EA: Occlusal caries: pathology, diagnosis and logical management. Dent Update 2001;28:380–387.
5 Gängler P: Pathogenesis of dental caries and periodontal diseases – the concept of progression and stagnation. Zahn Mund Kieferheilkd Zentralbl 1985;73: 477–483.
6 Nyvad B, Machiulskiene V, Baelum V: Reliability of a new caries diagnostic system differentiating between active and inactive caries lesions. Caries Res 1999;33:252–260.
7 Nyvad B, Machiulskiene V, Baelum V: Construct and predictive validity of clinical caries diagnostic criteria assessing lesion activity. J Dent Res 2003;82:117–122.
8 Baelum V, Hintze H, Wenzel A, Danielsen B, Nyvad B: Implications of caries diagnostic strategies for clinical management decisions. Community Dent Oral Epidemiol 2012;40:257–266.
9 Chandler NP, Gray AR, Murray CM: Eyesight: a study of the staff of a dental school. BDJ Open 2017;3:17008.
10 Eichenberger M, Perrin P, Neuhaus KW, Bringolf U, Lussi A: Influence of loupes and age on the near visual acuity of practicing dentists. J Biomed Opt 2011; 16:035003.
11 Eichenberger M, Perrin P, Neuhaus KW, Bringolf U, Lussi A: Visual acuity of dentists under simulated clinical conditions. Clin Oral Investig 2013;17:725–729.
12 Mitropoulos P, Rahiotis C, Kakaboura A, Vougiouklakis G: The impact of magnification on occlusal caries diagnosis with implementation of the ICDAS II criteria. Caries Res 2012;46:82–86.
13 Neuhaus KW, Jost F, Perrin P, Lussi A: Impact of different magnification levels on visual caries detection with ICDAS. J Dent 2015;43:1559–1564.
14 Neuhaus KW, Jasarevic E, Lussi A: Impact of different illumination conditions on visual caries detection with ICDAS. Caries Res 2015;49:633–636.

15 Ismail AI, Sohn W, Tellez M, Amaya A, Sen A, Hasson H, Pitts NB: The International Caries Detection and Assessment System (ICDAS): an integrated system for measuring dental caries. Community Dent Oral Epidemiol 2007;35:170–178.
16 Frencken JE, de Amorim RG, Faber J, Leal SC: The Caries Assessment Spectrum and Treatment (CAST) index: rationale and development. Int Dent J 2011;61:117–123.
17 Alberg AJ, Park JW, Hager BW, Brock MV, Diener-West M: The use of "overall accuracy" to evaluate the validity of screening or diagnostic tests. J Gen Intern Med 2004;19:460–465.
18 Machiulskiene V, Nyvad B, Baelum V: A comparison of clinical and radiographic caries diagnoses in posterior teeth of 12-year-old Lithuanian children. Caries Res 1999;33:340–348.
19 Machiulskiene V, Nyvad B, Baelum V: Comparison of diagnostic yields of clinical and radiographic caries examinations in children of different age. Eur J Paediatr Dent 2004;5:157–162.
20 Gimenez T, Piovesan C, Braga MM, Raggio DP, Deery C, Ricketts DN, Ekstrand KR, Mendes FM: Visual inspection for caries detection: a systematic review and meta-analysis. J Dent Res 2015;94:895–904.
21 Ricketts D, Kidd E, Weerheijm K, de Soet H: Hidden caries: what is it? Does it exist? Does it matter? Int Dent J 1997; 47:259–265.
22 Ando M, Eckert GJ, Zero DT: Preliminary study to establish a relationship between tactile sensation and surface roughness. Caries Res 2010;44:24–28.
23 Kühnisch J, Dietz W, Stösser L, Hickel R, Heinrich-Weltzien R: Effects of dental probing on occlusal surfaces – a scanning electron microscopy evaluation. Caries Res 2007;41:43–48.
24 Topping GVA, Pitts NB: Clinical visual caries detection. Monogr Oral Sci 2009; 21:15–41.
25 Pitts NB, Longbottom C: Temporary tooth separation with special reference to the diagnosis and preventive management of equivocal approximal carious lesions. Quintessence Int 1987;18:563–573.
26 Seddon RP: The detection of cavitation in carious approximal surfaces in vivo by tooth separation, impression and scanning electron microscopy. J Dent 1989;17:117–120.
27 Lussi A, Hotz P: Approximal and smooth-surface caries: their diagnosis and therapeutic principles. Schweiz Monatsschr Zahnmed 1995;105:1438–1445.
28 Lussi A, Hotz P, Stich H: Fissure caries: their diagnosis and therapeutic principles. Schweiz Monatsschr Zahnmed 1995;105:1164–1173.
29 de Almeida Rodrigues J, de Vita TM, Cordeiro Rde C: In vitro evaluation of the influence of air abrasion on detection of occlusal caries lesions in primary teeth. Pediatr Dent 2008;30:15–18.
30 Neuhaus KW, Ciucchi P, Donnet M, Lussi A: Removal of enamel caries with an air abrasion powder. Oper Dent 2010; 35:538–546.
31 Bühler J, Amato M, Weiger R, Walter C: A systematic review on the effects of air polishing devices on oral tissues. Int J Dent Hyg 2016;14:15–28.
32 Sculean A, Bastendorf KD, Becker C, Bush B, Einwag J, Lanoway C, Platzer U, Schmage P, Schoeneich B, Walter C, Wennström JL, Flemmig TF: A paradigm shift in mechanical biofilm management? Subgingival air polishing: a new way to improve mechanical biofilm management in the dental practice. Quintessence Int 2013;44:475–477.
33 Wenzel A: Radiographic display of carious lesions and cavitation in approximal surfaces: advantages and drawbacks of conventional and advanced modalities. Acta Odontol Scand 2014;72:251–264.
34 Schwendicke F, Tzschoppe M, Paris S: Radiographic caries detection: a systematic review and meta-analysis. J Dent 2015;43:924–933.
35 European Commission: Radiation protection: European guidelines on radiation protection in dental radiology. Luxembourg, European Communities, 2004, issue 136.
36 Pendlebury ME, Horner K, Eaton KA (eds): Good Practice Guidelines: Selection Criteria for Dental Radiography. London, Faculty of General Dental Practitioners, 2004.
37 Espelid I, Mejàre I, Weerheijm K: EAPD guidelines for use of radiographs in children. Eur J Paediatr Dent 2003;4:40–48.
38 American Dental Association: Dental radiographic examinations: recommendations for patient selection and limiting radiation exposure. Chicago, ADA, 2012.
39 Tarım Ertas E, Küçükyılmaz E, Ertaş H, Savaş S, Yırcalı Atıcı M: A comparative study of different radiographic methods for detecting occlusal caries lesions. Caries Res 2014;48:556–574.
40 Akdeniz BG, Gröndahl HG, Magnusson B: Accuracy of proximal caries depth measurements: comparison between limited cone beam computed tomography, storage phosphor and film radiography. Caries Res 2006;40:202–207.
41 Young SM, Lee JT, Hodges RJ, Chang TL, Elashoff DA, White SC: A comparative study of high-resolution cone beam computed tomography and charge-coupled device sensors for detecting caries. Dentomaxillofac Radiol 2009;38:445–451.
42 Gaalaas L, Tyndall D, Mol A, Everett ET, Bangdiwala A: Ex vivo evaluation of new 2D and 3D dental radiographic technology for detecting caries. Dentomaxillofac Radiol 2016;45:20150281.
43 Dula K, Benic GI, Bornstein M, Dagassan-Berndt D, Filippi A, Hicklin S, Kissling-Jeger F, Luebbers HT, Sculean A, Sequeira-Byron P, Walter C, Zehnder M: SADMFR guidelines for the use of cone-beam computed tomography/digital volume tomography. Swiss Dent J 2015;125:945–953.
44 Karlsson L: Caries detection methods based on changes in optical properties between healthy and carious tissue. Int J Dent 2010;2010:270729.
45 Buchalla W, Attin T, Niedmann Y, Niedmann PD: Porphyrins are the cause of red fluorescence of carious dentine: verified by gradient reversed-phase HPLC. Caries Res 2008;42:223.
46 Lussi A, Hellwig E: Performance of a new laser fluorescence device for the detection of occlusal caries in vitro. J Dent 2006;34:467–471.
47 Lussi A, Imwinkelried S, Pitts N, Longbottom C, Reich E: Performance and reproducibility of a laser fluorescence system for detection of occlusal caries in vitro. Caries Res 1999;33:261–266.
48 Lussi A, Megert B, Longbottom C, Reich E, Francescut P: Clinical performance of a laser fluorescence device for detection of occlusal caries lesions. Eur J Oral Sci 2001;109:14–19.
49 Lussi A, Hack A, Hug I, Heckenberger H, Megert B, Stich H: Detection of approximal caries with a new laser fluorescence device. Caries Res 2006;40:97–103.

50 Neuhaus KW, Rodrigues JA, Hug I, Stich H, Lussi A: Performance of laser fluorescence devices, visual and radiographic examination for the detection of occlusal caries in primary molars. Clin Oral Investig 2011;15:635–641.
51 de Almeida Rodrigues J, Hug I, Diniz MB, Cordeiro RC, Lussi A: The influence of zero-value subtraction on the performance of two laser fluorescence devices for detecting occlusal caries in vitro. J Am Dent Assoc 2008;139:1105–1112.
52 Twetman S, Axelsson S, Dahlén G, Espelid I, Mejàre I, Norlund A, Tranæus S: Adjunct methods for caries detection: a systematic review of literature. Acta Odontol Scand 2013;71:388–397.
53 Huth KC, Lussi A, Gygax M, Thum M, Crispin A, Paschos E, Hickel R, Neuhaus KW: In vivo performance of a laser fluorescence device for the approximal detection of caries in permanent molars. J Dent 2010;38:1019–1026.
54 Huth KC, Neuhaus KW, Gygax M, Bucher K, Crispin A, Paschos E, Hickel R, Lussi A: Clinical performance of a new laser fluorescence device for detection of occlusal caries lesions in permanent molars. J Dent 2008;36:1033–1040.
55 Jablonski-Momeni A, Heinzel-Gutenbrunner M, Klein SM: In vivo performance of the VistaProof fluorescence-based camera for detection of occlusal lesions. Clin Oral Investig 2014;18:1757–1762.
56 Jablonski-Momeni A, Liebegall F, Stoll R, Heinzel-Gutenbrunner M, Pieper K: Performance of a new fluorescence camera for detection of occlusal caries in vitro. Lasers Med Sci 2013;28:101–109.
57 Jablonski-Momeni A, Schipper HM, Rosen SM, Heinzel-Gutenbrunner M, Roggendorf MJ, Stoll R, Stachniss V, Pieper K: Performance of a fluorescence camera for detection of occlusal caries in vitro. Odontology 2011;99:55–61.
58 Jablonski-Momeni A, Stucke J, Steinberg T, Heinzel-Gutenbrunner M: Use of ICDAS-II, fluorescence-based methods, and radiography in detection and treatment decision of occlusal caries lesions: an in vitro study. Int J Dent 2012;2012:371595.
59 Rechmann P, Charland D, Rechmann BM, Featherstone JD: Performance of laser fluorescence devices and visual examination for the detection of occlusal caries in permanent molars. J Biomed Opt 2012;17:036006.
60 Rechmann P, Liou SW, Rechmann BM, Featherstone JD: Performance of a light fluorescence device for the detection of microbial plaque and gingival inflammation. Clin Oral Investig 2016;20:151–159.
61 Mendes FM, Novaes TF, Matos R, Bittar DG, Piovesan C, Gimenez T, Imparato JC, Raggio DP, Braga MM: Radiographic and laser fluorescence methods have no benefits for detecting caries in primary teeth. Caries Res 2012;46:536–543.
62 Lussi A, Reich E: The influence of toothpastes and prophylaxis pastes on fluorescence measurements for caries detection in vitro. Eur J Oral Sci 2005;113:141–144.
63 Neuhaus KW, Rodrigues JA, Seemann R, Lussi A: Detection of proximal secondary caries at cervical class II-amalgam restoration margins in vitro. J Dent 2012;40:493–499.
64 Rodrigues JA, Neuhaus KW, Hug I, Stich H, Seemann R, Lussi A: In vitro detection of secondary caries associated with composite restorations on approximal surfaces using laser fluorescence. Oper Dent 2010;35:564–571.
65 Astvaldsdottir A, Ahlund K, Holbrook WP, de Verdier B, Tranæus S: Approximal caries detection by DIFOTI: in vitro comparison of diagnostic accuracy/efficacy with film and digital radiography. Int J Dent 2012;2012:326401.
66 Neuhaus KW, Longbottom C, Ellwood R, Lussi A: Novel lesion detection aids. Monogr Oral Sci 2009;21:52–62.
67 Söchtig F, Hickel R, Kühnisch J: Caries detection and diagnostics with near-infrared light transillumination: clinical experiences. Quintessence Int 2014;45:531–538.
68 Kühnisch J, Söchtig F, Pitchika V, Laubender R, Neuhaus KW, Lussi A, Hickel R: In vivo validation of near-infrared light transillumination for interproximal dentin caries detection. Clin Oral Investig 2016;20:821–829.
69 Jost F, Kühnisch J, Lussi A, Neuhaus K: Reproducibility of near-infrared light transillumination for approximal enamel caries: a clinical controlled trial. Clin Oral Investig 2015;19:1752.
70 Guedes RS, Piovesan C, Ardenghi TM, Emmanuelli B, Braga MM, Ekstrand KR, Mendes FM: Validation of visual caries activity assessment: a 2-yr cohort study. J Dent Res 2014;93:101S–107S.
71 Neuhaus KW, Schlafer S, Lussi A, Nyvad B: Infiltration of natural caries lesions in relation to their activity status and acid pretreatment in vitro. Caries Res 2013;47:203–210.
72 Neuhaus KW, Nyvad B, Lussi A, Jaruszewski L: Evaluation of perpendicular reflection intensity for assessment of caries lesion activity/inactivity. Caries Res 2011;45:408–414.
73 Jablonski-Momeni A, Kneib L: Assessment of caries activity using the Calcivis® caries activity imaging system. Open Access J Sci Technol 2016;4:101241.
74 Braga MM, de Benedetto MS, Imparato JC, Mendes FM: New methodology to assess activity status of occlusal caries in primary teeth using laser fluorescence device. J Biomed Opt 2010;15:047005.

Klaus W. Neuhaus
Department of Preventive, Restorative and Pediatric Dentistry
Freiburgstrasse 7
CH–3010 Bern (Switzerland)
E-Mail klaus.neuhaus@zmk.unibe.ch

Schwendicke F, Frencken J, Innes N (eds): Caries Excavation: Evolution of Treating Cavitated Carious Lesions.
Monogr Oral Sci. Basel, Karger, 2018, vol 27, pp 32–41 (DOI: 10.1159/000487829)

Removing or Controlling? How Caries Management Impacts on the Lifetime of Teeth

Falk Schwendicke[a] • Thomas Lamont[b] • Nicola Innes[b]

[a]Operative and Preventive Dentistry, Charité – Universitätsmedizin Berlin, Corporate Member of Freie Universität Berlin, Humboldt-Universität zu Berlin, and Berlin Institute of Health, Berlin, Germany; [b]School of Dentistry, University of Dundee, Dundee, UK

Abstract

Historically, traditional carious lesion management focused on the importance of removal of all carious tissue, with little thought to the lesion origins. The surgical removal of any sign of a carious lesion was prioritised with little, or no, consideration to pulp vitality, loss of tooth structure, or caries disease management. This symptomatic approach concentrating on lesions rather than on the cause of the disease, focused on preventing secondary carious lesion development. Early detection and improved understanding of the caries process – that lesion progress can be arrested or slowed – has led to preventive measures and less destructive management as a focus. The choice of lesion management depends on: whether a primary or permanent tooth is involved; which tooth surface(s) is/are involved; whether the lesion is confined to enamel or extends into dentine; the lesion depth, and lesion cleansability. Use of preventive and minimally invasive operative strategies is complicated by the lack of predictable ways of recording lesions' status to allow early detection of failed strategies and early intervention. Because re-restoration usually makes the cavity larger and, consequently, the tooth weaker, the clinician should be certain about initiating the repeat restoration cycle, delaying the first restoration as much as possible. The 3 main principles that support preventing or slowing the repeat restoration cycle are: (1) avoid restoration placement until there is no other option; (2) place them for maximum longevity; (3) if re-restoration is necessary, repair or refurbishment is preferable to replacement of a defective restoration.

Traditional Management (Removal) of Caries

The dental profession's understanding of the aetiology of carious lesions has developed (and continues to do so) tremendously since G.V. Black first described cavity preparation at the beginning of the last century. The historic – or traditional – management of dental caries involves the complete removal of carious tissue to leave only hard tissue behind. Indeed, it used to be recommended that cavity preparation should be extended throughout the fissure anatomy and that margins be placed in a cleansable area proximally to "prevent" further carious lesion development, termed "extension for prevention" [1]. Detection of any lesion resulted in a diagnosis of dental caries and intervention would be initiated at the first signs of decay or a "sticky" fissure, diagnosed with a sharp dental probe [2], often causing cavitation [3, 4]. The traditional management of caries and carious lesions stressed the importance of removal of all carious tissue, without paying any attention to the origins of the lesion. The surgical removal of any sign of a carious lesion was prioritised and little or no consideration given to pulp vitality, loss of tooth structure, or the management of the disease dental caries; the focus was on the symptoms, i.e., lesions rather than the cause of the disease. The basis for diagnosing and treating dental caries historically was logical thinking and practitioners' personal experience rather than the results of research.

Carious Lesions and Factors Impacting on Lesion Management

Understanding of the biological process of caries [as outlined in the chapter by Conrads and About; this vol., pp. 1–10] and improved detection methods for early lesion diagnosis has led to management strategies which aim to treat carious lesions without the necessity for removal of carious tissue. These management strategies involve techniques that aim to tip the balance of the caries process towards "remineralisation" rather than further "demineralisation." Successful control and prevention of further lesion development requires patient involvement. The starting point for professionals to achieve this is encouraging effective home care: toothbrushing with fluoride toothpaste. This preventive action should be combined with dietary investigation and advice, stressing the importance of reduced intake of refined carbohydrates. Professional interventions include the application of preventive agents that contain a high dose of fluoride (e.g., fluoride varnish, silver nitrate or silver diamine fluoride) and applying sealants to act as barriers.

There are several factors associated with carious lesions that will impact on the clinical decision making when considering their management:

- Primary or permanent teeth. Management may vary depending on the tooth type involved. With all other lesion factors being equal, the management of primary teeth may involve more minimally invasive options than those available for permanent teeth. With the average lifespan of primary teeth expected to be much shorter than permanent teeth, prevention alone strategies may be sufficient to allow natural tooth exfoliation without undesirable sequelae, such as pain or sepsis. Additionally, very young patients may be less able to cope with invasive treatment than adults, making operative intervention in primary teeth less likely to be successful.
- Tooth surface. Management strategy choice will also be affected by the tooth surface involved. Preventive strategies like fissure sealants, which aim to seal a high-risk caries surface lesion and prevent further progression, can be provided more easily and reliably on occlusal and palatal/buccal surfaces compared to proximal surfaces.
- Enamel/Dentine. Enamel lesions present at the earlier stages of the caries process, and prevention and minimally invasive operative management strategies should be the first line of treatment. The deeper dentinal lesions, visible on bitewing radiographs, may contain large numbers of bacteria and be heavily contaminated. These lesions, especially in permanent teeth, may be more suitably treated with operative management [5].
- Lesion depth. Deep carious lesions are those close to the pulp, i.e., radiographically extending into the inner third or quarter of the pulp, or clinically are in proximity to the pulp car-

rying a risk of pulp exposure during invasive interventions. With carious tissue removal strategies which involve the historic approach, where the carious lesion is completely removed to leave only hard dentine, there is an increased risk of pulp exposure [6]. More conservative treatment, including selective caries removal [outlined in the chapter by Ricketts et al.; this vol., pp. 82–91] has the added benefit of preserving tooth structure whilst also giving the dental pulp time to protect itself [7]. Maintaining pulpal vitality should be prioritised when dealing with deep lesions [as described in the chapter by Conrads and About [this vol., pp. 1–10]. For shallow or moderately deep lesions, the restoration longevity is the focus and cavity preparation and carious tissue removal should be performed pulpally to firm dentine and peripherally to hard dentine [see the chapter by Göstemeyer et al.; this vol., pp. 42–55].
- Lesion cleansability. The ability of the patient to adequately clean a dentine lesion will influence the management options. Frequent disruption of the plaque biofilm tips the caries process balance towards remineralisation and can lead to the arrest of the dentine carious lesion [8]. The critical point in deciding on the need for operative intervention is often linked to the cleansability of the lesion. Surface breakdown, or cavitation, can prevent the adequate disruption of the plaque biofilm, leading to a shift in microbiota which favours further demineralisation and lesion progression [5, 9].

Intervention Thresholds: Lesion Changes over Time

Unfortunately, even with early detection and implementation of control and preventive strategies, carious lesions can continue to progress. Historically, the perspective was that all lesions would progress regardless of any change in the lesion's environment or in the behaviour and improvement of the cleaning skills of the patient. This meant that all lesions, even if limited to the enamel and not extending into dentine, would be removed and a restoration placed. Now, however, an understanding of the dynamic nature of de- and remineralisation has meant that enamel lesions should only be treated with remineralisation strategies or sealed in to prevent progression. Even cleansable dentinal lesions or those considered not to be heavily contaminated may be sealed [10–12]. However, a recent systematic review [13] has shown that a large number of dental professionals continue to carry out the removal of non-cavitated lesions confined to enamel. These would potentially be reversible without destructive surgical intervention.

Dental professionals and patients need to be vigilant of carious lesions that are being managed with a prevention strategy to remineralise them, to ensure that failure to arrest the lesion, i.e., its continued progression, is picked up quickly and timely provision of a more intensive level of prevention or restorative care can be implemented. The difficulties with watchful vigilance of these lesions should not be underestimated [14]. Traditional record keeping with circles drawn on charts do not support the comparison of lesions over time to detect their progression. Even more in-depth recording systems such as ICDAS or Nyvad's system still do not easily allow subtle changes in lesion progression to be noted and the instigation of early action. Early detection of changes in carious lesion progression is also difficult with radiographic monitoring, especially when radiographs are not standardised. Individualised bitewing holders are helpful in trying to standardise repeated radiographs from the same tooth or area, allowing better comparisons with time.

There are two possible methods to improve the comparison of lesions over time (increasing the accuracy of detecting any changes). These are clinical photography to visually record lesion stages avoiding reliance on memory, and digital subtraction radiography (DSR; Fig. 1), which is also useful for detecting subtle changes in lesion progression as well as success in remineralisation strategies where lesions regress [15].

However, both DSR and clinical photography are time-consuming, expensive, beyond the usual treatment practices for most dentists and, in the case of DSR, the technology is not commercially available at the moment. So, monitoring lesion progression/regression over time remains difficult.

Differences between Lesions: Impact of Surface Cavitation

The important point in deciding whether a lesion is reversible, from a pathophysiological point of view, is whether the lesion is cavitated or not. Once coronal caries cavitation occurs, the lesion is usually no longer easily cleansable (Fig. 2). If the cavity opening remains unchanged, the carious biofilm has a sheltered environment in which to develop and mature. Such a situation makes lesion arrest or reversal difficult and often not even possible. However, if the cavity can be opened further or is large, which is mainly applicable in primary teeth, the biofilm can be removed with a toothbrush and fluoride toothpaste.

In sheltered cavities, it is much more difficult for saliva, food, and oral structures (tongue and cheeks) to disrupt the biofilm. This then becomes the time when a more interventional strategy may be needed. Note that root surfaces often do not show such "cavitation" and, even if they do, these lesions can often still be cleansable and therefore amenable to preventative measures delivered professionally (e.g., fluoride varnish or silver diamine fluoride) or oral hygiene measures implemented by the motivated and capable patient [8, 16].

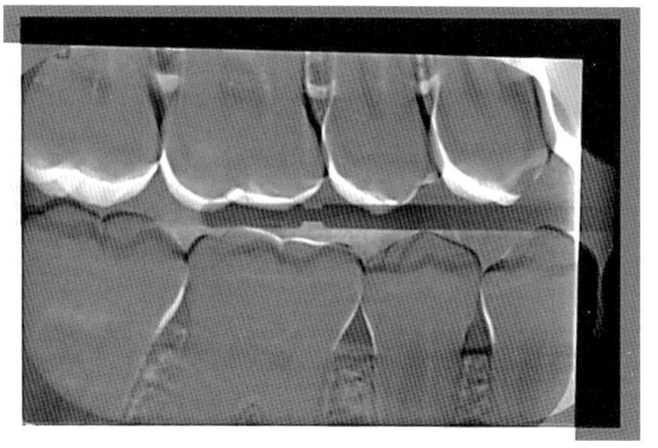

Fig. 1. Digital subtraction of 2 radiographs of the lower right first permanent molar (2 years apart). The radiographs have been manipulated to allow the lower first permanent molars to overlie with the "best fit" and to accentuate any differences between them using subtraction of the greyscales. Rather than simply showing the presence of lesions, DSR allows subtle changes in the lesion time to show up. In this radiograph, the mesial and distal lesions appear darker than the rest of the tooth, indicating the lesions have changed between the first and second radiograph.

The diagnosis of lesions is more difficult for tooth surfaces that are not visible [as mentioned in Neuhaus and Lussi, this vol., pp. 26–27]. Whilst radiographs and other diagnostic adjuncts can give additional information to judge the lesion depth, they do not always help inform whether the lesion is cavitated on proximal surfaces [17, 18]. Orthodontic separators can help in visualising the surfaces (Fig. 3 [see also Fig. 3 in Fontana and Innes, this vol., p. 107]), but these rings seem to be infrequently used because of the disadvantage of having to get the patient to return for another appointment several days later after space has been created.

It can also be difficult to judge whether there is microcavitation in the bases of deep fissures [19, 20]. Where radiography indicates dentine involvement of such occlusal lesions, bacterial contamination is present. This might be a case where, despite cavitation not being visible, invasive management is needed and carious tissue removal is required to allow the placement of long-lasting restorations. This is sometimes known as "hidden caries." Only sealing such lesions using an unfilled or low filled resin fissure sealant may not be sufficiently long-lasting and can, at present, not be recommended [21–23].

In summary, cavitated lesions usually require invasive interventions to reproduce the surface integrity and thus cleansability of the restoration and tooth surface, but also to restore functionality and aesthetics. For certain lesions (root surface caries or large cleansable cavities in primary teeth), invasive interventions may not be needed even in cases where the surfaces are no longer intact. If we need to place restorations, i.e., perform invasive therapy, for such cavitated lesions, then one may ask: why not restore all lesions – as has been done for decades, as described above? Answering this question will be the focus of the next sections.

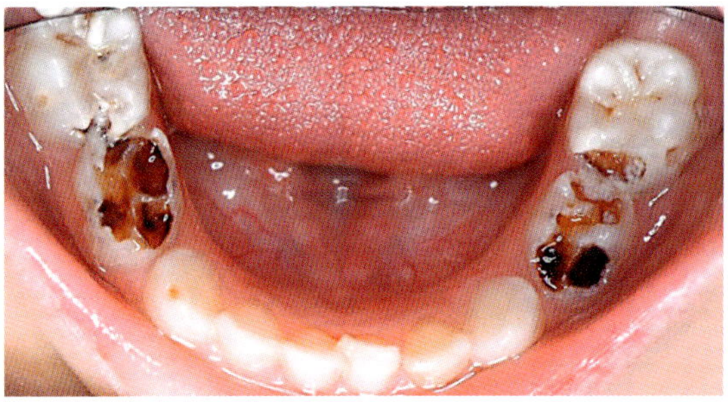

Fig. 2. Both lower first primary molar teeth lesions can be cleaned. Lower second primary molars have cavitated lesions on the mesial surfaces. The one on the right (tooth 85) is probably the least cleansable. A toothbrush would not fit into it to clean it. There are other lesions with plaque that would be difficult to clean. Some of the lesions that are more cleansable are hard and the carious lesion is more likely to be arrested.

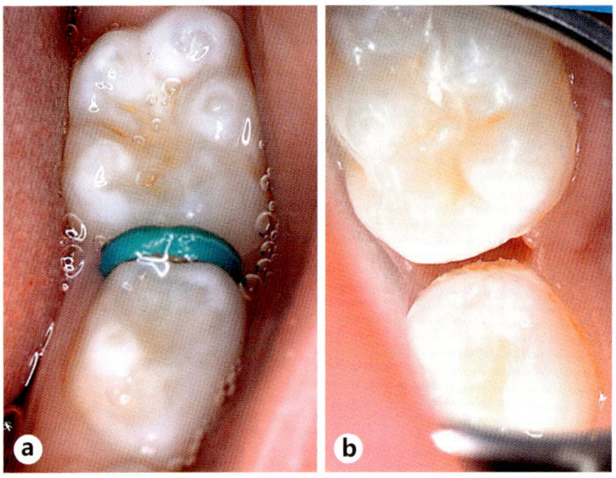

Fig. 3. Lower first and second primary molars with an orthodontic separator in place (**a**), and 3 days later after removal of the separator (**b**). The space created allows the proximal surfaces of the teeth to be viewed directly.

The Problem with Invasive Therapies

Today's dentists have a large and increasing number of restorative materials to choose from when restoring cavities. These materials come with ever improved chemicophysical and biomedical properties. Modern composite resins, for example, are highly aesthetic, show similar physical properties as dentine, have high bond strengths to both enamel and dentine, and a number of restorative materials are even beneficially bioactive (remineralising, antibacterial), like glass-ionomer. Nevertheless, all dental restorations show a finite lifespan. Under optimal conditions – often found in university/secondary care/specialist practice-based trials and selected groups of patients – one can find a <2% annual failure rate for resin composite restorations on average [24–27]. If we make an assumption of linearity of failure rate, this means after roughly 25 years the average restoration is replaced. Under everyday clinical practice conditions, these annual failure rates are much higher, from 5% to even 15% or more [28–30]. Although there is little hard data to predict failure rates, by basing conjecture on the previous information, it could be that after only 3–10 years the average restoration is replaced.

There are a number of reasons for high failure rates and why these are not represented in the rates published in the literature. Firstly, restorations are challenged both physically and biologically to different extents depending on the patient and the oral environment. For example, patients with parafunctional habits show very high masticatory forces and are usually excluded from many studies on restorative material performance. The same applies to high-risk caries patients where there is an increased chance of carious lesion development adjacent to restorations or new ones on other tooth surfaces. These patients are often irregular attenders and also excluded from controlled trials, yet they represent the reality of daily practice [31]. Secondly, general dentists often have to work in suboptimal conditions and financial drivers can be essential to business survival: optimal materials may not be available, appointment times can be short, and pressure can lead to compromising what are perceived as less-important treatment steps (including, not exhaustively, moisture control, or light-curing). As a result, no treatment should be considered "permanent" – restoration failure needs to be accepted as a fact and considered when making treatment plans and informing patients.

The Repeat Restoration Cycle

Restoration failure would not be a problem if the average lifetime of our patients was only 2 years. If this were the case, most restorations would survive longer and "outlive" them! However, many patients who receive restorations for managing (coronal) carious lesions are young adults, who retain their teeth for longer as well as having longer lifespans themselves. If a restoration is placed in an average 10-year-old today, it needs to survive for over 70 years. This, as described above, is unrealistic in most cases and the first restoration placed in a tooth is just that. It will seldom be the last and is simply the stepping stone for further larger, deeper direct restorations placed over the patient's lifecycle. Given the 70-year period mentioned, and assuming a "normal" restoration lasts 10 years, it could theoretically be replaced up to 7 times over this period based on the assumption of a 10-year restoration lifespan [32].

This, again, would not be problematic if an identical restoration could be placed each subsequent time (like buying the exact same car again if your old one breaks down). However, numerous studies show that with each renewal restorations are enlarged, with increasing hard tissue loss during this process [33, 34]. The reasons underpinning this include further disease, tooth fracture from weakened areas, and aesthetic concerns necessitating enlarging the cavity:

- The most frequent causes of failure for resin composite restorations are secondary caries or fracture which automatically result in a loss of additional hard tissue [35–37]. The consequence is that the new restoration to treat secondary caries will extend beyond the edge of the previous restoration (including the new carious lesion parts).
- Similarly, if fractures occur, they often include parts of the tooth too, again hard tissue is lost and will need replacement with the new restoration. This is particularly the case for resin composite but not for glass-ionomer, which tends to fracture cohesively.
- If restoration replacement is due to the wear or loss of surface lustre (aesthetic reasons), removing it is often not easy. The resin composite restorations are especially hard to remove as they are bonded to the tooth tissue, which makes removal technically difficult and they are hard to distinguish from the sound tooth tissue (which is why they are highly aesthetic). Glass-ionomer restorations do not present such a problem. Their colour matches that of dentine and enamel, but the material is sufficiently distinguishable from the tooth structures.

Together, these factors lead to removal of tooth substance as part of the replacement exercise, increasing the size of the restoration and structurally weakening the tooth as well as increasing the chance of compromising the pulp. Amalgam or other metal restorations are retained macromechanically and clearly distinguished from the tooth; after reducing their retention, removal is easier.

In summary, the limited lifespan of restorations essentially means that in most patients they are replaced several times, each time involving increased tooth tissue loss. This is called the repeat restoration cycle [32, 33]. Often, at some point re-restoration is no longer possible and teeth are deemed to require extraction due to restorative reasons – the teeth are "unrestorable" (Fig. 4), which has, perhaps somewhat dramatically, been known as the "death spiral" [34]. Regardless of its name, many teeth experiencing such restorative re-treatments will also require additional therapies associated with the repeated restoration failure, including endodontic therapy or surgical treatments (like pre-restorative crown lengthening, or surgical endodontics). These additional therapies are expensive and complex.

Therefore, avoiding restorations wherever possible and managing caries and carious lesions preventively and biologically has long-term importance. Modelling studies show that, over an individual's lifetime, early treatment decisions (placing a restoration for a small primary carious lesion or not) have profound consequences over time [38–44].

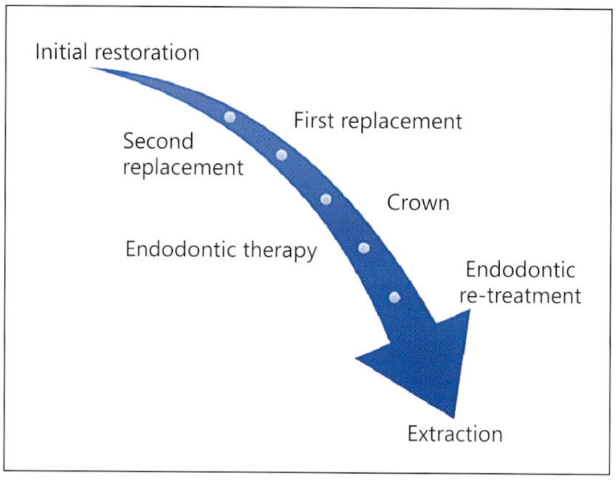

Fig. 4. A visual representation of the repeat restoration cycle, or "death spiral" of restorative intervention. The first restorations may be direct restorations of amalgam or an adhesive material, but with each replacement the cavity will increase in size. The treatments required can be seen to increase in invasiveness as the death spiral continues.

Principles to Avoid or Slow Down the Repeat Restoration Cycle

There are 3 main principles that should be adhered to, in order to avoid or slow down the repeat restoration cycle:

1 The initial and probably most important thing is to prevent placing a restoration if at all possible. Only place one if there is no alternative. Restoring a carious lesion does not cure the disease of dental caries; instead, it serves to locally manage the symptoms of the disease, the carious lesion. Restorative care can largely be avoided for non-cavitated lesions; these can and should, where feasible, be managed preventively or, where necessary, microinvasively. Only cavitated lesions require further invasive therapy, mainly restorations (we will discuss exemptions from this rule later in this book). Restorations are placed to reconstruct the tooth surface and thus allow the removal of biofilm from the tooth surface. They serve to support additional general caries prevention strategies (which could involve dietary or biofilm control, or remineralisation therapies) [5, 45].

2 When restorations are unavoidable, they should be placed in such a way that maximises their longevity. Careful moisture control (for adhesive restorations), an appropriate concept for dealing with carious tissue (the core concept of this book and discussed in detail later on), cautious restorative procedures during placement, and, most importantly, managing the caries dis-

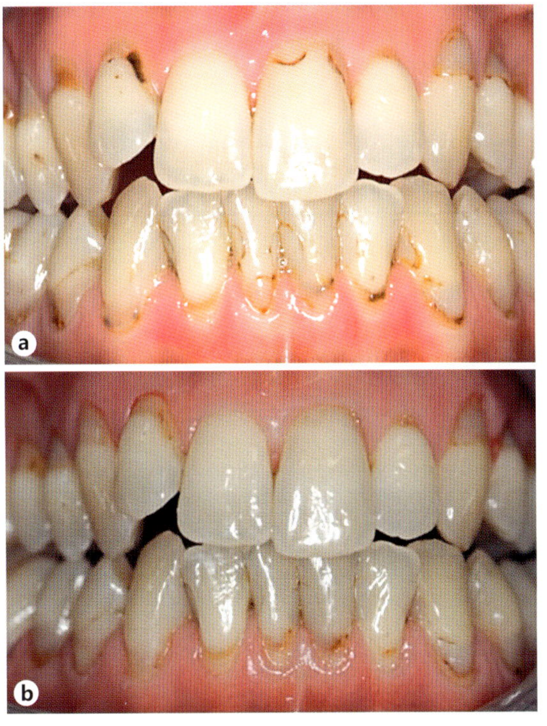

Fig. 5. a This 35-year-old patient presented with a large number of cervical composite restorations or initial cervical carious lesions. **b** After managing her caries risk, it was decided not to replace most of the restorations, which showed margin imperfections and discolourations, but to recontour or repolish them. The patient was highly satisfied with the aesthetic result and was happy to not have the restorations replaced.

ease by ensuring optimal preventive strategies are implemented with the patient will reduce the risk of secondary dentine carious lesions. These factors will all support the optimisation of restoration survival.

3 Re-interventions should be avoided or their negative consequences reduced as much as possible. Dentists should use meaningful decision criteria and re-intervene very cautiously on existing restorations. Marginal discolourations, but also wear or imperfect margin adaptation can be acceptable in many cases; in fact, marginal integrity might be of little importance if the risk of secondary dentine carious lesion development is managed successfully (Fig. 5) [31, 46].

If re-interventions are needed, it is now a recommended standard that complete replacement of partially faulty restorations is avoided by carrying out repairs, re-polishing, or refurbishing instead. This is known to increase the lifetime of teeth, as it significantly slows down the repeat restoration cycle, even if the repaired restoration is less long-lasting than a new restoration [47–51].

Conclusions

Placing restorations after removing carious tissues does not manage dental caries or carious lesions, it merely removes the symptoms of the disease. Restorations are likely to be needed for cavitated dentine lesions (although in some cases preventive strategies may be chosen for cleansable lesions on root surfaces or for medium/large cavities in primary teeth). When restorative interventions are necessary, the restoration should be placed to a high standard and according to the material's protocol as their placement initiates a long-lasting and escalating cycle of re-interventions. If re-intervention does become necessary, it should be performed in a way that is as minimally invasive as possible to reduce the associated damage of sound hard tissue.

References

1 Black GV: The pathology of hard tissues of the teeth: oral diagnosis. Part III. Treatment of caries; in Operative Dentistry. London, Medico-Dental Publishing, 1936, vol 1.

2 Gibson GB, Richardson AS: Sticky fissure management: 30-month report. J Can Dent Assoc 1980;46:255–258.

3 Penning C, van Amerongen JP, Seef RE, ten Cate JM: Validity of probing for fissure caries diagnosis. Caries Res 1992; 26:445–449.

4 Kuhnisch J, Dietz W, Stosser L, Hickel R, Heinrich-Weltzien R: Effects of dental probing on occlusal surfaces – a scanning electron microscopy evaluation. Caries Res 2007;41:43–48.
5 Schwendicke F, Frencken JE, Bjorndal L, Maltz M, Manton DJ, Ricketts D, van Landuyt K, Banerjee A, Campus G, Domejean S, Fontana M, Leal S, Lo E, Machiulskiene V, Schulte A, Splieth C, Zandona AF, Innes NP: Managing carious lesions: consensus recommendations on carious tissue removal. Adv Dent Res 2016;28:58–67.
6 Schwendicke F, Paris S, Tu Y: Effects of using different criteria and methods for caries removal: a systematic review and network meta-analysis. J Dent 2015;43:1–15.
7 Ricketts D, Lamont T, Innes NP, Kidd E, Clarkson JE: Operative caries management in adults and children. Cochrane Database Syst Rev 2013;28:CD003808.
8 Nyvad B, Fejerskov O: Active root surface caries converted into inactive caries as a response to oral hygiene. Scand J Dent Res 1986;94:281–284.
9 Bjorndal L, Demant S, Dabelsteen S: Depth and activity of carious lesions as indicators for the regenerative potential of dental pulp after intervention. J Endod 2014;40(4 suppl):S76–S81.
10 Griffin SO, Oong E, Kohn W, Vidakovic B, Gooch BF, Bader J, Clarkson J, Fontana MR, Meyer DM, Rozier RG, Weintraub JA, Zero DT: The effectiveness of sealants in managing caries lesions. J Dent Res 2008;87:169–174.
11 Oong EM, Griffin SO, Kohn WG, Gooch BF, Caufield PW: The effect of dental sealants on bacteria levels in caries lesions. J Am Dent Assoc 2008;139:271–278.
12 Mertz-Fairhurst EJ, Curtis JW, Ergle JW, Rueggeberg FA, Adair SM: Ultraconservative and cariostatic sealed restorations: results at year 10. J Am Dent Assoc 1998;129:55–66.
13 Innes N, Schwendicke F: Dentists' thresholds for restorative intervention in carious lesions: systematic review and meta-analysis. J Dent Res 2017;96:501–508.
14 Gruythuysen R: Non-restorative cavity treatment: managing rather than masking caries activity. Ned Tijdschr Tandheelkd 2010;117:173–180.
15 Maggio JJ, Hausmann EM, Allen K, Potts TV: A model for dentinal caries progression by digital subtraction radiography. J Prosthet Dent 1990;64:727–732.
16 Lopez R, Smith PC, Gostemeyer G, Schwendicke F: Ageing, dental caries and periodontal diseases. J Clin Periodontol 2017;44(suppl 18):S145–S152.
17 Baelum V, Hintze H, Wenzel A, Danielsen B, Nyvad B: Implications of caries diagnostic strategies for clinical management decisions. Community Dent Oral Epidemiol 2012;40:257–266.
18 Ratledge DK, Kidd EA, Beighton D: A clinical and microbiological study of approximal carious lesions. Part 1: the relationship between cavitation, radiographic lesion depth, the site-specific gingival index and the level of infection of the dentine. Caries Res 2001;35:3–7.
19 Ricketts DN, Ekstrand KR, Kidd EA, Larsen T: Relating visual and radiographic ranked scoring systems for occlusal caries detection to histological and microbiological evidence. Oper Dent 2002;27:231–237.
20 Ricketts DN, Kidd EA, Beighton D: Operative and microbiological validation of visual, radiographic and electronic diagnosis of occlusal caries in non-cavitated teeth judged to be in need of operative care. Br Dent J 1995;179:214–220.
21 Bakhshandeh A, Qvist V, Ekstrand K: Sealing occlusal caries lesions in adults referred for restorative treatment: 2–3 years of follow-up. Clin Oral Investig 2012;16:521–529.
22 Hesse D, Bonifacio CC, Mendes FM, Braga MM, Imparato JC, Raggio DP: Sealing versus partial caries removal in primary molars: a randomized clinical trial. BMC Oral Health 2014;14:58.
23 Schwendicke F, Jäger AM, Paris S, Hsu L-Y, Tu Y-K: Treating pit-and-fissure caries: a systematic review and network meta-analysis. J Dent Res 2015;94:124–137.
24 Schwendicke F, Gostemeyer G, Blunck U, Paris S, Hsu LY, Tu YK: Directly placed restorative materials: review and network meta-analysis. J Dent Res 2016;95:613–622.
25 Angeletaki F, Gkogkos A, Papazoglou E, Kloukos D: Direct versus indirect inlay/onlay composite restorations in posterior teeth: a systematic review and meta-analysis. J Dent 2016;53:12–21.
26 Opdam NJ, van de Sande FH, Bronkhorst E, Cenci MS, Bottenberg P, Pallesen U, Gaengler P, Lindberg A, Huysmans MC, van Dijken JW: Longevity of posterior composite restorations: a systematic review and meta-analysis. J Dent Res 2014;93:943–949.
27 Hickel R, Manhart J: Longevity of restorations in posterior teeth and reasons for failure. J Adhes Dent 2001;3:45–64.
28 Raedel M, Hartmann A, Priess HW, Bohm S, Samietz S, Konstantinidis I, Walter MH: Re-interventions after restoring teeth – mining an insurance database. J Dent 2017;57:14–19.
29 Burke FJ, Lucarotti PS, Holder RL: Outcome of direct restorations placed within the general dental services in England and Wales (part 2): variation by patients' characteristics. J Dent 2005;33:817–826.
30 Schwendicke F, Kruger H, Schlattmann P, Paris S: Restoration outcomes after restoring vital teeth with advanced caries lesions: a practice-based retrospective study. Clin Oral Investig 2016;20:1675–1681.
31 Opdam NJM, Collares K, Hickel R, Bayne SC, Loomans BA, Cenci MS, Lynch CD, Correa MB, Demarco F, Schwendicke F, Wilson NHF: Clinical studies in restorative dentistry: new directions and new demands. Dent Mater 2018;34:1–12.
32 Elderton RJ: Clinical studies concerning re-restoration of teeth. Adv Dent Res 1990;4:4–9.
33 Brantley C, Bader J, Shugars D, Nesbit S: Does the cycle of rerestoration lead to larger restorations? J Am Dent Assoc 1995;126:1407–1413.
34 Qvist V: Longevity of restorations: the "death spiral"; in Fejerskov O, Kidd EAM (eds): Dental Caries: The Disease and Its Clinical Management. Oxford, Blackwell Munksgaard, 2008, pp 444–455.
35 Demarco FF, Correa MB, Cenci MS, Moraes RR, Opdam NJ: Longevity of posterior composite restorations: not only a matter of materials. Dent Mater 2012;28:87–101.
36 Opdam NJ, Bronkhorst EM, Cenci MS, Huysmans MC, Wilson NH: Age of failed restorations: a deceptive longevity parameter. J Dent 2011;39:225–230.
37 Brunthaler A, Konig F, Lucas T, Sperr W, Schedle A: Longevity of direct resin composite restorations in posterior teeth. Clin Oral Investig 2003;7:63–70.

38 Schwendicke F, Gostemeyer G: Cost-effectiveness of root caries preventive treatments. J Dent 2017;56:58–64.
39 Schwendicke F, Meyer-Lueckel H, Stolpe M, Dorfer CE, Paris S: Costs and effectiveness of treatment alternatives for proximal caries lesions. PLoS One 2014; 9:e86992.
40 Schwendicke F, Paris S, Stolpe M: Detection and treatment of proximal caries lesions: milieu-specific cost-effectiveness analysis. J Dent 2015;43:647–655.
41 Schwendicke F, Splieth CH, Thomson W, Reda S, Stolpe M, Foster Page LA: Cost-effectiveness of caries-preventive fluoride varnish applications in clinic settings among patients of low, moderate, and high risk. Community Dent Oral Epidemiol 2018;46:8–16.
42 Schwendicke F, Stolpe M: In-office application of fluoride gel or varnish: cost-effectiveness and expected value of perfect information analysis. Caries Res 2017;51:231–239.
43 Schwendicke F, Stolpe M, Innes N: Conventional treatment, Hall Technique or immediate pulpotomy for carious primary molars: a cost-effectiveness analysis. Int Endod J 2016;49:817–826.
44 Schwendicke F, Stolpe M, Meyer-Lueckel H, Paris S: Detecting and treating occlusal caries lesions: a cost-effectiveness analysis. J Dent Res 2014;94:272–280.
45 Innes NP, Frencken JE, Bjorndal L, Maltz M, Manton DJ, Ricketts D, van Landuyt K, Banerjee A, Campus G, Domejean S, Fontana M, Leal S, Lo E, Machiulskiene V, Schulte A, Splieth C, Zandona A, Schwendicke F: Managing carious lesions: consensus recommendations on terminology. Adv Dent Res 2016;28:49–57.
46 Schwendicke F, Opdam N: Clinical studies in restorative dentistry: design, conduct, analysis. Dent Mater 2017;34:29–39.
47 Hickel R, Brushaver K, Ilie N: Repair of restorations – criteria for decision making and clinical recommendations. Dent Mater 2013;29:28–50.
48 Mjor IA, Gordan VV: Failure, repair, refurbishing and longevity of restorations. Oper Dent 2002;27:528–534.
49 Gordan VV, Riley JL, Blaser PK, Mondragon E, Garvan CW, Mjor IA: Alternative treatments to replacement of defective amalgam restorations: results of a seven-year clinical study. J Am Dent Assoc 2011;142:842–849.
50 Opdam NJ, Bronkhorst EM, Loomans BA, Huysmans MC: Longevity of repaired restorations: a practice based study. J Dent Child 2012;40:889–835.
51 Kanzow P, Wiegand A, Schwendicke F: Cost-effectiveness of repairing versus replacing composite or amalgam restorations. J Dent 2016;54:41–47.

Falk Schwendicke
Operative and Preventive Dentistry, Charité – Universitätsmedizin Berlin
Corporate Member of Freie Universität Berlin
Humboldt-Universität zu Berlin, and Berlin Institute of Health
Assmannshauser Strasse 4-6
DE–14197 Berlin (Germany)
E-Mail falk.schwendicke@charite.de

Schwendicke F, Frencken J, Innes N (eds): Caries Excavation: Evolution of Treating Cavitated Carious Lesions.
Monogr Oral Sci. Basel, Karger, 2018, vol 27, pp 42–55 (DOI: 10.1159/000487831)

Restoring the Carious Lesion

Gerd Göstemeyer · Falk Schwendicke · Uwe Blunck

Operative and Preventive Dentistry, Charité – Universitätsmedizin Berlin, Corporate Member of Freie Universität Berlin, Humboldt-Universität zu Berlin, and Berlin Institute of Health, Berlin, Germany

Abstract

Restoring carious lesions can be challenging, especially for deep lesions in proximity to the pulp. A number of factors can influence restoration longevity. This chapter will discuss aspects that should be considered when restoring carious lesions. In the first part, factors that might have an effect on the pulp such as preparation trauma, tooth hypersensitivity, and the use of liners will be described. In the second part, the challenges and limitations of adhesive bonding to (sound and carious) dentine will be discussed. Lastly, recommendations on the suitability of different bonding techniques and restorative materials in different situations will be given.

Faced with a carious lesion, dentists will – in line with the chapters of this book – first need to decide which therapy to choose (non-, micro-, or invasive therapy), and then – if needed – how to remove carious tissue (selective removal, stepwise removal, etc.). Eventually, in this case, the carious lesion and the resulting cavity will need to be restored. This chapter will deal with the challenges when restoring dentine carious lesions, especially deep ones, using resin-based and glass-ionomer-based restoratives, and how these challenges might be overcome.

Restorative Risks for the Pulp

Pulpal Trauma due to Preparation

It is well known that even carious lesions restricted to enamel lead to some form of pulpal reaction, mainly inflammation, and that the deeper the carious lesion progresses the more pulpal inflammation occurs [1]. Preparation of a tooth, mainly with diamonds and rotary burs, additionally results in a release of inflammatory mediators in the pulp due to physical irritations (mostly heat development) [2]. Depending on the clearance by pulpal blood circulation, which can additionally be affected by adrenaline-containing local anaesthesia, the concentration of these mediators can increase to a level resulting in severe pulp haemorrhage and, eventually, pulp necrosis [3]. Water cooling during preparation reduces heat generation; the recommended flow rate of the water coolant should be at about 35–50 mL/min [4]. In order to keep the risk of pulpal irritation to a minimum and for determining whether the dentine is soft, firm, or hard, the International Caries Consensus Collaboration (ICCC) recommends the use of the hand excavator for removing carious tissue from within the cavity during the selective removal process. The use of excavators is also associated to the ICCC's guiding principle of carious tissue removal: "avoiding pain/discomfort and dental anxiety" [5].

Tooth Hypersensitivity

Tooth hypersensitivity after restoring the carious lesion can be the result of pulpal irritations due to preparation, but also due to incomplete bonding between the resin-based restoration material and dentine near the pulp, as well as insufficient curing of a large volume of the resin-based restoratives.

Incomplete bonding can be the result of inadequate handling of the adhesive systems. When using an etch-and-rinse system, an unintentionally long phosphoric acid etching period can lead to a deep demineralised dentine layer, which cannot be fully penetrated by the primer, hence resulting in an incomplete hybrid layer. Similarly, neglecting the wet bonding technique followed by a too short and only passive primer application can result in incomplete infiltration of the monomers into the collagen network [6]. When using self-etching adhesives, only passively applying them (omitting agitation) or not fully evaporating the solvent can also lead to such incomplete hybrid layers [6]. For both adhesives systems it is clear that saliva and/or blood contamination can compromise a stable adhesion to the cavity floor [7]. Based on such incomplete hybrid layers and reduced bond strengths, the polymerisation shrinkage of the applied composite resin can pull the restorative material off the dentine surface, resulting in a gap formation at the cavity floor. This gap is filled with dentinal liquid, which can then be pressed by mechanical loading back into the tubules, stimulating the A-δ-fibres and creating a sharp pain [8]. Insufficient conversion of resin-based materials because of curing devices that emit too low energy and do not reach the deeper part of the material or a layer of resin-based material that is too voluminous may lead to the leaking of unreacted monomer from the resin-based material into a pulpal direction, causing adverse effects [9, 10].

Tooth hypersensitivity after the placement of a restoration can disappear after weeks or months. However, these attacks can also overload the healing capacity of the individual pulp, resulting in irreversible pulpitis or eventually necrosis. Whilst hypersensitivity due to incomplete bonding can already be a challenge for the pulp in "normal" cavities [11], it might be even more harmful for the pulp in deep carious lesions with already compromised pulpal tissue.

Use of Liners

Aiming to reduce hypersensitivity, but also assuming a number of positive effects of such therapy (see below), dental practitioners usually place cavity liners (commonly based on calcium hydroxide) onto pulpal walls of the cavity floor in deep cavities prior to restoration. This procedure is commonly called indirect pulp capping (Fig. 1) [12]. Given the described changes in the understanding of dental caries and the restorative options when using adhesive restoration materials, the relevance and need for such liners can be questioned [13].

Cavity liners were supposed to have a positive effect on the pulp for a number of reasons. First, they were thought to be antibacterial, i.e., to significantly reduce the number of bacteria remaining in the dentine around the pulp. This antibacterial effect, however, might be irrelevant given that the sealing itself and the resulting deprivation from dietary carbohydrates will result in the

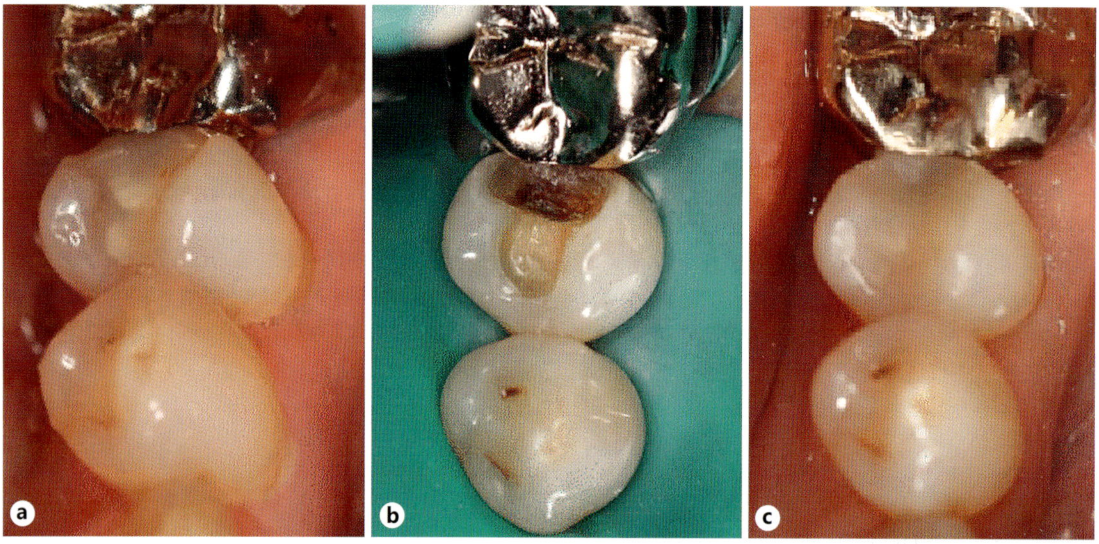

Fig. 1. Replacement of a lined composite restoration. **a** The restoration had been washed out and showed signs of secondary caries at the cervical margin. Beneath the composite, a calcium hydroxide liner had been used, which is shining through the occlusal box. The liner inhibits any bonding in this area and additionally weakens the restoration. **b** After removal of the restoration and the liner, selective excavation to firm dentine was performed. Discoloured but firm or hard dentine was not removed. **c** The final restoration.

vast majority of bacteria dying beneath the restoration in the long-term (as previously discussed) [14]. In addition, the specific antibacterial effects of calcium hydroxide in comparison with other liners are increasingly doubted. Calcium hydroxide was supposed to be antibacterial via releasing hydroxyl ions given its alkaline pH [15], as has been demonstrated by a number of – predominantly older – studies [16, 17]. More recent studies, however, have not necessarily confirmed any antibacterial effect of calcium hydroxide [13, 18], and other materials such as calcium silicates (mineral trioxide aggregate, Biodentine) [19] or resin-modified glass-ionomer cements have been found to have similar or even more potent antibacterial properties [20].

Second, cavity liners were placed to block harmful (toxic) ingredients from the restorative materials to avoid irritating pulpal tissue. Remineralising potential has been attributed to liners not only to calcium hydroxide and glass ionomer-based cement, but also to MTA and other calcium silicates [21]. It remains unclear if the observed mineral gains truly restore the physical parameters (mainly hardness and elastic modulus of the dentine), i.e., remineralise the lesion biomimetically, or if the mineral is accumulated between, instead of within, the collagen fibres, thereby only limitedly adding to the strength of the dentine [22]. Moreover, mineral gains in sealed carious lesions have also been found when no liners were used at all, which might serve as an indication that the minerals are delivered not necessarily by the lining material, but the pulp (either actively mediated by odontoblasts or as passive transudation from pulp vessels into the tubules) [23]. Such mineral gain from the pulp has been confirmed after only a few months, as detected radiographically but also when analysing dentine ex vivo [24].

A third aspect is the induction of reactionary dentine when calcium hydroxide is applied. This induction has been confirmed by a number of animal experiments [25, 26]. It has also been hypothesised to reduce pulp inflammation after restoring the cavity, possibly by isolation of the pulp against chemical components of adhesives (like hydroxyethyl methacrylate) or the acid of glass-ionomer cements (GICs) [27]. The resulting theoretical advantages – less pain, reduced incidence of postoperative hypersensitivities – might be one major reason for the popularity of cavity liners [28], but have not been unambiguously confirmed in clinical trials [29, 30]. Instead, there is increasing evidence that in both permanent and primary teeth, use of liners might not necessarily have only benefits, but could possibly also do harm [31–33]. The reason might be that conventional liners – mainly calcium hydroxide – do not allow any bonding to dentine and therefore lack in mechanical support of the restoration. Newer lining materials like calcium silicates might have some advantages here [34].

Cavity liners seem to have little or no significant effect for the pulp due to their assumed modes of action. For reducing postoperative pulpal complications, the seal of the cavity might be a more important factor [32]. This can mainly be ensured by creation of a sufficient bond of the restorative material to the cavity walls.

Challenges for Bonding Resin-Based Materials to Different Dentine Surfaces

With the advent of bonding systems that offer the potential to lute resin-based restorative materials adhesively to tooth structures, the principles of cavity design have been altered. As it is no longer necessary to prepare macroretentive groves in order to hold the restoration in place, carious lesions can be restored with minimal invasion, mainly involving opening of the cavity, carious tissue removal and, if needed, rounding off and/or bevelling sharp margins [35].

However, in contrast to enamel, achievement of a sustainable bond to dentine with resin-based materials remains challenging. Dentine is a mineralised vital tissue consisting of about 70% by weight (40–45% by volume) inorganic components (mainly hydroxyapatite), 20% by weight (30% by volume) organic components (mainly collagen fibrils), and 10% by weight (20–25% by volume) in water [36]. Therefore, dentine cavity surfaces are hydrophilic in nature and impede the bonding of hydrophobic resins. This phenomenon is not present in the bonding process of the hydrophilic glass-ionomers to dentine. Local alterations of the dentine substrate as a pulpal response to environmental stimuli further complicate the creation of a sufficient bond to dentine with resin-based materials. The composition and structure of the dentine surface can considerably differ within the same cavity [35, 37].

Effective bonding of restorative materials to any substrate requires: (1) a microretentive and (2) wettable surface, as well as (3) a lowly viscous adhesive. The traditional bonding strategies to dentine involve etching the dentinal surface and application of low viscous primer/bonding agents, which infiltrate into the demineralised dentine and form the hybrid layer [38]. Conditioning the dentine with acids can be achieved by phosphoric acid, which is washed away by water after demineralising the dentine surface (etch-and-rinse technique) or acidic monomers incorporated into the adhesive where the solvent is evaporated after application (self-etch technique) [39].

The phosphoric acid demineralises the dentine surface, resulting in an exposed dentine collagen matrix with nanometre-sized porosities. This porous dentine matrix requires water to prevent the collapse of the exposed collagen promoting the monomers to infiltrate into the microretentive surface. It has been shown that the resin monomers are not always able to fully infiltrate the demineralised dentine, and a part of demineralised dentine remains susceptible to hydrolytic degradation [40].

Acidic monomers in the self-etching approach dissolve the smear layer – created by mechanical pretreatment of dentine, including carious tissue removal [41] – and demineralise the superficial dentine while simultaneously penetrating into the exposed collagen network. The resulting hybrid layer of dentine and hydrophilic resin monomers is essentially a semipermeable membrane, which allows water diffusion. One fear resulting from this water diffusion is that hydrolytic dentine enzymes, which are only active in a water-containing environment, eventually degrade the resin layer and exposed collagen fibres, thereby destroying the formed interface in the long term [42].

Adhesion of Glass-Ionomer-Based Materials to Tooth Tissue

A GIC is the only true adhesive restorative material. Its bonding mechanism to tooth tissue is based on a substitution reaction. The carboxylate group from the glass-ionomer mixture substitutes with the hydroxyl groups, and calcium and phosphate from the apatite. As enamel has a higher calcium content than dentine, the adhesion to enamel is stronger than to dentine. The process of adhesion results in the development of a hypermineralised ion-exchange layer at the interface of glass-ionomer and tooth tissue. This layer is more resistant to acid attack than the surrounding glass-ionomer material and tooth tissue [43]. It secures a strong bond between the glass-ionomer material and tooth tissue. The values for adhesion of glass-ionomer to tooth tissue are not as high as achieved for resin-based systems, because of cohesive failures of the glass ionomer itself before the adhesion to the tooth substrate fails. This is proven in microleakage and clinical studies [44, 45]. Restoring non-carious cervical lesions with various types of adhesive materials showed that the material with the highest clinical retention rate after 6 years was glass-ionomer, followed by the 3-step etch-and-rinse adhesive.

Factors Limiting Durability of Resin Bonding to Dentine

Complete infiltration of resin monomers into the demineralised dentine matrix, albeit desired, can still not be achieved and the resulting hybrid-layer might have several imperfections. These imperfections are the origin for the occurrence of different phenomena leading to limited durability of resin-dentine bonds [46]. The main factors that reduce the durability of resin-dentine bonding are:

- Incomplete infiltration of resin monomers. Neither the etch-and-rinse nor the self-etch approaches are capable of completely replacing water from the internal and external water compartments of the collagen network. In fact, nanoleakage within the water-rich zones of the hybrid layer and the adhesive can frequently be detected [46]. Additionally, highly hydrated proteoglycans, which are present in acid-etched dentine, form a hydrogel within the interfibrillar spaces of the collagen network. These hydrogels may be responsible for "molecular sieving" by retaining larger acrylates like Bis-GMA and allowing smaller molecules like HEMA to penetrate into the base of the hybrid layer. As HEMA does not cross-link during polymerisation, the formed resin layer is less durable than a layer containing Bis-GMA. Both nanoleakage and HEMA-rich regions in the hybrid layer are prone to failure of the adhesive bond [46].
- Hydrophilic monomers have been incorporated into adhesive systems in order to increase the compatibility of the hydrophobic resins and the moist, acid-etched dentine surfaces. However, creating a hydrophilic dentine-resin interface has several disadvantages. High concentrations of hydrophilic monomers hamper the evapora-

tion of water, which serves as a solvent in many adhesives. As a result, water can be entrapped into the adhesive layer, which might deteriorate the mechanical properties of the bond. The water can also lead to nano-phase separation of the adhesive components, which further decreases the mechanical properties and increases their susceptibility to hydrolysis [46]. Due to the presence of ester linkages, hydrophilic monomers are highly vulnerable to hydrolysis. Matrix metalloproteinases (MMPs) are host-derived proteases that are trapped in mineralised dentine. They can be activated by acid exposure and lead to the degradation of collagen. In the pathogenesis of dentine caries they contribute to the breakdown of collagen matrices. However, they can also be activated by the application of acid etching gels or acidic self-etch systems, and lead to the degradation of resin-sparse collagen fibrils of the hybrid layer [46, 47]. Cysteine cathepsins are another family of proteases that can contribute to the breakdown of collagens. They can be expressed by odontoblasts in intact dentine, but also carious dentine. They can be activated in mildly acid environments (e.g., by acids from adhesive systems), which can result in the degradation of collagens and can also further result in the activation of MMPs [46].

In the aftermath of the Minamata Treaty on the use of mercury, which resulted in the phase-down of dental amalgam worldwide, the level of toxicity of dental materials was a widely discussed topic. Notably, the monomers in resin-based materials are a concern. It prompted the World Dental Association (FDI) to issue a policy statement in 2013 that called upon the manufacturers to produce bisphenol A (derivate)-free resin-based materials. By 2016, the percentage of bisphenol A (derivate)-free resin composite in Europe was still low, but was increasing [48]. The changes in the composition of the resin-based materials (adhesives and resin composites) resulted in new materials and, subsequently, in studies that have tested these.

Alterations of Dentine

The abovementioned challenges related to resin-based materials to create a durable adhesion to dentine become even more important when one considers that restoring carious lesions does not usually mean to bond to normal, unaltered dentine. Before we discuss the problems of bonding to carious dentine, however, we would like to highlight that even physiologically developed ("sound") dentine is not a homogenous substrate. For example, peritubular dentine is harder than intertubular dentine [49]. The number of tubules ranges from 45,000 to 65,000/mm^2 close to the pulp, and from 29,500 to 35,000/mm^2 near the enamel-dentine junction. Tubule diameters range from 2 to 3 μm at the pulpal side, to less than 1 μm at the dentinoenamel junction [50].

Restoring carious lesions after selective or stepwise carious tissue removal means to bond to demineralised or bacterially contaminated dentine, as described in the chapter by Schwendicke [this vol., pp. 56–67; 37, 51]. Demineralised dentine has a lower hardness and modulus of elasticity than sound dentine, primarily as the mineral content of the dentine is reduced [35, 52]. While for demineralised dentine the collagen matrix remains mostly intact and is believed to still be able to remineralise [47], bacterially contaminated dentine may also involve collagen which is not intact (cross-linked) and hence not remineralisable any longer. It is clear that, clinically, dentists are only limitedly able to discriminate such "layers" or "zones" of carious dentine, which means that for bonding various dentine qualities (sound, demineralised, contaminated) may be present in the same cavity.

The bond strength of both etch-and-rinse and self-etch adhesives to demineralised and contaminated dentine is generally lower compared to sound dentine, which may be a result of the reduced hardness (Fig. 2) [37, 51, 52]. Also, the hybrid layers formed in demineralised or contaminated dentine are thicker and more porous compared to those in sound dentine [37, 51, 52]. This

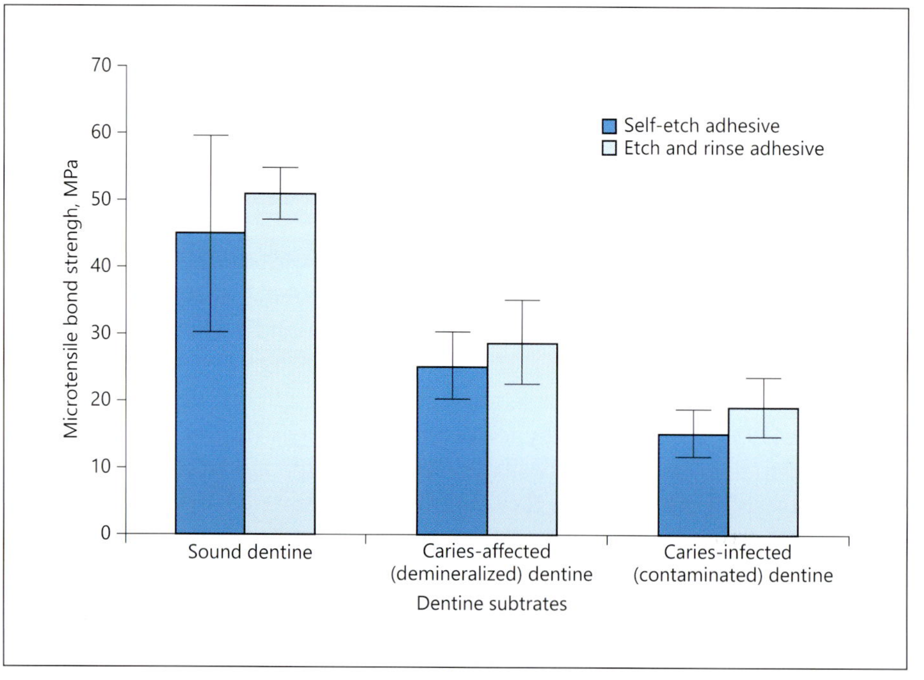

Fig. 2. Bond strength of self-etch and etch and rinse adhesive to different dentine substrates. Adhesive bond strength for both self-etch and etch and rinse adhesives is increasingly reduced the more the caries process has led to alterations of dentine. From Yoshiyama et al. [52].

might be the result of the deeper diffusion of the applied acidic conditioners (phosphoric acids, acidic monomers) into the more porous and demineralised dentine. Such deeper demineralised layers are harder to fully penetrate with the adhesives in the subsequent bonding step, resulting in incomplete penetration [52]. Deposition of mineral casts in the dentine tubules in demineralised or contaminated dentine might also reduce the penetration of monomers into the tubules, and therefore hampers the formation of resin tags [35]. Besides reduced stability of the bonding interface, these irregularities might lead to increased vulnerability to degradation of the hybrid layer [51], especially when considering that carious dentine contains higher concentrations of active MMPs and cathepsins [47].

Prior to placing a glass-ionomer restorative, the cavity is conditioned with an organic acid, usually a polyacrylic acid in a concentration of 10–20%. The conditioner removes the smear layer, pre-activates calcium ions in enamel and dentine, and renders them more available for ion exchange with the carboxylate ions from the glass-ionomer mixture. The conditioner also exposes collagen fibrils into which glass-ionomer components diffuse [53]. In cavities that are cleaned according to the selective removal to soft and to firm methods, the bonding of glass-ionomers to dentine will be lower than to dentine, with a higher level of hydroxyapatite. Nevertheless, an ex vivo study that assessed the interface of dentine and glass-ionomer placed in cavities of primary molars that had been cleaned using selective removal to firm dentine (atraumatic restorative treatment, ART, method) concluded that, using electron probe microanalysis, fluoride and strontium from the glass-ionomer had penetrated into the residual dentine. In places where the removal of carious dentine was incomplete, the glass-ionomer remained adherent to the dentine tissue in all 4 specimens on the basis of SEM images [54].

It should be highlighted that the resulting bond strengths when applying adhesives and glass-ionomers to contaminated dentine are lower than to clean dentine; a sustainable bond is not always possible and, in many cases (especially when thicker layers of soft, contaminated dentine are left in proximity to the pulp), even impossible. On the other hand, it needs emphasising that the reduced bond strengths to demineralised and, more so, to contaminated dentine might not be clinically relevant, as long as the cavity is surrounded by sufficient surfaces of sound enamel or (hard) dentine [5, 52]. So far, there is no clinical evidence available that shows that leaving limited amounts of carious dentine beneath an adhesively placed resin-based restoration leads to a higher risk of restoration failure. The previous chapters have outlined in detail the limits of sealing carious tissue, and it should always be emphasised that leaving carious tissue in a cavity prior to restoration is not an aim by itself – it serves the purpose of maintaining pulp vitality. In areas where pulp vitality is not at risk, there is no argument to be made for why (at least contaminated) carious dentine should be left.

Different Bonding Systems and Their Suitability for Different Lesions

Bonding Systems

As already mentioned before, there are 2 different approaches for bonding resin composite to enamel and dentine: the etch-and-rinse technique and the self-etch technique. Both include the 4 fundamental steps of: (1) conditioning the enamel, (2) conditioning the dentine, (3) the application of small hydrophilic monomers (primers), and (4) the application of longer cross-linking monomers (adhesives), which create a stabile interface to dental hard tissue in order to withstand the stress from polymerisation shrinkage and mechanical loading [40]. These 4 steps can be combined in different ways, thus a high number of different products are available on the dental market. The development of new products has gone in the direction of easier handling with less application steps. However, in vitro and clinical studies showed that the so-called gold standard products, launched decades ago, remain those yielding the highest bond strengths and the highest restoration longevity.

A number of adhesives nowadays contain the monomer 10-methacryloyloxydecyl dihydrogen phosphate (MDP), which allows the additional creation of nanolayers within the exposed collagen network where not only micromechanical retention occurs, but also a chemical bond between dentine calcium and the resin adhesives is established [55]. MDP also bonds chemically to sandblasted metal and oxide ceramic, especially zirconia. Adhesives containing MDP are therefore usually marketed as "universal" adhesives. Although this term is not 100% correct (these adhesives do not universally promote adhesion to all substrates; for example, the long-term bond strength to glass-based ceramic is low), these adhesives have in fact a wide applicability [56, 57]. They can be used to bond to both enamel and dentine, and can be used in an etch-and-rinse as well as a self-etching mode.

They are especially interesting when one wants to perform "selective enamel etching" using phosphoric acid, followed by the application of self-etch adhesives to enamel and dentine. This approach combines the high bond strengths in enamel yielded by etching with phosphoric acid (self-etch adhesives are too mild and bond strengths remain inferior when no separate phosphoric acid etching is performed in enamel) with the ease of handling and advantages of self-etch adhesives in dentine bonding. However, when such selective etching in enamel is performed also acid-etch of the dentine cannot absolutely be avoided. When now applying conventional self-etching adhesive systems (without MDP), the dentine bond strength in these over-etched dentine areas is inferior [58]. Universal adhesives do not show this disadvantage and are thus recommended when selective etching is performed [59].

Another advantage is that these universal adhesives can handle dried acid-etched dentine, as their solvent is – at least in parts – water (otherwise they would not be self-etching). The application of these adhesives to dried dentine hence works as a rewetting procedure (when they are actively applied, i.e., rubbed into the dentine). Lastly, as these universal adhesives create sustainable bonds to many restoration materials (except for glass-based ceramics), they can also be recommended when restoring (repairing etc.) partially failed restorations [59].

Restorative Materials

Restorative materials are placed in order to restore the form, function, and aesthetics of the tooth, and thereby aid biofilm control and protect the pulp-dentine while causing no unnecessary harm. The resulting restoration should guarantee durability and postpone or even avoid the need for repair or replacement [5]. Directly placed restorative materials that are suitable for this purpose are usually based on GICs or composite resins.

Resin Composite Restorative Materials

Resin composites have replaced traditionally used amalgams as the main dental restorative material in many countries, while their longevity is not necessarily higher, especially in high-risk caries patients [60, 61]. Placement of a resin composite restoration usually requires more time and is more technique sensitive than placing other restorative materials. Due to their hydrophobic character, resin-based materials are prone to water contamination. Therefore, they require higher efforts in contamination control compared to, for example, amalgams and glass-ionomers. Most resin composites have to be incrementally applied and polymerised (at least in larger cavities) in order to reduce polymerisation stresses, which additionally requires time. To ensure retention of the filling without relying on macroretentive preparation, resin composites need to be bonded adhesively to the tooth. Such adhesive bonding is also important to seal the restoration margins and to withstand polymerisation shrinkage stress [5].

As previously discussed, the bond strength of all available adhesives is significantly reduced to demineralised dentine and even more on bacterially contaminated dentine compared to sound tooth surfaces. Clinically, this seems to be acceptable if only limited amounts of carious dentine are left beneath a restoration. However, in order to ensure a sufficient seal of the restoration it is important to have the cavity margins located in sound tooth structures and carious dentine that is left to preserve pulpal health should be limited to areas proximate to the dental pulp [62].

As in adhesives, a recent trend in resin composite development has been focused on improving handling and reducing application time. This has led to the introduction of "bulk-fill" composites as a new composite class. By reducing polymerisation shrinkage stress and increasing sensitivity to the curing light, these materials allow for application in larger increments (up to 5 mm) compared to conventional composites (thus, placement in bulk is often possible) [63, 64]. The marginal adaptation of bulk-fill composites placed in load-bearing cavities is similar to that of conventional composites [65]. However, clinical data on long-term performance of bulk-fills is scarce so far. Application of bulk-fill composites in large cavities or cavities with high C-factor results in less polymerisation-shrinkage stress than when placing conventional composites in bulk; placement of bulk fill composites might further improve the fracture resistance of the restored tooth [66]. However, it should be noted that this might apply to highly viscous bulk-fills, but not to the frequently used flowable bulk-fill composites, which exhibit inferior mechanical properties compared to conventional composites [67]. Therefore, the application of an additional layer of conventional composite on top of a flowable bulk-fill is recommended to increase the load stability of the restoration [68]. Primarily in extensive cavities, bulk-fill composites might be an economic alternative to conventional composites [69].

Resin composites can be used in clinical situations where sufficient contamination control can be assured. Due to their good aesthetic and mechanical properties, these materials might be preferred in visible areas and in larger cavities where multiple surfaces are involved. As resin composites can adhesively be bonded to both tooth structures and different kinds of restorative materials, they are the ideal material for the repair of defective restorations.

Glass-Ionomer Cement

GICs are increasingly becoming an alternative to amalgam and resin composites. Although GICs, in general, are less aesthetic, recently launched GICs have improved aesthetics, although not yet to the level achieved with resin composite. GICs have inferior mechanical properties (mainly flexural strength) compared with composites, and show an increased solubility in an erosive environment, similar to enamel. However, GICs offer some advantages:

- They are highly biocompatible. In the aftermath of the Minamata Treaty, the replacement for amalgam should be biomimetic [70]. GIC restoratives come closest to this requirement.
- As they are less moisture sensitive than composite resins, GICs can also be placed in situations where perfect moisture control cannot be ensured, such as in cervical cavities.
- Polymerisation shrinkage is absent and the restorative can therefore be applied in bulk.
- The ability of fluoride and calcium/strontium diffusion from GICs into demineralised dentine and enamel remineralises these tissues. It supports the ICCC recommendations of selective carious tissue removal to firm dentine.
- Placement of GIC restorations is generally less technique sensitive and time consuming than the placement of resin composites. GICs are often used in clinical situations where resin composites are not indicated, like paediatric dentistry, the restoration of root carious lesions or, generally, treatment of disabled or immobile patients [71].
- Survival percentages of single-surface glass-ionomer restorations in both primary and permanent teeth, produced according to the ART method, do not differ from comparable resin composite and amalgam restorations [65, 66; see the chapter by Leal et al.; this vol., pp. 92–102].
- Secondary dentine carious lesion development at the margins of single surface ART restorations in both primary and permanent teeth are very low, at 0.5% per annum [72].

The Problem of Carious Dentine – The Mechanics of Teeth with Deep Lesions

As described, carious dentine is less elastic and supportive for dental restorations. This seems to have an impact on fracture resistance, if certain factors come together. First, the masticatory load must be directed onto the carious dentine, i.e., the lesions. In vitro studies showed that in occlusally located lesions, where the load is directed perpendicularly onto the dentine surface, the fracture resistance of the restorations decreased [73]. In proximal cavities, where the lesion is located on the cavoproximal surface, and the load is directed in parallel to the dentine, this decrease in fracture resistance seems to be significantly lower [74, 75]. Moreover, the quality of the dentine remaining after carious tissue removal plays a significant role. If very soft dentine is left beneath restorations, this might significantly decrease the fracture resistance of the restoration, as a number of studies on sealing dentine carious lesions have found [76, 77]. If, in contrast, only small surface areas with leathery or only minimally soft dentine are left, the impact on restoration stability is likely to be minimal [75]. Using more flexurally strong materials, for example fibre-enforced composites, may further improve the restoration longevity when larger areas of soft dentine are left beneath the restoration [74].

Conclusion

Restoring a carious lesion can be challenging. Especially if the lesion has progressed closely to the pulp and has led to extended cavities, some factors should be considered. The following recommendations can be given:

- To avoid pulpal trauma due to preparation, in central pulp-proximal parts of the cavity, careful carious tissue removal, for example using hand instruments, should be performed. In any case, and in all parts of the cavity, high-speed preparation should be performed with sufficient water cooling.
- To reduce the risk of pulpal postoperative hypersensitivity due to incomplete bonding, all application steps of the adhesive should be precisely performed with sufficient contamination control, and proper light curing of the resin composite should be guaranteed.

The possible beneficial effects of cavity liners have not been clinically confirmed. Therefore, the use of liners as cavity pretreatment can be questioned.

The bond strengths of adhesives are decreased when bonding to demineralised and even more so to bacterially contaminated instead of sound dentine. Hence, such carious dentine should only be left in limited areas of a cavity before restoring it, mainly following selective carious tissue removal to soft or leathery dentine in deep lesions. In shallow lesions, where pulpal exposure is unlikely during excavation, there is no reason to leave substantial amounts of soft carious dentine in the cavity.

Resin composites combined with an adhesive are commonly used as directly placed restorative materials. Recent developments in adhesives and composites aimed to increase the simplicity of application.

GICs are increasingly relevant as an alternative to resin-based materials and amalgam. However, given their inferior mechanical properties (mainly flexural strength and abrasion resistance) compared to resin composites, their indication remains limited to single-surface cavities in primary and permanent teeth and to very small multiple-surface cavities in primary teeth.

Materials with high flexural strength might be advantageous for the restoration of cavities where larger areas of carious dentine have been left (especially in loaded areas).

References

1 Reeves R, Stanley HR: The relationship of bacterial penetration and pulpal pathosis in carious teeth. Oral Surg Oral Med Oral Pathol 1966;22:59–65.

2 Kim S, Edwall L, Trowbridge H, Chien S: Effects of local anesthetics on pulpal blood flow in dogs. J Dent Res 1984;63:650–652.

3 Pashley DH: The influence of dentin permeability and pulpal blood flow on pulpal solute concentrations. J Endod 1979;5:355–361.

4 von Fraunhofer JA, Siegel SC, Feldman S: Handpiece coolant flow rates and dental cutting. Oper Dent 2000;25:544–548.

5 Schwendicke F, Frencken JE, Bjorndal L, Maltz M, Manton DJ, Ricketts D, van Landuyt K, Banerjee A, Campus G, Domejean S, Fontana M, Leal S, Lo E, Machiulskiene V, Schulte A, Splieth C, Zandona AF, Innes NP: Managing carious lesions: consensus recommendations on carious tissue removal. Adv Dent Res 2016;28:58–67.

6 Giannini M, Makishi P, Ayres AP, Vermelho PM, Fronza BM, Nikaido T, Tagami J: Self-etch adhesive systems: a literature review. Braz Dent J 2015;26: 3–10.
7 Powers JM, Farah JW: Technique sensitivity in bonding to enamel and dentin. Compend Contin Educ Dent 2010;31: 1–9.
8 Brannstrom M: The hydrodynamic theory of dentinal pain: sensation in preparations, Caries, and the dentinal crack syndrome. J Endod 1986;12:453–457.
9 Bakopoulou A, Papadopoulos T, Garefis P: Molecular toxicology of substances released from resin-based dental restorative materials. Int J Mol Sci 2009;10: 3861–3899.
10 Lagocka R, Jakubowska K, Chlubek D, Buczkowska-Radlinska J: The influence of irradiation time and layer thickness on elution of triethylene glycol dimethacrylate from SDR® bulk-fill composite. Biomed Res Int 2016;2016:3481723.
11 Reis A, Dourado Loguercio A, Schroeder M, Luque-Martinez I, Masterson D, Cople Maia L: Does the adhesive strategy influence the post-operative sensitivity in adult patients with posterior resin composite restorations? A systematic review and meta-analysis. Dent Mater 2015;31:1052–1067.
12 Weiner R: Liners and bases in general dentistry. Aust Dent J 2011;56(suppl 1):11–22.
13 Corralo DJ, Maltz M: Clinical and ultrastructural effects of different liners/restorative materials on deep carious dentin: a randomized clinical trial. Caries Res 2013;47:243–250.
14 Oong EM, Griffin SO, Kohn WG, Gooch BF, Caufield PW: The effect of dental sealants on bacteria levels in caries lesions: a review of the evidence. J Am Dent Assoc 2008;139:271–278, quiz 357–358.
15 McComb D, Ericson D: Antimicrobial action of new, proprietary lining cements. J Dent Res 1987;66:1025–1028.
16 King JB Jr, Crawford JJ, Lindahl RL: Indirect pulp capping: a bacteriologic study of deep carious dentine in human teeth. Oral Surg Oral Med Oral Pathol 1965;20:663–669.
17 Leung RL, Loesche WJ, Charbeneau GT: Effect of Dycal on bacteria in deep carious lesions. J Am Dent Assoc 1980;100: 193–197.
18 Bressani AE, Mariath AA, Haas AN, Garcia-Godoy F, de Araujo FB: Incomplete caries removal and indirect pulp capping in primary molars: a randomized controlled trial. Am J Dent 2013;26: 196–200.
19 Neelakantan P, Rao CV, Indramohan J: Bacteriology of deep carious lesions underneath amalgam restorations with different pulp-capping materials – an in vivo analysis. J Appl Oral Sci 2012;20: 139–145.
20 Duque C, Negrini Tde C, Sacono NT, Spolidorio DM, de Souza Costa CA, Hebling J: Clinical and microbiological performance of resin-modified glass-ionomer liners after incomplete dentine caries removal. Clin Oral Investig 2009; 13:465–471.
21 Kuhn E, Chibinski AC, Reis A, Wambier DS: The role of glass ionomer cement on the remineralization of infected dentin: an in vivo study. Pediatr Dent 2014; 36:E118–E124.
22 Al-Abdi A, Paris S, Schwendicke F: Glass hybrid, but not calcium hydroxide, remineralized artificial residual caries lesions in vitro. Clin Oral Investig 2017; 21:389–396.
23 Schwendicke F, Al-Abdi A, Meyer-Lueckel H, Paris S: Pulpal remineralisation of artificial residual caries lesions in vitro. Caries Res 2015;49:591–594.
24 Alves LS, Fontanella V, Damo AC, Ferreira de Oliveira E, Maltz M: Qualitative and quantitative radiographic assessment of sealed carious dentin: a 10-year prospective study. Oral Surg Oral Med Oral Pathol Oral Radiol Endod 2010; 109:135–141.
25 Schroder U: Effects of calcium hydroxide-containing pulp-capping agents on pulp cell migration, proliferation, and differentiation. J Dent Res 1985;64:541–548.
26 Ivanovic V, Santini A: Rate of formation of tertiary dentin in dogs' teeth in response to lining materials. Oral Surg Oral Med Oral Pathol 1989;67:684–688.
27 Krifka S, Spagnuolo G, Schmalz G, Schweikl H: A review of adaptive mechanisms in cell responses towards oxidative stress caused by dental resin monomers. Biomaterials 2013;34:4555–4563.
28 Schwendicke F, Meyer-Lueckel H, Dorfer C, Paris S: Attitudes and behaviour regarding deep dentin caries removal: a survey among German dentists. Caries Res 2013;47:566–573.
29 Wegehaupt F, Betke H, Solloch N, Musch U, Wiegand A, Attin T: Influence of cavity lining and remaining dentin thickness on the occurrence of postoperative hypersensitivity of composite restorations. J Adhes Dent 2009;11:137–141.
30 Franzon R, Casagrande L, Pinto AS, Garcia-Godoy F, Maltz M, de Araujo FB: Clinical and radiographic evaluation of indirect pulp treatment in primary molars: 36 months follow-up. Am J Dent 2007;20:189–192.
31 Schenkel AB, Peltz I, Veitz-Keenan A: Dental cavity liners for class I and class II resin-based composite restorations. Cochrane Database Syst Rev 2016; 10:CD010526.
32 Schwendicke F, Gostemeyer G, Gluud C: Cavity lining after excavating caries lesions: meta-analysis and trial sequential analysis of randomized clinical trials. J Dent 2015;43:1291–1297.
33 Opdam NJ, van de Sande FH, Bronkhorst E, Cenci MS, Bottenberg P, Pallesen U, Gaengler P, Lindberg A, Huysmans MC, van Dijken JW: Longevity of posterior composite restorations: a systematic review and meta-analysis. J Dent Res 2014;93:943–949.
34 Vural UK, Kiremitci A, Gokalp S: Clinical assessment of mineral trioxide aggregate in the treatment of deep carious lesions. Niger J Clin Pract 2017;20:600–604.
35 de Almeida Neves A, Coutinho E, Cardoso MV, Lambrechts P, van Meerbeek B: Current concepts and techniques for caries excavation and adhesion to residual dentin. J Adhes Dent 2011;13: 7–22.
36 Goldberg M, Kulkarni AB, Young M, Boskey A: Dentin: structure, composition and mineralization. Front Biosci 2011;3:711–735.
37 Perdigao J: Dentin bonding-variables related to the clinical situation and the substrate treatment. Dent Mater 2010; 26:e24–e37.
38 Nakabayashi N, Nakamura M, Yasuda N: Hybrid layer as a dentin-bonding mechanism. J Esthet Dent 1991;3:133–138.

39 Cardoso MV, de Almeida Neves A, Mine A, Coutinho E, Van Landuyt K, De Munck J, van Meerbeek B: Current aspects on bonding effectiveness and stability in adhesive dentistry. Aust Dent J 2011;56(suppl 1):31–44.
40 Pashley DH, Tay FR, Breschi L, Tjaderhane L, Carvalho RM, Carrilho M, Tezvergil-Mutluay A: State of the art etch-and-rinse adhesives. Dent Mater 2011; 27:1–16.
41 Pashley DH: Smear layer: overview of structure and function. Proc Finn Dent Soc 1992;88(suppl 1):215–224.
42 Tay FR, Pashley DH, Suh BI, Carvalho RM, Itthagarun A: Single-step adhesives are permeable membranes. J Dent 2002; 30:371–382.
43 Ngo H, Mount GJ, Peters MC: A study of glass-ionomer cement and its interface with enamel and dentin using a low-temperature, high-resolution scanning electron microscopic technique. Quintessence Int 1997;28:63–69.
44 Peumans M, Kanumilli P, de Munck J, van Landuyt K, Lambrechts P, van Meerbeek B: Clinical effectiveness of contemporary adhesives: a systematic review of current clinical trials. Dent Mater 2005;21:864–881.
45 Santos MJ, Ari N, Steele S, Costella J, Banting D: Retention of tooth-colored restorations in non-carious cervical lesions – a systematic review. Clin Oral Investig 2014;18:1369–1381.
46 Liu Y, Tjaderhane L, Breschi L, Mazzoni A, Li N, Mao J, Pashley DH, Tay FR: Limitations in bonding to dentin and experimental strategies to prevent bond degradation. J Dent Res 2011;90:953–968.
47 Mazzoni A, Tjaderhane L, Checchi V, Di Lenarda R, Salo T, Tay FR, Pashley DH, Breschi L: Role of dentin MMPs in caries progression and bond stability. J Dent Res 2015;94:241–251.
48 Dursun E, Fron-Chabouis H, Attal JP, Raskin A: Bisphenol a release: survey of the composition of dental composite resins. Open Dent J 2016;10:446–453.
49 Kinney JH, Balooch M, Marshall SJ, Marshall GW Jr, Weihs TP: Hardness and Young's modulus of human peritubular and intertubular dentine. Arch Oral Biol 1996;41:9–13.
50 Brannstrom M, Garberoglio R: The dentinal tubules and the odontoblast processes: a scanning electron microscopic study. Acta Odontol Scand 1972;30: 291–311.
51 Erhardt MC, Toledano M, Osorio R, Pimenta LA: Histomorphologic characterization and bond strength evaluation of caries-affected dentin/resin interfaces: effects of long-term water exposure. Dent Mater 2008;24:786–798.
52 Yoshiyama M, Tay FR, Doi J, Nishitani Y, Yamada T, Itou K, Carvalho RM, Nakajima M, Pashley DH: Bonding of self-etch and total-etch adhesives to carious dentin. J Dent Res 2002;81:556–560.
53 Inoue S, van Meerbeek B, Abe Y, Yoshida Y, Lambrechts P, Vanherle G, Sano H: Effect of remaining dentin thickness and the use of conditioner on micro-tensile bond strength of a glass-ionomer adhesive. Dent Mater 2001;17:445–455.
54 Smales RJ, Ngo HC, Yip KH, Yu C: Clinical effects of glass ionomer restorations on residual carious dentin in primary molars. Am J Dent 2005;18:188–193.
55 Yoshida Y, Yoshihara K, Nagaoka N, Hayakawa S, Torii Y, Ogawa T, Osaka A, Meerbeek BV: Self-assembled nano-layering at the adhesive interface. J Dent Res 2012;91:376–381.
56 Elsayed A, Younes F, Lehmann F, Kern M: Tensile bond strength of so-called universal primers and universal multi-mode adhesives to zirconia and lithium disilicate ceramics. J Adhes Dent 2017; 19:221–228.
57 Cardenas AM, Siqueira F, Hass V, Malaquias P, Gutierrez MF, Reis A, Perdigao J, Loguercio A: Effect of MDP-containing silane and adhesive used alone or in combination on the long-term bond strength and chemical interaction with lithium disilicate ceramics. J Adhes Dent 2017;19:203–212.
58 Frankenberger R, Lohbauer U, Roggendorf MJ, Naumann M, Taschner M: Selective enamel etching reconsidered: better than etch-and-rinse and self-etch? J Adhes Dent 2008;10:339–344.
59 Rosa WL, Piva E, Silva AF: Bond strength of universal adhesives: a systematic review and meta-analysis. J Dent 2015;43:765–776.
60 Opdam NJ, Bronkhorst EM, Loomans BA, Huysmans MC: 12-year survival of composite vs. amalgam restorations. J Dent Res 2010;89:1063–1067.
61 Rasines Alcaraz MG, Veitz-Keenan A, Sahrmann P, Schmidlin PR, Davis D, Iheozor-Ejiofor Z: Direct composite resin fillings versus amalgam fillings for permanent or adult posterior teeth. Cochrane Database Syst Rev 2014:CD005620.
62 Schwendicke F, Meyer-Lueckel H, Dorfer C, Paris S: Failure of incompletely excavated teeth – a systematic review. J Dent 2013;41:569–580.
63 Jang JH, Park SH, Hwang IN: Polymerization shrinkage and depth of cure of bulk-fill resin composites and highly filled flowable resin. Oper Dent 2015;40: 172–180.
64 Ilie N, Kessler A, Durner J: Influence of various irradiation processes on the mechanical properties and polymerisation kinetics of bulk-fill resin based composites. J Dent 2013;41:695–702.
65 Schwendicke F, Gostemeyer G, Blunck U, Paris S, Hsu LY, Tu YK: Directly placed restorative materials: review and network meta-analysis. J Dent Res 2016; 95:613–622.
66 Rosatto CM, Bicalho AA, Verissimo C, Braganca GF, Rodrigues MP, Tantbirojn D, Versluis A, Soares CJ: Mechanical properties, shrinkage stress, cuspal strain and fracture resistance of molars restored with bulk-fill composites and incremental filling technique. J Dent 2015;43:1519–1528.
67 Leprince JG, Palin WM, Vanacker J, Sabbagh J, Devaux J, Leloup G: Physico-mechanical characteristics of commercially available bulk-fill composites. J Dent 2014;42:993–1000.
68 van Dijken JW, Pallesen U: A randomized controlled three year evaluation of "bulk-filled" posterior resin restorations based on stress decreasing resin technology. Dent Mater 2014;30:e245–e251.
69 Vianna-de-Pinho MG, Rego GF, Vidal ML, Alonso RCB, Schneider LFJ, Cavalcante LM: Clinical time required and internal adaptation in cavities restored with bulk-fill composites. J Contemp Dent Pract 2017;18:1107–1111.
70 Frencken JE, Peters MC, Manton DJ, Leal SC, Gordan VV, Eden E: Minimal intervention dentistry for managing dental caries – a review: report of a FDI task group. Int Dent J 2012;62:223–243.
71 Berg JH, Croll TP: Glass ionomer restorative cement systems: an update. Pediatr Dent 2015;37:116–124.

72 Frencken JE: Atraumatic restorative treatment and minimal intervention dentistry. Br Dent J 2017;223:183–189.
73 Hevinga MA, Opdam NJ, Frencken JE, Truin GJ, Huysmans MC: Does incomplete caries removal reduce strength of restored teeth? J Dent Res 2010;89: 1270–1275.
74 Schwendicke F, Kern M, Dorfer C, Kleemann-Lupkes J, Paris S, Blunck U: Influence of using different bonding systems and composites on the margin integrity and the mechanical properties of selectively excavated teeth in vitro. J Dent 2015;43:327–334.
75 Schwendicke F, Kern M, Meyer-Lueckel H, Boels A, Doerfer C, Paris S: Fracture resistance and cuspal deflection of incompletely excavated teeth. J Dent 2014; 42:107–113.
76 Hesse D, Bonifacio CC, Mendes FM, Braga MM, Imparato JC, Raggio DP: Sealing versus partial caries removal in primary molars: a randomized clinical trial. BMC Oral Health 2014;14:58.
77 Bakhshandeh A, Qvist V, Ekstrand KR: Sealing occlusal caries lesions in adults referred for restorative treatment: 2–3 years of follow-up. Clin Oral Investig 2012;16:521–529.

Gerd Göstemeyer
Department of Operative and Preventive Dentistry
Charité – Universitätsmedizin Berlin
Corporate Member of Freie Universität Berlin
Humboldt-Universität zu Berlin, and Berlin Institute of Health
Assmannshauser Strasse 4-6
DE–14197 Berlin (Germany)
E-Mail Gerd.Goestemeyer@charite.de

Schwendicke F, Frencken J, Innes N (eds): Caries Excavation: Evolution of Treating Cavitated Carious Lesions.
Monogr Oral Sci. Basel, Karger, 2018, vol 27, pp 56–67 (DOI: 10.1159/000487832)

Removing Carious Tissue: Why and How?

Falk Schwendicke

Operative and Preventive Dentistry, Charité – Universitätsmedizin Berlin, Corporate Member of Freie Universität Berlin, Humboldt-Universität zu Berlin, and Berlin Institute of Health, Berlin, Germany

Abstract

Caries is no longer seen as an infectious disease, and the aim of treating carious lesions is to control their activity, not to remove the lesion itself. Such control can be implemented by sealing off the lesion from the environment, with sealed bacteria being deprived from carbohydrates and thus inactivated. For cavitated lesions, controlling them usually involves the placement of restorations to rebuild the cleansability of the surface. In this case, dental practitioners have traditionally removed carious tissues prior to the restoration. This has historically been for a number of reasons, while today the main reason for restoring a cavity is to maximise restoration longevity. In shallow lesions, dental practitioners should aim to remove as much carious tissue as possible (to allow adequate depth for the restorative material) without unnecessarily removing sound or remineralisable dentine. This means removal to hard dentine around the periphery, to firm dentine centrally for optimising restoration longevity and allowing a tight cavity seal. For deep lesions in teeth with vital pulps (without irreversible pulpitis), maintaining pulp vitality is critical. Dental practitioners should aim to avoid pulp exposure, leaving soft or leathery dentine in pulpoproximal areas. Peripherally, hard tissue is left, again to ensure a tight seal and sufficient mechanical support of the restoration. As an alternative to the selective removal to soft dentine, stepwise removal can be used. With this approach, the soft dentine is temporarily rather than permanently sealed in, and removed in a second step after 6–12 months. Strategies where carious tissue in cavitated lesions is not removed at all, but sealed or managed non-restoratively, are currently restricted to primary teeth.

The Aims of Carious Tissue Removal

As discussed in the first part of this book, understandings of what caries disease is and how it is caused have changed over the last 30 years. Traditionally, caries has been regarded as an infectious disease, with a specific bacterium or bacterial species – mainly streptococci (especially *Streptococcus mutans*) – being associated with the presence and severity of caries and its symptoms, the carious lesions. This understanding has been termed "specific plaque hypothesis" [1]. Consequently, to "cure" caries, it was necessary to remove all these causative bacteria from the mouth (this was the reason why antibacterial therapies including vaccinations were long-sought for managing caries). According to Black [2], dental practitioners needed to remove all cariogenic bacteria from the "infected" dental hard tissues, with subsequent placement of a plastic restoration. Thus, one historical aim of carious tissue removal prior to placing a restoration was to remove all bacteria.

As described, this no longer matches the current understanding of caries being the result of an ecological imbalance, mainly triggered by an abundant intake of fermentable carbohydrates, leading to an imbalance in the biofilm composition and activity, and a net mineral loss caused by bacterial acids (produced by metabolising the carbohydrates) [3]. Following this understanding, there is no need to remove all or specific bacteria from the mouth to control caries and arrest carious lesions. During invasive/restorative therapies, dental practitioners do not need to remove all bacteria from the contaminated dental hard tissues, but can seal bacteria under the subsequently placed restorations, as this deprives the bacteria from nutrition, leading to their inactivation [4]. The great majority of the bacteria are unable to withstand this starvation for long, and in the long term only negligible numbers of viable bacteria remain. As a consequence, there is no need to remove all contaminated tissue prior to placing a restoration.

Another historical aim was to remove all demineralised dentine, as this dentine was found to be softer than sound dentine and not to support restorations as well as sound dentine [5, 6]. The removal of demineralised dentine was thus thought to be needed to place long-lasting restorations. However, conventionally, dentists used to place cavity liners beneath restorations, which are also soft and do not support the restoration. Nevertheless, restorations lasted relatively long. This shows that very limited areas of soft substrate beneath restorations might be acceptable, as long as restoration support is available in large parts of the cavity. Moreover, the collagen backbone of demineralised dentine remains to some degree as long as the dentine is not heavily contaminated with bacteria. For such demineralised dentine, remineralisation and functional "healing" (including restitution of the mechanical properties of the dentine) is possible [7–9].

Finally, with traditional amalgam restorations, carious tissue removal created undercuts, which were desirable for macroretention of the restoration. Such undercuts are not required today when using adhesive restorative materials; so this historical aim no longer applies.

In theory, and based on what was described above, there should be no need to remove any carious tissue prior to placing a restoration. To control a carious lesion, a hermetic seal of the bacteria should be sufficient. However, there are 2 arguments to be explored against this. Firstly, as discussed above, carious dentine is softer than sound dentine, and leaving it everywhere in the cavity has been found to certainly affect the stability (fracture resistance) of the restoration. Moreover, carious dentine does not function as well as a base layer for modern dental resin-based adhesives; bond strengths to carious dentine are reduced to less than 50% compared with sound dentine. Thus, placing restorations on nothing but carious tissue will severely impact on restoration stability [6, 10–14]. As a consequence, from the point of view of achieving a securely based restoration, some carious tissue removal is needed prior to placing a restoration. A main aim of carious tissue removal which applies today is to increase the longevity of the subsequently placed restoration through creating sufficient wall space to bond to.

The second argument targets the bacteria which are sealed. Large numbers of bacteria may be sealed in and inactivated. However, they will continue to release virulence factors until starvation leads to their inactivation, and when they eventually starve, they may release a number of toxic products. Both could severely irritate the pulp. Only limited research is available to support this hypothesis, and clinical data indicate that it does not seem to produce associated clinical problems and, therefore, does not apply (as will be discussed later on).

However, removing carious tissue at least in wide parts of the cavity to reduce the bacterial load seems sensible.

The Principles of Carious Tissue Removal

As described, carious tissue removal is not carried out mainly to remove bacteria, or to remove demineralised dentine, or to create undercuts, but rather to place a long-lasting restoration, as this will ensure that the cycle of restorations is slowed down and pulpal health maintained (see the first part of this book). Slowing down the repeat restoration cycle will eventually allow long-term retention of the tooth (which should be the supreme aim). Following this logic, a number of principles for carious tissue removal have been agreed upon [15, 16]:

"1. avoid discomfort/pain and dental anxiety (...)

2. preserve non-demineralised as well as remineralisable tissue (...)

3. achieve an adequate seal by placing the peripheral restoration onto sound dentine and/or enamel, thus controlling the lesion and inactivating remaining bacteria (...)

4. maintain pulpal health by preserving residual dentine (avoiding unnecessary pulpal irritation/insult) and preventing pulp exposure (...)

5. maximise longevity of the restoration by removing enough soft dentine to place a durable restoration of sufficient bulk and resilience [16].

Avoiding discomfort and pain is central for most of our patients and will also help to avoid dental anxiety, which is a main reason for dental non-attendance and lack of treatment [17–19]".

Preserving non-demineralised (sound) and demineralised but remineralisable tissue helps to reduce the hard tissue loss from carious tissue removal. It helps to limit the size of the cavities and slow down the cycle of restorations [20–22].

Achieving an adequate seal is essential to allow the remaining bacteria to be tolerated beneath restorations [23]. This seal is not needed everywhere in the cavity; it seems sufficient to achieve a tight seal peripherally, with some bacteria remaining centrally under a restoration, where carious tissue is left and the bond strength of the restorative material to the dentine is limited. Removing carious tissue in the large peripheral parts of a cavity will also ensure that restoration longevity is optimised because of an enlarged clean area to bond to.

Maintaining pulpal health will, in deep lesions extending close to the pulp, come down to avoiding pulp exposure. Why is avoiding pulp exposure relevant? Pulp exposure can (conventionally) be treated with 1 of 2 therapies: either a direct pulp cap is performed, which has been shown to have a poor long-term prognosis (except when the exposure occurs in teeth without carious lesions being present, mainly during dental trauma), or a root-canal treatment is initiated ("vital extirpation"), which is highly invasive, increasing the risk of tooth fracture, and shortening the lifespan of teeth [24–30]. Admittedly, in specialised settings and using specific medications or techniques, direct capping might achieve higher success rates [31–34], but so far the available literature indicates that these techniques and materials are not common and that success rates are poor in most daily dental settings [26, 35, 36]. This can also be said about root-canal treatment: there are studies where such procedures yielded long-term success rates far above 90%, which means that teeth can be retained in the long term. In practice, however, success rates seem far lower, with a significant proportion of teeth not being retained after 10 years post-treatment [37, 38]. Avoiding pulp exposure and therefore avoiding any endodontic therapy is thus a most relevant principle during carious tissue removal.

The last 2 principles – maintaining pulpal health by preserving residual dentine, and maximising restoration longevity by removing as much dentine as possible – seem to be in conflict with each other. On the one hand, it is demanded to maximise restoration longevity. On the other hand, removing all carious tissue in deep lesions will often (in around 30–40% of the cases where lesions extend radiographically into the inner third or quarter of the dentine) lead to pulp exposure [39].

Thus, a pragmatic decision will need to be taken, based on the priorities for the specific tooth and situation. For lesions that are not at risk of pulp exposure, i.e., those which do not extend into the pulp areas (inner third or quarter of dentine radiographically), dentists should aim to maximise restoration longevity and remove as much carious dentine as possible. As discussed, this will certainly include removing carious tissues from the periphery of the cavity (to achieve a tight seal). In lesions that are close to the pulp, dentists should prioritise avoiding pulp exposure, and should leave carious dentine in proximity to the pulp. Nevertheless, peripherally, a zone which allows sufficient support and a tight seal of the restoration needs to be provided.

Note that all these considerations only apply to teeth with pulps which can be maintained. In teeth with pulps that are irreversibly inflamed (showing permanent or long-lasting pain) or necrotic (no positive response to any sensitivity testing, possibly even with signs of periapical inflammation), maintaining pulp vitality and avoiding pulp exposure is not appropriate. In these teeth, root-canal treatment is needed anyway, and in preparation for this all carious tissue should be removed from the cavity.

To perform carious tissue removal according to these principles, dentists should thus know the status of the pulp and the expected depth of the carious lesion, and then tailor the carious tissue removal accordingly. Four removal strategies are available, which will be discussed further below. All 4 strategies are characterised by how exactly they are performed (i.e., in descriptive terms), mainly as to the carious dentine that is left and what is removed. Thus, before explaining these 4 strategies in some detail (more details will be given in the next chapters of this book), it is necessary to learn how carious tissue removal can be assessed.

The Problems of Assessing Carious Tissue Removal

Assessing carious tissue removal objectively and reliably has been challenging operative dentistry since it was first performed. This is due to a number of reasons: first, the clinical appearance of dentine during carious tissue removal does not correlate with any histologic findings; one cannot, for example, relate carious tissue removal to histologic dentine layers. The latter would be, in theory, desirable, as layers like "contaminated" or "demineralised" (but not bacterially contaminated) dentine have been histologically described. Especially during the period when removing bacteria was the main aim of carious tissue removal, it would have been relevant to identify the "contaminated dentine" layer clinically. However, these layers are artificial zones; clinically, they merge into each other, often gradually (Fig. 1). Thus, histology is also only arbitrarily able to discern these layers, and clinicians (who do not have the option of histology at hand) cannot readily distinguish bacteria-containing dentine from demineralised dentine, for example. As discussed above, and more relevantly, it seems currently not too important to know these layers clinically, as removing all contaminated or all demineralised dentine from a cavity is not in line with the current principles of carious tissue removal.

This brings us to a large misunderstanding when dealing with carious tissue removal. For decades, researchers and dental practitioners alike have termed carious tissue removal strategies as to what one aimed to remove from (or leave in) the cavity. Two antagonistic strategies of "complete" and "incomplete" removal were developed; one where carious tissue was removed "completely" and one where one actively left carious tissue in the cavity. However, following the descriptions above, it is clinically unclear what exactly is "completely" or "incompletely" removed and how this is supposed to be measured – is it bacteria being removed – which is clinically only possible using

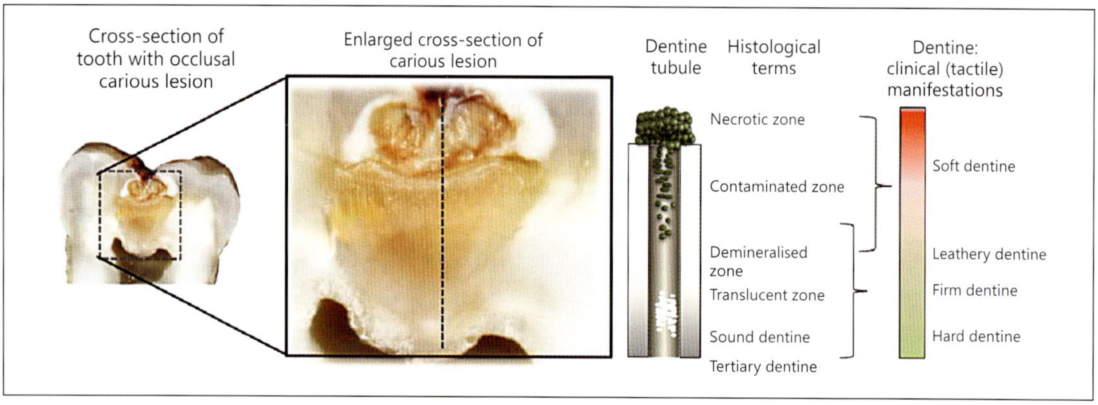

Fig. 1. Carious lesions: histology and clinical manifestation. From Innes et al. [15]. Reprinted by Permission of SAGE Publications, Inc.

certain detection aids, or is it soft dentine being removed – which is highly subjective; is it discoloured dentine or degraded dentine? Based on these considerations, it is unlikely that any carious tissue removal was ever perfectly "complete" or "incomplete" (regardless of which criterion is chosen), as the gradual changes throughout the discussed zones of carious dentine make it very hard to determine what exactly was removed or left.

In summary, carious tissue removal should not be described (or termed) according to what one aims to remove or leave (completely or incompletely remove carious dentine), but how exactly the removal is performed (until soft dentine is removed, etc.). This was the conclusion of a recent consensus conference and will be discussed further in this book [15]. We will now describe the different methods for assessing carious tissue removal.

The criterion that has been consistently used in both daily practice and dental research is the hardness of the dentine that is either removed or retained [40]. The hardness of the remaining dentine is clinically meaningful as it has implications for the restoration longevity (see above). It can be assessed using probes (usually straight probes are better suited than curved ones), or via tactile feedback during removal with an excavator or a bur. Hardness can be described using a number of terms, the most common ones are briefly defined below [15].

- Hard dentine (Fig. 2): "A pushing force needs to be used with a hard instrument to engage the dentine and only a sharp cutting edge or a bur will lift it. A scratchy sound or 'cri dentinaire' can be heard when a straight probe is taken across the dentine."
- Firm dentine (Fig. 3): "Firm dentine is physically resistant to hand excavation and some pressure needs to be exerted through an instrument to lift it."
- Leathery dentine (Fig. 4): "Although the dentine does not deform when an instrument is pressed onto it, leathery dentine can still be easily lifted without much force being required."
- Soft dentine (Fig. 5): "Soft dentine will deform when a hard instrument is pressed onto it, and can be easily scooped up (e.g., with a sharp hand excavator) with little force being required."

A range of other criteria for assessing the removed and retained dentine have been described, including moisture, colour, dye stainability, etc. Most of them have not been or not comprehensively been validated in clinical studies, and some (like dye stainability) have even been found to be clinically harmful (removing all stainable dentine in deeper parts of the cavity increases the risk of pulp exposure). Moreover, neither of them comes with a great advantage (being more reliable or easier to use) over hardness (for example, dentine stainability follows the gradual degradation of the collagen, and is thus also clinically gradual; dental practitioners can therefore also assess the hardness gradient instead of using a dye) [41–45]. Thus, we will mainly build on hardness as the criterion for assessing carious tissue removal in this book.

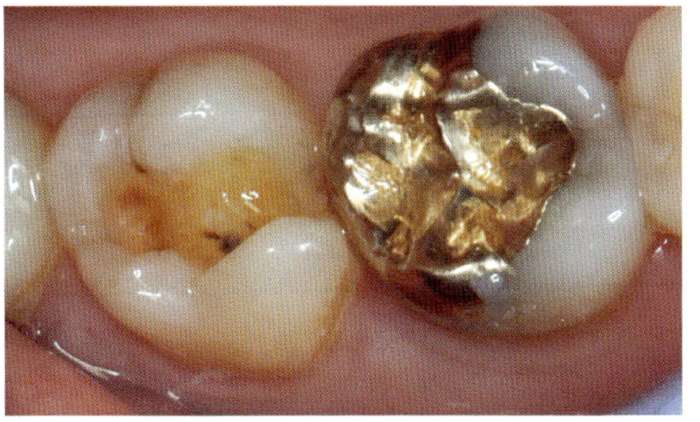

Fig. 2. Hard dentine. The dentine can only be lifted under forces; scratching over it with a straight probe induces the "cri dentinaire." Here, the dentine is additionally coloured identically to sound dentine. The situation emerged after loss of a gold inlay, which was subsequently recemented.

Overview of Removal Strategies

The 4 main removal strategies will be discussed in detail in the next chapters. Here, we will start with a brief overview. The 4 strategies extend from the conventional approach of non-selectively removing all presumably carious dentine (assessed via hardness; carious tissue removal until hard dentine) over more selective removal strategies to no carious tissue removal at all (sealing carious tissue or controlling carious lesions non-restoratively).

Non-Selective Removal to Hard Dentine
Non-selective removal to hard dentine (formerly also known as "complete removal") is the removal of all softened dentine, stopping when only hard dentine (see above; similar to sound dentine) is reached. This is done everywhere in the cavity (non-selectively), both in the periphery and in proximity to the pulp [15]. As such, removal of all softened, even firm, dentine also means the removal of demineralised dentine. By removing demineralised dentine, the tooth defence mechanism of remineralisation is not used. Hence, non-selective removal is nowadays considered overtreatment and no longer recommended. This is even more so for deep carious lesions with vital painless pulps, as non-selective removal to hard dentine comes with significant risks of pulp exposure [16, 40, 46].

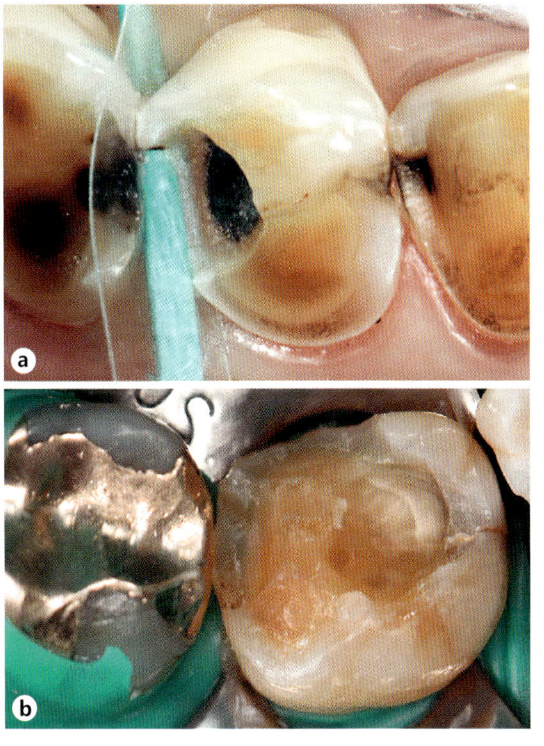

Fig. 3. Firm dentine. Firm dentine can be lifted under limited force. Scratching will not lead to the "cri dentinaire." Firm dentine can be heavily stained (**a**), but is usually dry (**b**). Image **a** courtesy of Diana Wald, Berlin.

Selective Removal to Firm Dentine

When performing selective removal (Fig. 6), different criteria for assessing (and stopping) carious tissue removal are used in the different areas of the cavity (removal is performed selectively). As one of the principles of carious tissue removal, the periphery of a cavity should be prepared (via carious tissue removal) to allow an optimal (and hermetic) seal of the restoration. Thus, in these areas (and also wide parts of the cavity, where maintaining the pulp vitality is not at stake), hard dentine is left. In the pulpal area of the cavity, however, firm dentine can be left [15]. This approach is recommended for shallow or moderately deep lesions; it prioritises restoration survival. For deep lesions (i.e., involving the inner third or quarter of the dentine radiographically, or those clinically extending close to the pulp, with pulp exposure being a conceived risk) in teeth with vital pulps, selective removal to firm dentine comes with considerable risks of pulp exposure and harm. Thus, other techniques are needed.

Selective Removal to Soft Dentine

One such technique is selective removal to soft dentine (Fig. 7), which is recommended for deep carious lesions in teeth with a vital (and not irreversibly inflamed) pulp. While, again, peripherally, achieving a good seal and a long-lasting restoration are aimed for and removal to hard tissue is performed, the pulpal area of a cavity is not treated as invasively. Instead, the aim is to avoid pulp exposure and to maintain the residual thickness of dentine. To achieve this, it is acceptable that leathery or soft carious dentine remains. Selective removal to soft dentine has been shown to reduce the risk of pulpal exposure compared with non-selective removal to hard or selective removal to firm dentine [40, 46, 47]. Selective removal to soft dentine has also been known as partial or incomplete removal in the past. These terms, as discussed, are not very helpful as it is unclear what is partially or incompletely removed.

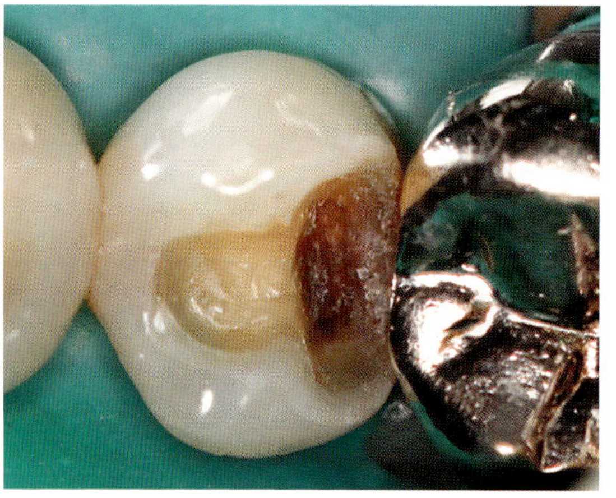

Fig. 4. Leathery dentine. In the central parts of the cavity, leathery dentine is left. Using a sharp excavator, this dentine could be lifted, often in larger flakes.

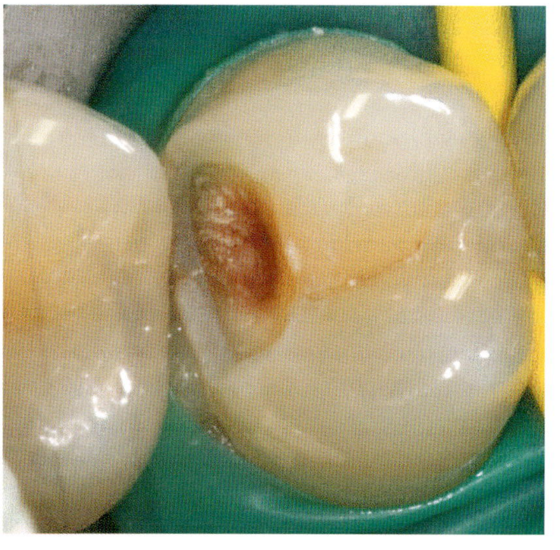

Fig. 5. Soft dentine. In the pulpoproximal aspect of the cavity, soft dentine was left. It can be easily scooped up using an excavator.

Stepwise Removal

Stepwise removal is carious tissue removal in 2 steps (visits) [48–50]. It combines selective removal to soft dentine in the first step and, after 6–12 months, selective removal to firm dentine in the second step. Between these 2 visits, soft or leathery carious dentine is sealed beneath a temporary restoration. This allows the odontoblasts time to lay down reactionary dentine (which reduces the risk of pulp exposure during the second step), to remineralise and dry the carious dentine, and to inactivate bacteria by sealing them. For the temporary restoration, a very "temporary" material has traditionally been used. However, studies have found the failure of this temporary restoration to be the major complication of stepwise removal, often leading to progression of the carious lesion – it allows substrate to reach the lesion through microleakage. Thus, a restorative material that is durable for at least 12 months, like glass-ionomer cement [51], is recommended. Alternatively, composite or compomer might be used; however, a colour should be chosen which allows the temporary material to be easily differentiated from tooth substance. Stepwise removal has been shown to have higher risks of pulp exposure than selective removal to soft dentine. Given the additional efforts needed for the second treatment step and the associated costs, stepwise removal is mainly recommended for very deep lesions (those involving the inner quarter of the dentine), as will be discussed in the chapter by Bjørndal [this vol., pp. 68–81; 39, 40, 51].

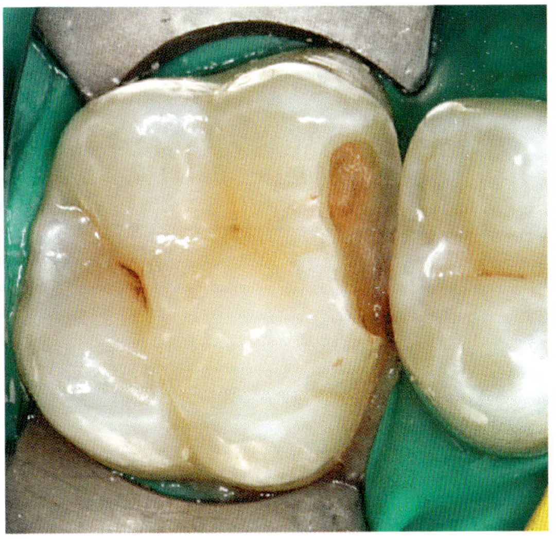

Fig. 6. Selective removal to firm dentine. In the periphery, enamel and dentine are hard, while centrally, firm dentine is left.

No Removal at All

Sealing in Strategies

There are 2 types of strategies where carious tissues are not removed at all, but sealed beneath a plastic dental material. The first one, which has been studied since the 1970s, is sealing over carious lesions using a plastic material (usually resin, but also glass-ionomer cements or variations on these materials). A growing body of research supports this strategy [47, 52]. However, placing sealants onto carious lesions is obviously limited by the sealant's material strength [53]. No plastic sealant material can withstand biting forces if it is not somewhat supported by sound or at least firm tissue. This is why this strategy is not advocated for cavitated lesions, where the sealant would be mainly supported by dentine, and would fracture at some point. Instead, non-cavitated lesions in both permanent or primary teeth can be sealed, on occlusal and also on buccal or oral surfaces. For proximal surfaces, sealing-in strategies for non-cavitated lesions (including caries infiltration) have also been investigated by a number of studies and have been found to be efficacious [54].

The second strategy involves sealing in lesions using stainless steel crowns (the Hall Technique). This technique is used for primary molars, where crowns designed for primary teeth are placed onto the tooth without any preparation. The advantage of this type of sealing is that it does not only biologically control lesion activity, but also restores the cavity well. Especially in primary teeth, most other direct restorations (on a composite, compomer, or glass-ionomer cement basis) show poor results [55], while stainless steel crowns achieve survival rates similar to restorations placed in permanent teeth. Using a stainless steel crown for

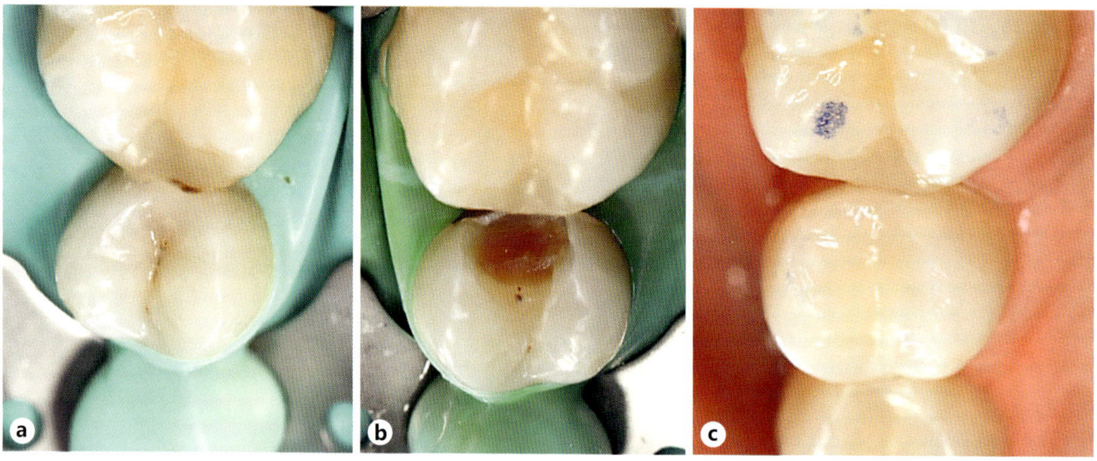

Fig. 7. Selective removal to soft dentine. **a** A cavitated carious lesion is present distally. **b** Soft carious dentine is left centrally, while in the periphery, hard dentine is left. **c** The cavity is restored adhesively.

sealing cavitated lesions overcomes the previously discussed issues of poor mechanical strength. More details on the indications and how to perform the Hall Technique will be given. However, it is notable that the Hall Technique, by completely sealing in lesions with no removal and achieving high success rates through a predictable hermetic seal, exemplifies the successes that can be achieved from sealing in lesions [56, 57].

Non-Restorative Cavity Control

As discussed in the first part of the book, managing caries and also managing non-cavitated carious lesions does not necessarily require any restorative element. Restorative therapy is only needed to reinstate the surface integrity in case of cavitated lesions, thereby allowing cleansability of the tooth surface again. One therapy that has been suggested to achieve the same without placing a restoration is non-restorative cavity control [58]. It works by making cavitated carious lesions cleansable again but does not attempt to restore the surface integrity. Although this treatment has a sound, logical, and pathophysiological basis, it is limited to primary teeth or to root surface caries, for example in special needs cases, high-risk children with limited compliance in a stabilisation phase, or immobile geriatric patients. The desire in permanent teeth and many of the cases previously mentioned is to restore the anatomy and integrity of the tooth to something resembling its former, precavitated glory. Non-restorative cavity control involves making cavities accessible via chiseling or drilling away the overhanging enamel or dentine, and maintaining an oral hygiene program including regular supply of fluoride toothpaste, silver diamine fluoride, or varnish for these accessible lesions, which are monitored over time for progression. This strategy will be discussed in detail in the chapter by van Strijp and van Loveren [this vol., pp. 124–136].

Conclusion

- Caries is no longer seen as an infectious disease. In parallel to this changing understanding, the philosophies around how to manage caries and carious lesions have also changed – the aim of treating carious lesions is to control their activity, not to remove them.

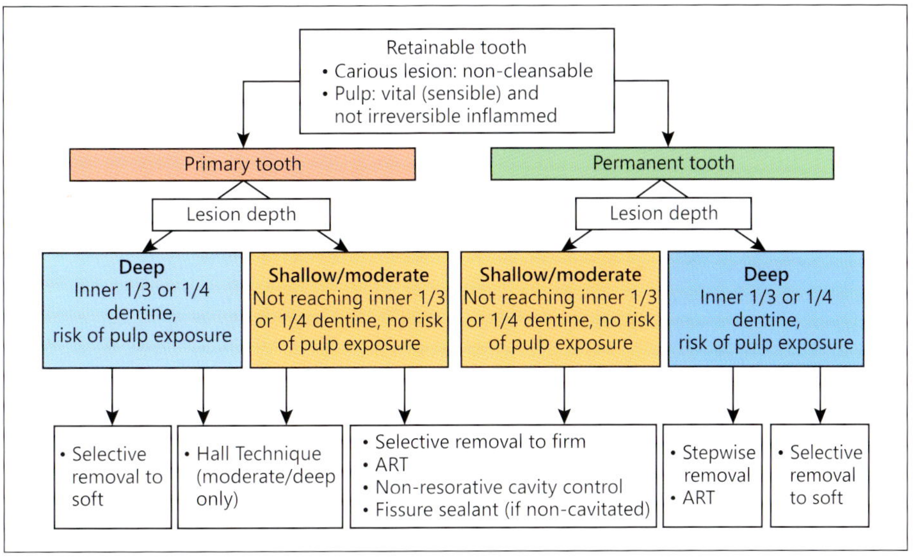

Fig. 8. Decision tree for cavitated carious lesions in teeth which can be retained and have vital, not irreversibly inflamed pulps. From Schwendicke et al. [16]. ART, Atraumatic Restorative Treatment. Reprinted by Permission of SAGE Publications, Inc.

- One option for controlling lesion activity is to seal in the lesion; this inhibits bacterial acids and dietary carbohydrates from diffusing into the dentine. For lesions that are bacterially contaminated, such sealing will deprive bacteria from their carbohydrate nutrition, which inactivates the sealed bacteria.
- For cavitated lesions, controlling them usually involves the placement of restorations to reinstall the cleansability of the surface. In this case, dental practitioners have traditionally removed carious tissues prior to restoration. This had a number of (historical) reasons, while today the main reason is to maximise restoration longevity and maintain pulpal health.
- In shallow lesions, dental practitioners should aim to remove as much carious tissue as possible without unnecessarily removing sound or demineralised but not bacterially contaminated dentine. Centrally, removal to firm dentine is carried out.
- For deep lesions in teeth with vital pulps (without irreversible pulpitis), maintaining pulp vitality is of greatest importance. Dentists should thus aim to avoid pulp exposure and pulp complications wherever possible.
- Consequently, in these lesions, in pulpoproximal areas soft or leathery dentine can be left. Peripherally, hard tissue is left, allowing a tight seal of any bacteria and sufficient mechanical support of the restoration.
- An alternative to the one-step selective removal to soft dentine is stepwise removal, where soft dentine is not permanently but temporarily sealed, and removed in a second step after 6–12 months.
- Strategies where carious tissue in cavitated lesions is not removed at all, but sealed or managed non-restoratively, are restricted to primary teeth.
- A decision tree summarising carious tissue removal is presented in Figure 8.

References

1 Loesche WJ: Clinical and microbiological aspects of chemotherapeutic agents used according to the specific plaque hypothesis. J Dent Res 1979;58:2404–2412.

2 Black GV: The pathology of hard tissues of the teeth. Part III. Treatment of caries; in Operative Dentistry. London, Medico-Dental Publishing, 1936, vol 1.

3 Marsh PD: Dental plaque as a biofilm and a microbial community – implications for health and disease. BMC Oral Health 2006;6:S14.

4 Oong EM, Griffin SO, Kohn WG, Gooch BF, Caufield PW: The effect of dental sealants on bacteria levels in caries lesions. J Amer Dent Assoc 2008;139:271–278.

5 Marshall GW, Habelitz S, Gallagher R, Balooch M, Balooch G, Marshall SJ: Nanomechanical properties of hydrated carious human dentin. J Dent Res 2001; 80:1768–1771.

6 Hevinga MA, Opdam NJ, Frencken JE, Truin GJ, Huysmans MC: Does incomplete caries removal reduce strength of restored teeth? J Dent Res 2010;89: 1270–1275.

7 Bertassoni LE, Habelitz S, Marshall SJ, Marshall GW: Mechanical recovery of dentin following remineralization in vitro – an indentation study. J Biomechanics 2011;44:176–181.

8 Tay FR, Pashley DH: Biomimetic remineralization of resin-bonded acid-etched dentin. J Dent Res 2009;88:719–724.

9 Schwendicke F, Meyer-Lückel H, Dörfer CE, Paris S: Pulpal remineralisation of artificial residual caries lesions in vitro. Caries Res 2015;49:591–594.

10 Schwendicke F, Kern M, Blunck U, Dorfer C, Drenck J, Paris S: Marginal integrity and secondary caries of selectively excavated teeth in vitro. J Dent 2014;42: 1261–1268.

11 Schwendicke F, Kern M, Meyer-Lueckel H, Boels A, Doerfer C, Paris S: Fracture resistance and cuspal deflection of incompletely excavated teeth. J Dent 2013; 42:107–113.

12 Bakhshandeh A, Qvist V, Ekstrand K: Sealing occlusal caries lesions in adults referred for restorative treatment: 2–3 years of follow-up. Clin Oral Investig 2012;16:521–529.

13 Mertz-Fairhurst EJ, Curtis JW, Ergle JW, Rueggeberg FA, Adair SM: Ultraconservative and cariostatic sealed restorations: results at year 10. J Am Dent Assoc 1998;129:55–66.

14 Hesse D, Bonifacio CC, Mendes FM, Braga MM, Imparato JC, Raggio DP: Sealing versus partial caries removal in primary molars: a randomized clinical trial. BMC Oral Health 2014;14:58.

15 Innes NP, Frencken JE, Bjorndal L, Maltz M, Manton DJ, Ricketts D, van Landuyt K, Banerjee A, Campus G, Domejean S, Fontana M, Leal S, Lo E, Machiulskiene V, Schulte A, Splieth C, Zandona A, Schwendicke F: Managing carious lesions: consensus recommendations on terminology. Adv Dent Res 2016;28:49–57.

16 Schwendicke F, Frencken JE, Bjorndal L, Maltz M, Manton DJ, Ricketts D, van Landuyt K, Banerjee A, Campus G, Domejean S, Fontana M, Leal S, Lo E, Machiulskiene V, Schulte A, Splieth C, Zandona AF, Innes NP: Managing carious lesions: consensus recommendations on carious tissue removal. Adv Dent Res 2016;28:58–67.

17 Armfield J: The avoidance and delaying of dental visits in Australia. Aust Dent J 2012;57:243–247.

18 Armfield JM: What goes around comes around: revisiting the hypothesized vicious cycle of dental fear and avoidance. Community Dent Oral Epidemiol 2013; 41:279–287.

19 Armfield JM, Mohan H, Luzzi L,Chrisopoulos S: Dental anxiety screening practices and self-reported training needs among Australian dentists. Aust Dent J 2014;59:464–472.

20 Banerjee A, Kidd EA, Watson TF: In vitro evaluation of five alternative methods of carious dentine excavation. Caries Res 2000;34:144–150.

21 de Almeida Neves A, Coutinho E, Cardoso MV, Lambrechts P, van Meerbeek B: Current concepts and techniques for caries excavation and adhesion to residual dentin. J Adhes Dent 2011;13:7–22.

22 Brantley C, Bader J, Shugars D, Nesbit S: Does the cycle of rerestoration lead to larger restorations? J Amer Dent Assoc 1995;126:1407–1413.

23 Schwendicke F, Diederich C, Paris S: Restoration gaps needed to exceed a threshold size to impede sealed lesion arrest in vitro. J Dent 2016;48:77–80.

24 Schwendicke F, Stolpe M, Meyer-Lueckel H, Paris S,Dörfer CE: Cost-effectiveness of one- and two-step incomplete and complete excavations. J Dent Res 2013;90:880–887.

25 Whitworth JM, Myers PM, Smith J, Walls AW, McCabe JF: Endodontic complications after plastic restorations in general practice. Int Endod J 2005;38: 409–416.

26 Bjørndal L, Reit C, Bruun G, Markvart M, Kjaeldgaard M, Nasman P, Thordrup M, Dige I, Nyvad B, Fransson H, Lager A, Ericson D, Petersson K, Olsson J, Santimano EM, Wennstrom A, Winkel P, Gluud C: Treatment of deep caries lesions in adults: randomized clinical trials comparing stepwise vs. direct complete excavation, and direct pulp capping vs. partial pulpotomy. Eur J Oral Sci 2010;118:290–297.

27 Cheung GS,Chan TK: Long-term survival of primary root canal treatment carried out in a dental teaching hospital. Int Endod J 2003;36:117–128.

28 Lucarotti PS, Lessani M, Lumley PJ, Burke FJ: Influence of root canal fillings on longevity of direct and indirect restorations placed within the general dental services in England and Wales. Br Dent J 2014;216:E14.

29 Molven O: Tooth mortality and endodontic status of a selected population group: observations before and after treatment. Acta Odontol Scand 1976;34: 107–116.

30 Aguilar P, Linsuwanont P: Vital pulp therapy in vital permanent teeth with cariously exposed pulp: a systematic review. J Endod 2011;37:581–587.

31 Bogen G, Kim JS, Bakland LK: Direct pulp capping with mineral trioxide aggregate: an observational study. J Am Dent Assoc 2008;139:305–315.

32 Hilton TJ, Ferracane JL, Mancl L; Northwest Practice-Based Research Collaborative in Evidence-based Dentistry (NWP): Comparison of CaOH with MTA for direct pulp capping: a PBRN randomized clinical trial. J Dent Res 2013;92:S16–S22.

33 Mente J, Geletneky B, Ohle M, Koch MJ, Friedrich Ding PG, Wolff D, Dreyhaupt J, Martin N, Staehle HJ, Pfefferle T: Mineral trioxide aggregate or calcium hydroxide direct pulp capping: an analysis of the clinical treatment outcome. J Endod 2010;36:806–813.
34 Marques MS, Wesselink PR, Shemesh H: Outcome of direct pulp capping with mineral trioxide aggregate: a prospective study. J Endod 2015;41:1026–1031.
35 Stangvaltaite L, Schwendicke F, Holmgren C, Finet M, Maltz M, Elhennawy K, Kerosuo E, Domejean S: Management of pulps exposed during carious tissue removal in adults: a multi-national questionnaire-based survey. Clin Oral Investig 2017;21:2303–2309.
36 Raedel M, Hartmann A, Bohm S, Konstantinidis I, Priess HW, Walter MH: Outcomes of direct pulp capping: interrogating an insurance database. Int Endod J 2016;49:1040–1047.
37 Raedel M, Hartmann A, Bohm S, Walter MH: Three-year outcomes of root canal treatment: mining an insurance database. J Dent 2015;43:412–417.
38 Ng YL, Mann V, Gulabivala K: Tooth survival following non-surgical root canal treatment: a systematic review of the literature. Int Endod J 2010;43:171–189.
39 Schwendicke F, Meyer-Lückel H, Dorfer C, Paris S: Failure of incompletely excavated teeth – a systematic review. J Dent 2013;41:569–580.
40 Ricketts D, Lamont T, Innes NP, Kidd E, Clarkson JE: Operative caries management in adults and children. Cochrane Database Syst Rev 2013;28:CD003808.
41 Hosoya Y, Taguchi T, Tay FR: Evaluation of a new caries detecting dye for primary and permanent carious dentin. J Dent 2007;35:137–143.
42 Itoh K, Kusunoki M, Oikawa M, Tani C, Hisamitsu H: In vitro comparison of three caries dyes. Am J Dent 2009;22:195–199.
43 Iwami Y, Hayashi N, Takeshige F, Ebisu S: Relationship between the color of carious dentin with varying lesion activity, and bacterial detection. J Dent 2008;36:143–151.
44 Iwami Y, Shimizu A, Hayashi M, Takeshige F, Ebisu S: Relationship between colors of carious dentin and laser fluorescence evaluations in caries diagnosis. Dent Mater J 2006;25:584–590.
45 Kidd EA, Joyston-Bechal S, Beighton D: The use of a caries detector dye during cavity preparation: a microbiological assessment. Br Dent J 1993;174:245–248.
46 Schwendicke F, Dorfer CE, Paris S: Incomplete caries removal: a systematic review and meta-analysis. J Dent Res 2013;92:306–314.
47 Schwendicke F, Paris S, Tu Y: Effects of using different criteria and methods for caries removal: a systematic review and network meta-analysis. J Dent 2015;43:1–15.
48 Bjørndal L, Larsen T, Thylstrup A: A clinical and microbiological study of deep carious lesions during stepwise excavation using long treatment intervals. Caries Res 1997;31:411–417.
49 Bjørndal L, Larsen T: Changes in the cultivable flora in deep carious lesions following a stepwise excavation procedure. Caries Res 2000;34:502–508.
50 Paddick JS, Brailsford SR, Kidd EA, Beighton D: Phenotypic and genotypic selection of microbiota surviving under dental restorations. Appl Environ Microbiol 2005;71:2467–2472.
51 Maltz M, Garcia R, Jardim JJ, de Paula LM, Yamaguti PM, Moura MS, Garcia F, Nascimento C, Oliveira A, Mestrinho HD: Randomized trial of partial vs stepwise caries removal: 3-year follow-up. J Dent Res 2012;91:1026–1031.
52 Fontana M, Platt JA, Eckert GJ, Gonzalez-Cabezas C, Yoder K, Zero DT, Ando M, Soto-Rojas AE, Peters MC: Monitoring of sound and carious surfaces under sealants over 44 months. J Dent Res 2014;93:1070–1075.
53 Wright JT, Crall JJ, Fontana M, Gillette EJ, Novy BB, Dhar V, Donly K, Hewlett ER, Quinonez RB, Chaffin J, Crespin M, Iafolla T, Siegal MD, Tampi MP, Graham L, Estrich C, Carrasco-Labra A: Evidence-based clinical practice guideline for the use of pit-and-fissure sealants: a report of the American Dental Association and the American Academy of Pediatric Dentistry. J Am Dent Assoc 2016;147:672–682.e12.
54 Dorri M, Dunn S, Sabbah W, Schwendicke F: Micro-invasive interventions for managing proximal dental decay in primary and permanent teeth. Cochrane Database Syst Rev 2015;11:CD010431.
55 Hickel R, Kaaden C, Paschos E, Buerkle V, García-Godoy F, Manhart J: Longevity of occlusally-stressed restorations in posterior primary teeth. Am J Dent 2005;18:198–211.
56 Santamaria RM, Innes NP, Machiulskiene V, Evans DJ, Splieth CH: Caries management strategies for primary molars: 1-year randomized control trial results. J Dent Res 2014;93:1062–1069.
57 Innes NP, Evans DJ, Stirrups DR: Sealing caries in primary molars: randomized control trial, 5-year results. J Dent Res 2011;90:1405–1410.
58 Gruythuysen R: Non-restorative cavity treatment: managing rather than masking caries activity. Ned Tijdschr Tandheelkd 2010;117:173–180.

Falk Schwendicke
Operative and Preventive Dentistry, Charité – Universitätsmedizin Berlin
Corporate Member of Freie Universität Berlin
Humboldt-Universität zu Berlin, and Berlin Institute of Health
Assmannshauser Strasse 4-6
DE–14197 Berlin (Germany)
E-Mail falk.schwendicke@charite.de

Schwendicke F, Frencken J, Innes N (eds): Caries Excavation: Evolution of Treating Cavitated Carious Lesions.
Monogr Oral Sci. Basel, Karger, 2018, vol 27, pp 68–81 (DOI: 10.1159/000487834)

Stepwise Excavation

Lars Bjørndal

Section of Cariology and Endodontics, Department of Odontology, Faculty of Health and Medical Sciences, University of Copenhagen, Copenhagen, Denmark

Abstract

The most recent inspiration for stepwise carious tissue removal in 2 stages originates from the knowhow on intralesion changes in deep carious lesions. The environmental change that takes place during the first stage of carious tissue removal is aiming for the arrest of the deep lesion, by placing a temporary restoration on top of the soft carious dentine. The cavity is optimised during the second stage for a final restoration, as potential shrinkage of the retained dentine may occur during the period of carious dentine arrestment. However, basic clinical limitations on the objective evaluation of pulp inflammation creates dilemmas in treating the deep lesions. Also, a global consensus is lacking for the definition of a so-called deep lesion. Finally, an optimal evidence goal for choosing the best approach for deep lesion treatment in adults has still not been fully defined. Taken together, it may not be a surprise that treatment variation is reported amongst general dental practitioners on deep caries treatment. Here, facts are presented supporting the treatment, including some drawbacks, as well as updated guidelines for the procedure. Recent clinical high evidence data from randomised clinical trials significantly favour the stepwise approach as a predictable and reliable treatment for well-defined deep carious lesions located in the pulpal quarter of the dentine in terms of avoiding pulp exposure, keeping the tooth vital and without the development of apical pathosis.

The Clinical Manipulation of Lesion Activity: The Key to Deep Lesion Management

The ecological plaque hypothesis provides the current platform for understanding the pathology of caries [1]. As a carious lesion grows in size, it is clinically more obvious why the lesion is progressing actively and when and why it may change and slow down its activity. Figure 1 depicts how an ecological plaque change of a lesion environment is visualised and tested. A deep nat-

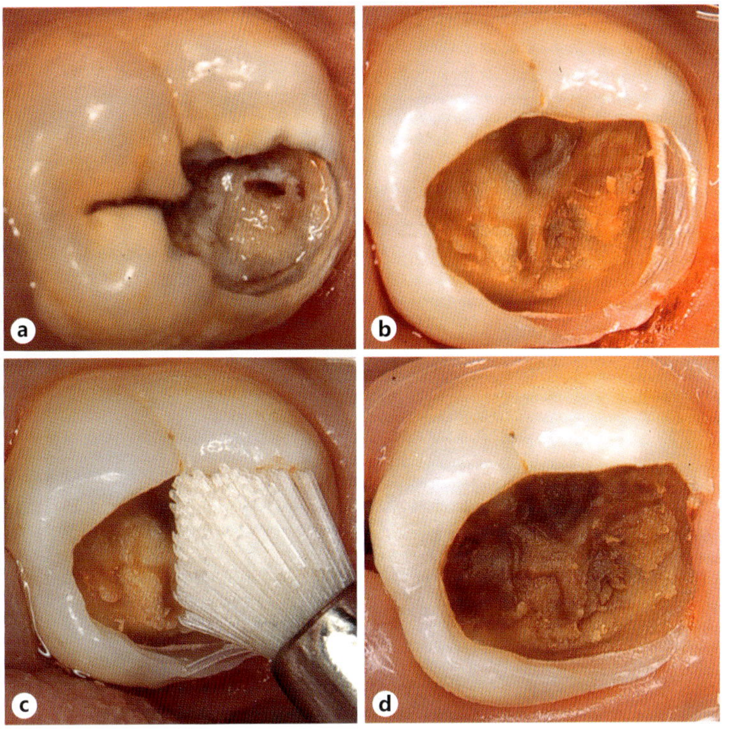

Fig. 1. A test demonstration shows the change of an active lesion environment converting into an arrested environment in a mandibular molar with a deep lesion. **a** The concept behind less invasive carious tissue removal procedures is shown. The undermined enamel and the surface biofilm has been professionally removed (**b**) and by using a rotating brush as well as hygiene instruction (**c**) the surface has been kept free from biofilm accumulation for 2 weeks (**d**). The test shows that the occlusal carious dentine clinically changes into a darker appearance after surface biofilm removal. Of course, a molar benefits from a coronal restoration, so this was only to test a short-term change following the removal of a surface biofilm. Lars Bjørndal ©.

ural untreated lesion environment is displayed in a lower mandibular molar with clear signs of a huge occlusal cavitation harbouring a well-defined cariogenic biofilm. The milky appearance of the enamel border surrounding the cavity reflects the progress of enamel demineralisation along the enamel-dentine junction at this late stage of lesion progress, also known as retrograde demineralisation. As seen from the conversion of lesion activity in root carious lesions [2], a control of the surface biofilm is an important factor in the arrestment of an active carious lesion. For this particular occlusal surface, the removal of undermined enamel (Fig. 1b) combined with a non-operative removal of the surface biofilm show clinical detectable changes over time that correspond to our clinical vision of an arrested carious lesion. The test treatment is carried out by the use of a professional rotating brush, removing the surface biofilm (Fig. 1c). Notably, to visualise the clinical changes no occlusal covering was made in this particular case scenario. The patient was told to keep the occlusal surface clean combined with a weekly professional clean. After 2 weeks, the clinical appearance of the exposed occlusal dentine cavity showed the classical signs of carious arrestment with a darkening of the soft dentine (Fig. 1d). Of course, this was only a test scenario as we would normally appreciate the presence of a functional restored occlusal surface. The important point of this introductory clinical case story is that the carious dentine reacts relatively quickly upon a marked change of a well-defined surface biofilm. After only a relatively short period of time the carious dentine shows the classical signs of so-called carious arrestment, turning darker and firm and to some extent exposing a less moist surface texture [3, 4]. The surface biofilm manipulation of the lesion environment is a key point for understanding the treatment concept of a less invasive carious removal procedure, such as the stepwise carious removal in 2 stages (Fig. 1d). Other treatment concepts, as described elsewhere in this book, do benefit from this concept as well.

The Dilemma: Issues for the Deep Carious Lesion

The description of the pulp and the deep carious lesions has a 2-fold concern. Firstly, the clinical community lacks the diagnostic tool of being able to measure a certain degree of inflammation in the pulp [5]. Thus, it is a clinical judgment based on indirect methods (i.e., dental history, vital pulp testing, paraclinical use of radiograph). Secondly, no effort has been made to make a clear definition of lesion penetration depths [6]. It is not at all obvious from various pulp-capping studies when and why the teeth were treated. In fact, what is meant by a deep lesion? On top of this, numerous studies and learned lessons have been used to develop a classification system comprising a standardised scoring scale of progressing stages of macroscopic and histological changes in order to detect and define signs of carious lesions with the aim of combining suggested treatment approaches [7–9]. However, as the system reaches and describes deeper lesion progress, details of the pulp are omitted and not described, which may be due to the reasons addressed above.

No Global Consensus

With the inspiration from the practitioner environment, the deep lesion can be defined as a lesion that is penetrating into the pulpal quarter or the entire dentine thickness when viewed radiographically [3]. Several questionnaire studies dealing with causes for treatment variation have used a threshold like this to show the concern from general dental practitioners (GDPs), when to expect a pulp exposure, and imaging a scenario with a non-selective carious removal [10–12]. Although the concept of using a non-selective approach today is interpreted as being overtreatment [13], the dental community is clearly carrying out much more invasive strategy and different treatments are suggested for the same clinical scenario. A recently documented review revealed that about half of the GDPs involved would not follow evidence-based guidelines on carious removal procedures [11]. Within the research environment, the lack of an overall consensus regarding how to treat a deep lesion was noted from some recent randomised clinical trials [14–17]. In principle, the same preoperative data are available but different clinical treatment endpoints are examined from invasive pulpotomy to indirect pulp capping and stepwise excavation. In reality, in 2 of the studies the actual outcome was material testing (Table 1).

No global consensus or tradition prevails in the treatment of a deep carious lesion with a vital pulp. One could argue whether or not this would be a realistic goal, knowing that GDPs find themselves in different environments with different possibilities and have different skills. However, variation caused by a lack of understanding of the pathology of caries should not be accepted. To solve these controversies, some details on lesion penetration will be presented.

The Deeper Stages of Lesion Progression: Definition and Subjacent Pathology

In order to obtain a better-defined portal for less invasive carious tissue removal procedures, as opposed to endodontic consideration of pulp treatments, some observations on deep stages of carious lesions are presented, also giving some consideration to the pulp response.

The current histological information of the inner pulpal quarter of carious dentine in deep lesions is that the infection has not yet reached the tertiary dentine as well as the pulp. The pulp may very well be chronically inflamed, but is typically

Table 1. Randomised clinical trials of pulp-preserving interventions with similarly preoperative status but with different treatment endpoints

Study	Tooth type and age, and preoperative status and diagnosis	Trial power and randomisation, and variables tested	Treatment protocol	Outcome assessment and follow-up	Success of analysed cases and conclusions
Jang et al. [17], 2015 (1-year) Comparing capping materials following pulpotomy	Permanent teeth (>19 years) Direct pulp exposure from trauma or dental caries (depth not further defined) Reversible pulpitis	*Trial:* intervention effect 15% Power 0.80%, $p < 0.5\%$ *Randomisation:* no concealed allocation sequence *Capping material:* ProRootMTA (control), $n = 23$, vs. Endocem, $n = 23$ *Stratification variable:* age and exposure site (occlusal or axial surfaces)	After complete caries excavation with a sterile spoon excavator exposed pulp was disinfected with 2.5% sodium hypochlorite Hemostasis should be reached within 10 min Thickness of the capping materials: 3 mm or as close as possible	*Blinded outcome assessment:* yes *Success:* positive response to pulp test; no evidence of irreversible pulpitis (not defined) and pulp necrosis, no well-defined apical radiolucency (not defined) *Follow-up:* 1, 2, 4 weeks, 3, 6 months, and 1 year	*Experimental* (Endocem): 87% success *Control* (ProRoot MTA): 85% success No significant difference between tested capping materials. Axial exposure site (class V cavity) showed significantly worse outcome
Hashem et al. [16], 2015 Comparing restorative procedure and paraclinical radiographical and CBCT assessments after indirect pulp capping/partial excavation	Permanent dentition (median 28 years) Carious dentine into pulpal quarter of the dentine), no signs of irreversible pulpitis (no widening of PDL or PA lesion)	*Trial:* intervention effect ~20%, power 0.80%, $p < 0.5\%$ *Randomisation:* concealed allocation (central procedure) *Material:* GIC (control), $n = 36$, vs. Biodentine, $n = 36$ *Stratification variable:* cavity size	Superficial soft infected dentine was removed by burr and deeper located areas by chemomechanical gel and hand instrumentation, but left at a residual level, whereby any added removal would lead to exposure	*Blinded outcome assessment:* unclear *Success:* positive response to pulp test at 12 moths; no irreversible pulpitis (defined); absence of PA radiographically (defined as >2 times width of PDL space); CBCT scan detecting so-called early PA lesions *Follow-up:* 1, 6, and 12 months	*Experimental* (Biodentine): 83% clinical success *Control* (GIC): 83% clinical success. No clinical and radiographical differences CBCT-PA alterations at baseline had a significantly higher failure rate at 1-year follow-up vs. teeth without CBCT-detected PA alterations
Bjørndal et al. [15], 2017 (5 years) Bjørndal et al. [14], 2010 (1.5 years) Comparing complete excavation vs. stepwise excavation, and subsequent pulp capping vs. partial pulpotomy if exposure occurred accidentally during the carious removal	Permanent dentition (median 29 years) Carious dentine into pulpal quarter of the dentine, no signs of irreversible pulpitis (no undisturbed night's sleep; no radiographical PA lesion)	*Trial:* intervention effect ~20%, power 0.90%, $p < 0.5\%$ *Randomisation:* concealed allocation (central procedure) *Intervention:* complete/non-selective excavation (control), $n = 158$, stepwise excavation, $n = 156$ *Stratification variable:* age and centre	*Stepwise excavation arm:* visit 1: removal of superficial necrotic and demineralised dentine, so a GIC temporary seal could be placed; visit 2 (8–12 weeks): final excavation leaving central yellowish or greyish hard dentine and a permanent seal and a resin restoration *Complete excavation arm:* final excavation leaving central yellowish or greyish hard dentine and a permanent seal; in case of perforation a nested trial; direct pulp capping vs. partial pulpotomy	*Blinded outcome assessment:* yes *Success:* possible response to pulp test at follow-up. No unbearable pain (no disturbed night's sleep); absence of PA radiographically (defined as >2 times width of PDL space) *Follow-up:* 1 and 5 years	Excavation trial (non-exposed treatment) at 5 years *Experimental* (stepwise): 60% success *Control* (complete excavation): 46% success Significant difference Nested pulp capping trial at 5 years: *Experimental* (partial pulpotomy): 11% success *Control* (direct pulp capping): 6% success No significant difference between capping interventions

PA, periapical; PDL, periodontal ligament; CBCT, cone beam computed tomography.

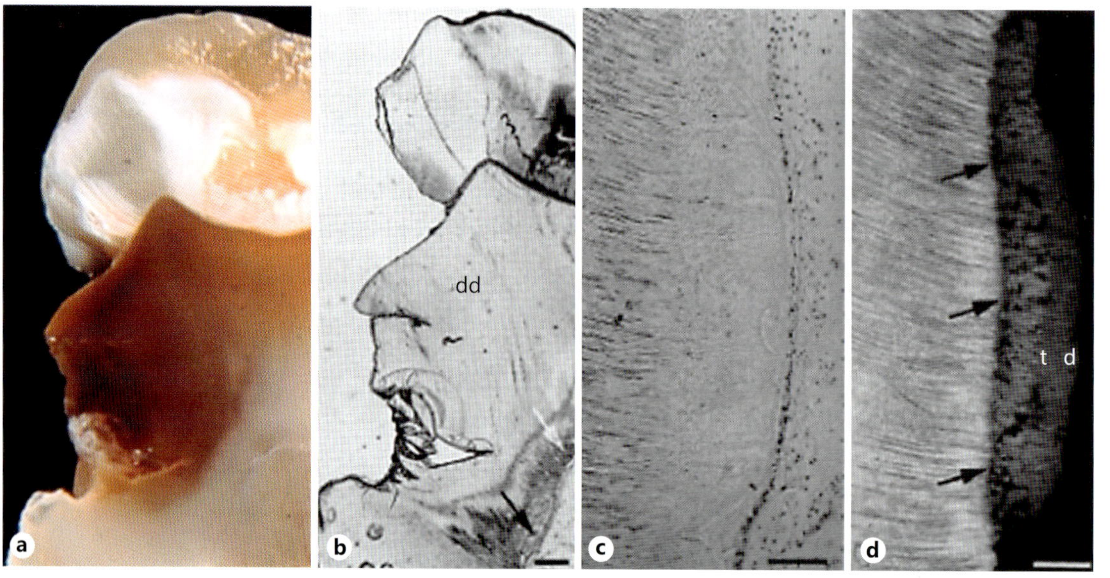

Fig. 2. a, **b** In natural untreated lesions the scenario of a change in lesion activity is noted when undermined enamel breaks off. The surface becomes darker and the pulp reacts with a reparative tertiary dentine formation. Lightmicroscopic (**c**) and microradiographic (**d**) overview of reparative tertiary dentine. The interface between dentine and tertiary dentine is calcospheritic (arrows) followed by formation of tubular dentine. dd, demineralised dentine; td, tubular dentine. Scale bars, 250 µm (**b**), 100 µm (**c**, **d**). Modified from Bjørndal and Darvann [58].

without an infection within the pulp [18]. The central part of a slow-progressing lesion with a total surface breakdown is noted with dark discoloured dentine and with a healing pulp with evidence of reparative tertiary dentine (Fig. 2). An updated interpretation of pulp inflammation includes the understanding of inflammation not only as a one-way route toward pulp cell impairment and subsequent necrosis and infection, but as a "double-edged sword" where a so-called wanted inflammation, given the right balance, will cause healing, whereas an unstable/unwanted inflammation will lead to pulp necrosis and an infected pulp cavity [19, 20] [see Conrads, this vol., pp. 5–7].

Deep Carious Lesion and Radiographical Definition

In the following, a brief explanation is given of the "infection scenario" for the deep carious lesion, compared to, for example, an infected wounded knee. The inflammatory cell reaches the pulp due to the influx of the cariogenic antigens, and most often a huge accumulation of inflammatory cells has occurred. As with scenarios in other parts of the body, these inflammatory cells will directly react towards the acute invading microorganisms. However, for the deep carious lesion involving the pulpal quarter of the dentine, but still with radiographically translucent dentine separating the pulp from the dentine demineralisation (Fig. 3), the inner parts of the dentine do not yet comprise bacteria per se, but in fact both a sclerotic (or hypermineralised) as well as a demineralised dentine normally borders the contaminated infected dentine [18]. The inflammatory cells are in proximity, but cannot establish a direct bacterial contact, as they normally would do following a wound of the skin. Therefore, the "deep carious lesion" affected pulp often features numerous inflammatory cells waiting to take care of the actual microorganisms. Concomitantly, the life-cycle of an ac-

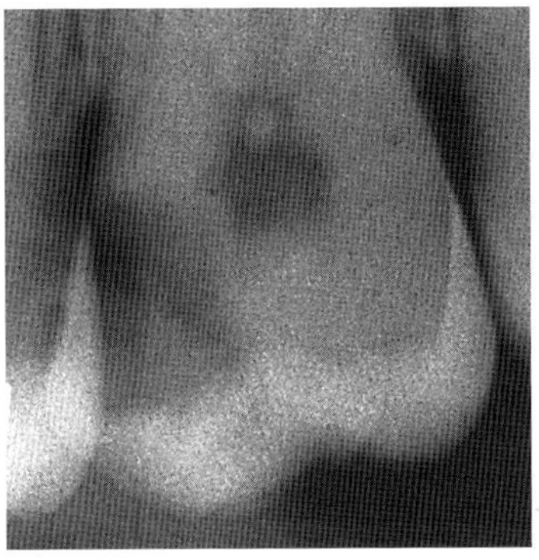

Fig. 3. A deep carious lesion defined as being in the pulpal quarter of the dentine with a radiodense zone separating the translucent zone from the pulp. Modified from Bjørndal and Ricucci [18] with permission from Springer.

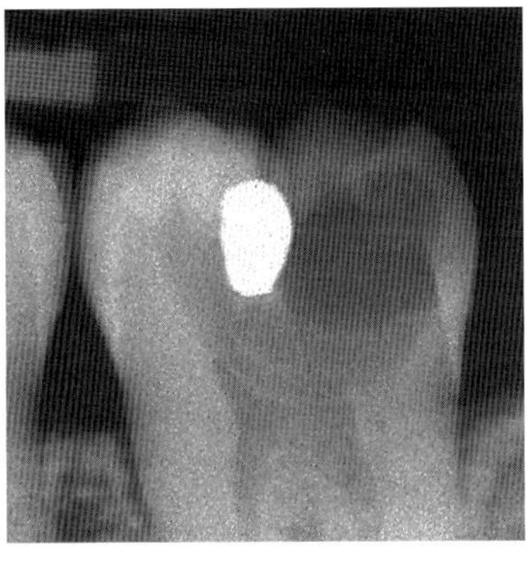

Fig. 4. The extremely deep lesion defines a penetration that involves the entire primary/secondary dentine, either with no radiodense zone separating the demineralised dentine from the pulp or with a radiodense zone located within the pulp chamber indicative of tertiary dentine. Modified from Bjørndal and Ricucci [18] with permission from Springer.

tive inflammatory cell is limited, leading to areas of focal necrosis. As long as the infection has not reached the pulp, this can be "taken care of" by other inflammatory cells, removing the elements of tissue necrosis. Taken together, the histological picture of a severely inflamed pulp may not be the sign of irreversibility in terms of infection. Moreover, if the carious-infected dentine is altered or removed, the pulp may eventually reach a threshold where a wanted inflammation can take over, eventually guiding the healing phase [18, 19]. Clinical data have confirmed that the treatment of lesions extending into the pulpal quarter of the dentine has a much better prognosis if the dentine barrier is kept intact as opposed to toward a broken dentine barrier [14].

Potential Reasons for Failures following Pulp Capping in Deep Lesions

In conjunction with the scenario of accumulated inflammatory cells and the development of pulp necrosis before the microorganisms are in contact with the pulp, the pulp represents a very sensible environment in cases where pulp exposure has taken place. Imagine a deep lesion exposure with fragments of infected carious dentine entrapped in the pulp with small focal areas of infected tissue. This "cocktail" will quite quickly lead toward total necrosis and infection of the entire pulp cavity, and with the possibility of severe accompanying pain. Pulp capping in deep lesions can be performed successfully, particularly when using magnification and enhanced illumination [21], but it seemingly becomes a critical procedure within a GDP environment where such equipment may be less common or not available at all.

Extremely Deep Carious Lesions and Subjacent Pulp Responses

To optimise the border of avoiding pulp exposure as well as the opportunity for an endodontic treatment procedure, it may be important to make a threshold for the penetration of deep lesions, from where the expectation of maintaining pulp vitality becomes less likely. An attempt to define the so-called extremely deep carious lesion illustrates such a threshold. As opposed to the deep pulpal quarter lesion, the extremely deep carious lesion is defined [6] as a carious lesion with a radiographical penetration depth involving the entire thickness of the dentine (Fig. 4). At this point, studies have shown that the tertiary dentine including the pulp chamber is infected, whereby the innermost dentine cannot be controlled by a non-invasive carious removal procedure [22]. This was recently confirmed at a clinical level – when infection advances to the pulp tissue it was a common finding in teeth with irreversible pulpitis, but was never observed in normal/reversibly inflamed pulps. This indicates that extremely deep carious lesions are not "candidates" for a less invasive carious removal procedure that attempts to avoid pulp exposure [23].

Microbial Data

What happens with the biofilm when a temporary filling is placed in retained carious dentine? A classical paper [24] addressed this topic by asking: "How clean must a cavity be?" The methods for investigating this were based on an indirect approach. The biofilm samples were provided by using a burr full of carious dentine [25], thereby testing the carious dentine before and after carious removal and before and after a treatment interval in order to detect the effect following intervention. Reports have noted a marked reduction on the basis of cultivable microorganisms before and after carious removal procedures [25–28], and not only for a limited period of time, but also for a period covering several months [29]. In addition, effort has been made to characterise the qualitative nature of biofilm in different well-defined carious lesions – is it a closed lesion environment (Fig. 5a–c) with features characterising a clinical active environment, or is it an open lesion environment (Fig. 5d–f)? In fact, a marked difference is noted between the 2 scenarios. The closed lesion environment comprises a biofilm with relatively few species, whereas the open lesion contains a much more complex composition. In particular, some of the bacteria seem to have potential properties that could influence the severity of the ongoing degradation of carious dentine, for example. However, within both scenarios (irrespective of the different biofilm complexity) the cultivable flora show, following a treatment interval during stepwise carious removal, that it can be compared to a biofilm resembling an arrested environment [26, 30, 31]. This emphasises the point depicted in Figure 1, showing that a surface control of the superficial part of a cavity not only creates a clinical change of the carious dentine, but this change is also reflected within the composition and number of the retained microorganisms in the carious dentine.

The dark colour of the demineralised carious dentine does not necessarily indicate low levels of microbial cultivable flora [32], it may also harbour complex biofilms that seem to decrease markedly following a treatment interval [29, 31]. Therefore, when evaluating lesion changes, it should always be evaluated as an intralesional measure [33], and it is the combined intralesional variables (colour, hardness, moisture) that over time can be noted in relation to lesional activity changes [3]. This strategy is used when evaluating the retained carious dentine at the second stage during stepwise carious tissue removal.

Why Does the Colour of Demineralised Dentine Change?

Besides external stain as well as the potential presence of black pigmented microorganisms [34], the clinical reported rehardening and darkening of the dentine after carious arrestment may partly by linked to generated AGE ("advanced glycation end-products"), which is the collective term for Maillard reaction products [35]. These products are the result of a non-enzymatic reaction between glucose or fructose (reducing sugars) contained in pulpal fluid that flows from the pulp to the enamel-dentine junction. The AGE only takes place in non-acidic environments and can be seen as the signs of slowly progressing carious lesions [36, 37]. The stepwise carious removal procedure benefits from these clinical detectable changes of carious dentine during intervention. This chapter will later revert to the clinical handling of carious dentine during a 2-stage selective carious removal in deep carious lesions.

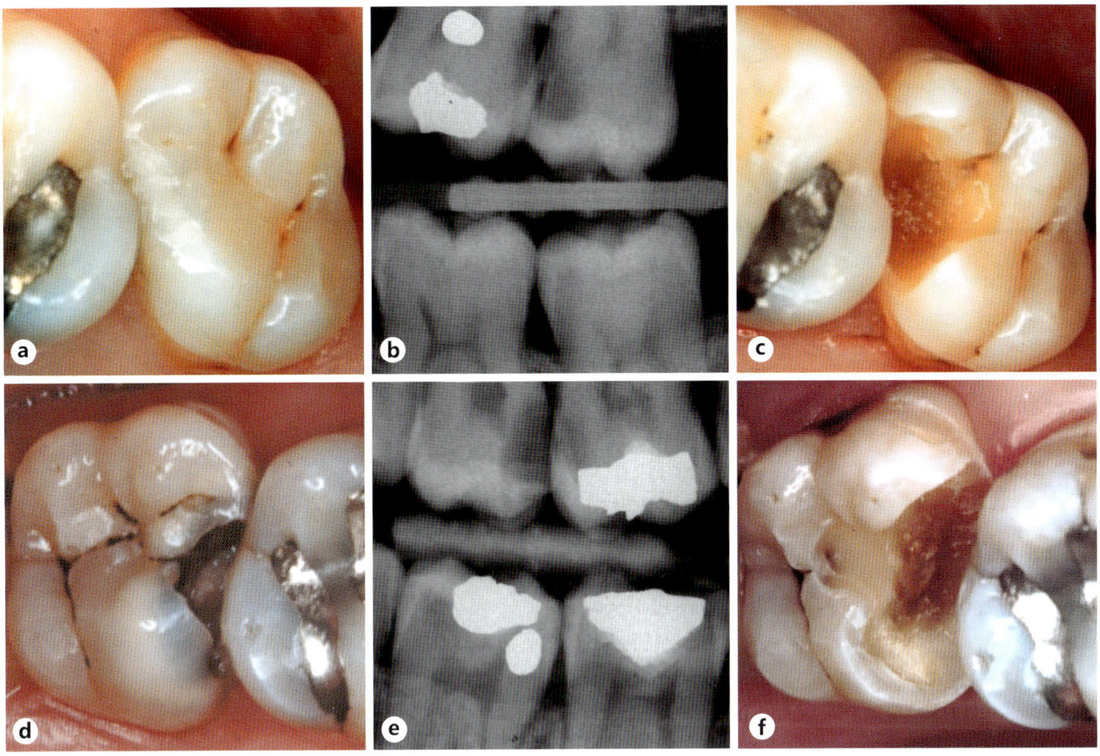

Fig. 5. Clinical and radiographical signs of deep proximal carious lesions. **a**, **b** A closed lesion environment in +7. During the first stage of carious tissue removal during stepwise excavation, the clinical expression of the carious dentine shows the signs of active progression, being light brown, soft, and wet (**c**), and with a homogeneous biofilm. **d**, **e** An open lesion environment is shown in 7+. The retained carious dentine looks darker after the first-stage carious removal (**f**), and contains a complex biofilm. In both scenarios, the biofilm converts to one known from arrested environments. Modified from Bjørndal and Larsen [26].

An Improved Evidence Platform Should Be the Solution to the Historical Dilemma

A lot of history is concerned with the "dilemma" in the treatment of deep carious lesions, and often with awe G.V. Black and Sir J. Tomes from formative years are cited for their opposing arguments about whether or not one should leave carious dentine behind [38, 39]. From the argumentation above, a simple element of lesion definition may provide less confusion and more consensuses. Imagine that the two professors above actually discussed two different lesion scenarios, we will never know! When G.V. Black was discussing the benefit of removing all carious dentine, he was perhaps already facing an extremely deep lesion, while Tomes was not. Nevertheless, the topic represents an area where clinical evidence has been sparse. From being a topic that is either handled by an invasive or a non-invasive approach based on various schools of opinion (Table 1), the goal is to arrive at an evidence-based platform.

The Evidence behind Avoiding Pulp Exposure

Recent clinical data have shown that the prognosis following pulp capping in deep lesions in adults is poor. Less than 10% of capped teeth maintain pulp vitality in the absence of pain and with sound apical parodontium after 5 years [15].

From a pulp protection view it seems quite clear that pulp exposure in deep lesions extending into the pulpal quarter of the dentine should be avoided within a GDP scenario. A 2-stage approach is a means of preventing exposure of the pulp, but only 5 studies have shown this trend. Two randomised trials have investigated the effects of a 2-stage stepwise carious removal versus a non-selective carious removal approach with respect to the treatment outcome of "pulp exposure" in deciduous teeth [40, 41], and only 3 trials in permanent teeth [14, 42, 43], of which 1 included both deciduous and permanent teeth [43]. A meta-analysis of the results from these 5 trials discloses that a 2-stage stepwise carious removal seems to reduce the risk of pulp exposure compared with a non-selective approach (Fig. 6). However, it should be noted that all these trials have a "high risk of bias," i.e., a high risk of overestimating a beneficial intervention effect. The high risk of bias is mainly caused by the fact that trial participants and personnel cannot be blinded. Moreover, only 1 of the trials conducted the randomisation procedure centrally [14]. Thus, firm evidence may not have been reached yet.

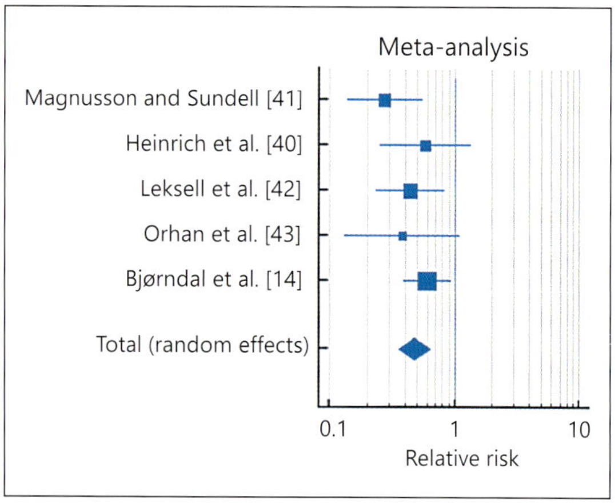

Fig. 6. The total relative risk ratio (95% confidence interval) of 0.47 (0.39–0.64) shows that it favours stepwise excavation ($p < 0.001$). Forest plot.

Clinical Trials and Stepwise Excavation

Although the number of systematic reviews [44–47] and narrative comments are increasing concerning selective carious removal on deep lesions [48], still relatively few clinical trials have examined the stepwise excavation concept in adults in permanent teeth using the definition of lesion depth being in the pulpal quarter of the dentine. Within deciduous teeth, one of the first studies in Scandinavia dealing with stepwise excavation versus a non-selective approach in molars had a split mouth design and showed a huge difference (close to 50%) in favour of the 2-stage procedure [41]. It was not a concealed randomised design and thus had a potential high risk of bias. More recent studies have been able to confirm a somewhat lower intervention effect, down to 15% [15, 42]. A clinical interpretation of this level of difference can be explained in the following way. Each time a dentist has treated 8 patients with a deep carious lesion, 1 pulp exposure has been prevented.

Stepwise Excavation and Some Critical Points

Some critical arguments have been addressed for a 2-stage approach. There is an economical issue due to the need for an extra visit, and it is also well known that additional pulp exposures may occur during the second stage, with a rate of approximately 15% [44, 48]. In the deciduous dentition in particular, studies have demonstrated that a 1-stage selective carious removal approach is successful [49, 50]. Also, the concept of sealing of the entire carious lesion with a stainless steel crown, also described as the Hall Technique [described by Santamaria and Innes, this vol., pp. 113–122], has proven to be beneficial [51–53]. For these approaches, a clear definition on lesion depth remains unclear.

Future Expectation of Clinical Evidence between Less Invasive Carious Removal Procedures

The evidence gained on deep carious lesions as defined here, as well as on an adult population, is still limited for a selective carious removal approach. Data have shown that on the basis of well-performed protocols between stepwise and selective carious removal the 2 approaches may be similar to a 1-stage approach [54], and appear suitable for treating deep carious lesions [47]. According to sound research methodology, however, firm evidence is still needed, mainly due to sparse data and repetitive testing within traditional meta-analyses leading to a high risk of type I errors [55, 56], suggesting that there may be a treatment effect, when in fact there is not.

A randomised clinical trial is the method to show which treatment is preferable for the scenario of preserving the vital pulp. The checklist below shows some essential rules for the comparison of, for example, stepwise versus selective carious tissue removal:

- well-defined inclusion and exclusion criteria (e.g., penetration depth of the carious lesion);
- power calculation reflecting the number of treatments needed to show a difference between control and experimental groups;
- a central randomisation of patients to control and experimental groups;
- a follow-up examination by an examiner who is not aware of which group the material or the patient belongs (blinded outcome evaluation).

Is Shrinkage of Retained Carious Dentine a Problem in Selective Carious Tissue Removal?

Clinically, it is unknown whether permanently retained carious dentine will shrink and impair the restoration. Perhaps there may be some influence with respect to cavity design and the longevity of the restoration when carious dentine in deep lesions is left permanently. It is known that insufficient temporary as well as permanent coronal seals during the less invasive carious removal strategies will lead to failure, including pulpal and apical pathosis [3, 54].

The Stepwise Carious Tissue Removal Principles and Protocol

In short, the inactivation and conversion of the outer cariogenic lesion environment is an important aspect explaining why a less invasive carious removal concept can be possible (Fig. 1), but also because the clinical arrestment of carious dentine after a treatment interval is associated with a reduction in the degree of infection [29, 31]. It is still unclear if these initial inactivation processes can last for years, as seen in less progressed stages of lesion formation [57], and therefore maintaining a 2-stage approach is currently suggested.

The first stage aims to convert the lesion activity into an arrested or slow progressing environment. Leaving behind carious dentine between 2 stages clinically turns an active deep carious environment from a soft, discoloured, and wet tissue (Fig. 7) to carious dentine with a darker, harder, and drier appearance (Fig. 8). The sealed period with a calcium hydroxide base material followed by a glass-ionomer restoration, for example, transforms carious dentine into a state where it is more clinically convenient to establish and finalise the final cavity for the permanent restoration. A gap between the temporary restoration and the retained carious dentine occurs (Fig. 9) due to shrinkage of active carious dentine that may take place during inactivation. Whether a persistent gap may impair the long-term outcome, in cases where it is not eliminated within a selective scenario, remains to be resolved.

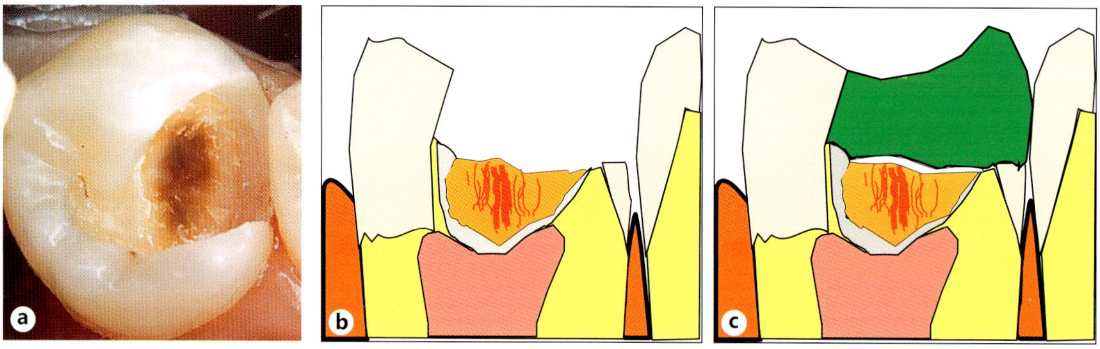

Fig. 7. First stage of the stepwise carious tissue removal. **a**, **b** Note the peripheral borders following non-selective removal. A properly performed temporary restoration should be placed. **c** A colouring of the temporary restoration makes the second-stage removal easier to perform without exposing the pulp. Photograph reproduced with permission (Bjørndal [4]).

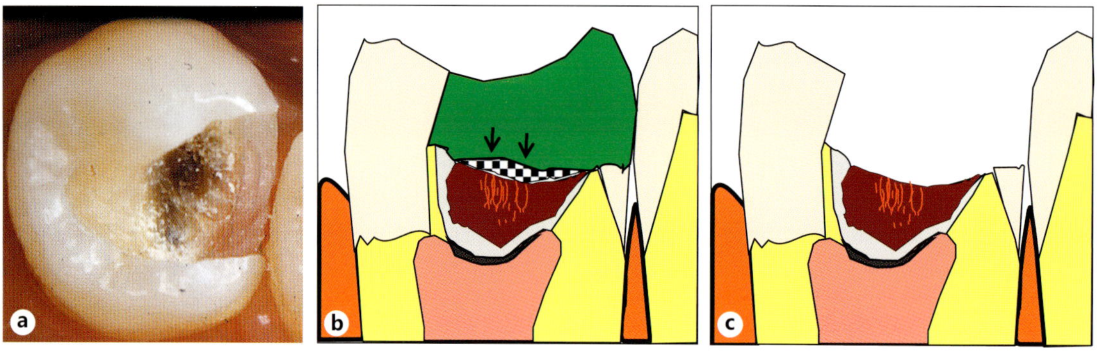

Fig. 8. After a 6-month treatment interval. **a** Removal of the temporary filling shows signs of lesion arrestment. A darker, harder, and dryer carious dentine appears. **b**, **c** A principal drawing of the scenario before and after removal of the temporary filling. The marked region (**b**) indicates the gap between restoration and the arrested carious dentine. Photograph reproduced with permission (Bjørndal [4]).

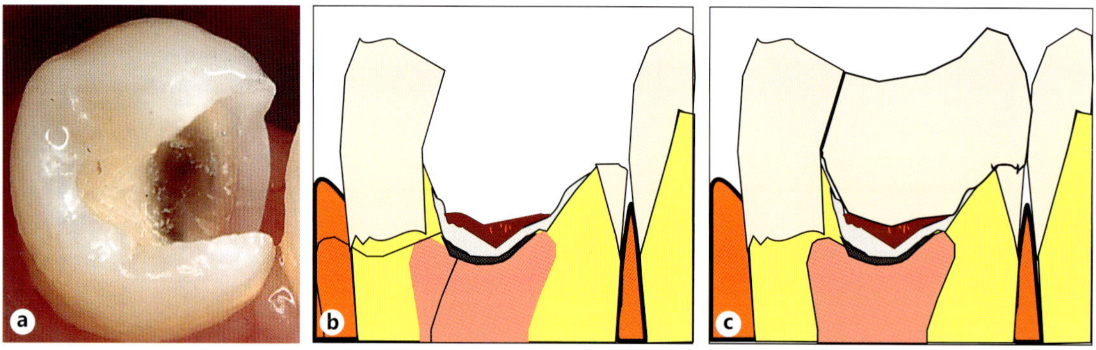

Fig. 9. a, **b** Hand excavators are used for the selective removal of carious-arrested dentine. The final permanent restoration has been placed and the potential gap between the temporary restoration and the retained carious dentine has been eliminated, whereby the cavity for a final long-lasting resin restoration is optimised (**c**). Photograph reproduced with permission (Bjørndal [4]).

The following steps should be taken into account using recent nomenclature for the stepwise carious removal procedure [13]:

- Two stages, i.e., 2 visits are used for the carious tissue removal procedure;
- First stage: selective removal to soft or firm dentine, carious tissue is left over the pulp, while peripheral dentine is prepared with a non-selective removal to hard dentine to accomplish a sufficient temporary restoration sealing of the retained carious dentine;
- The provisional restoration should be sufficiently durable to last up to 12 months and, if markedly coloured, the risk of iatrogenic pulp exposure is decreased;
- Second stage: selective removal to firm dentine;
- Permanent restoration.

References

1 Marsh PD: Microbial ecology of dental plaque and its significance in health and disease. Adv Dent Res 1994;8:263–271.

2 Nyvad B, Fejerskov O: Assessing the stage of caries lesion activity on the basis of clinical and microbiological examination. Community Dent Oral Epidemiol 1997;25:69–75.

3 Bjørndal L, Thylstrup A: A practice-based study on stepwise excavation of deep carious lesions in permanent teeth: a 1-year follow-up study. Community Dent Oral Epidemiol 1998;26:122–128.

4 Bjørndal L: Buonocore Memorial Lecture: dentin caries: progression and clinical management. Oper Dent 2002;27: 211–217.

5 Mejare IA, Axelsson S, Davidson T, Frisk F, Hakeberg M, Kvist T, Norlund A, Petersson A, Portenier I, Sandberg H, Tranaeus S, Bergenholtz G: Diagnosis of the condition of the dental pulp: a systematic review. Int Endod J 2012;45: 597–613.

6 Bjørndal L, Demant S, Dabelsteen S: Depth and activity of carious lesions as indicators for the regenerative potential of dental pulp after intervention. J Endod 2014;40:S76–S81.

7 Ekstrand KR, Martignon S, Ricketts DJ, Qvist V: Detection and activity assessment of primary coronal caries lesions: a methodologic study. Oper Dent 2007;32: 225–235.

8 Nyvad B, Machiulskiene V, Baelum V: Reliability of a new caries diagnostic system differentiating between active and inactive caries lesions. Caries Res 1999;33:252–260.

9 Ricketts DN, Ekstrand KR, Kidd EA, Larsen T: Relating visual and radiographic ranked scoring systems for occlusal caries detection to histological and microbiological evidence. Oper Dent 2002;27:231–237.

10 Oen KT, Thompson VP, Vena D, Caufield PW, Curro F, Dasanayake A, Ship JA, Lindblad A: Attitudes and expectations of treating deep caries: a PEARL Network survey. Gen Dent 2007;55:197–203.

11 Schwendicke F, Gostemeyer G: Understanding dentists' management of deep carious lesions in permanent teeth: a systematic review and meta-analysis. Implement Sci 2016;11:142.

12 Stangvaltaite L, Kundzina R, Eriksen HM, Kerosuo E: Treatment preferences of deep carious lesions in mature teeth: questionnaire study among dentists in Northern Norway. Acta Odontol Scand 2013;71:1532–1537.

13 Schwendicke F, Frencken JE, Bjørndal L, Maltz M, Manton DJ, Ricketts D, van Landuyt K, Banerjee A, Campus G, Domejean S, Fontana M, Leal S, Lo E, Machiulskiene V, Schulte A, Splieth C, Zandona AF, Innes NP: Managing carious lesions: consensus recommendations on carious tissue removal. Adv Dent Res 2016;28:58–67.

14 Bjørndal L, Reit C, Bruun G, Markvart M, Kjældgaard M, Näsman P, Thordrup M, Dige I, Nyvad B, Fransson H, Lager A, Ericson D, Petersson K, Olsson J, Santimano EM, Wennström A, Winkel P, Gluud C: Treatment of deep caries lesions in adults: randomized clinical trials comparing stepwise vs. direct complete excavation, and direct pulp capping vs. partial pulpotomy. Eur J Oral Sci 2010;118:290–297.

15 Bjørndal L, Fransson H, Bruun G, Markvart M, Kjældgaard M, Näsman P, Hedenbjörk-Lager A, Dige I, Thordrup M: Randomized clinical trials on deep carious lesions: 5-year follow-up. J Dent Res 2017;96:747–753.

16 Hashem D, Mannocci F, Patel S, Manoharan A, Brown JE, Watson TF, Banerjee A: Clinical and radiographic assessment of the efficacy of calcium silicate indirect pulp capping: a randomized controlled clinical trial. J Dent Res 2015; 94:562–568.

17 Jang Y, Song M, Yoo IS, Song Y, Roh BD, Kim E: A randomized controlled study of the use of ProRoot Mineral Trioxide Aggregate and Endocem as direct pulp capping materials: 3-month versus 1-year outcomes. J Endod 2015;41: 1201–1206.

18 Bjørndal L, Ricucci D: Pulp inflammation: from the reversible pulpitis to pulp necrosis during caries progression; in Goldberg M (ed): The Dental Pulp – Biology, Pathology and Regenerative Therapies. Heidelberg, Springer, 2016, pp 125–139.

19 Cooper PR, Takahashi Y, Graham LW, Simon S, Imazato S, Smith AJ: Inflammation-regeneration interplay in the dentine-pulp complex. J Dent 2010;38: 687–697.

20 Cooper PR, Holder MJ, Smith AJ: Inflammation and regeneration in the dentin-pulp complex: a double-edged sword. J Endod 2014;40:S46–S51.

21 Bogen G, Kim JS, Bakland LK: Direct pulp capping with mineral trioxide aggregate: an observational study. J Am Dent Assoc 2008;139:305–315.

22 Reeves R, Stanley HR: The relationship of bacterial penetration and pulpal pathosis in carious teeth. Oral Surg Oral Med Oral Pathol 1966;22:59–65.

23 Ricucci D, Loghin S, Siqueira JF Jr: Correlation between clinical and histologic pulp diagnoses. J Endod 2014;40:1932–1939.

24 Kidd EA. How "clean" must a cavity be before restoration? Caries Res 2004;38: 305–313.

25 Kidd EA, Joyston-Bechal S, Beighton D: Microbiological validation of assessments of caries activity during cavity preparation. Caries Res 1993;27:402–408.

26 Bjørndal L, Larsen T: Changes in the cultivable flora in deep carious lesions following a stepwise excavation procedure. Caries Res 2000;34:502–508.

27 Kidd EA, Joyston-Bechal S, Beighton D: The use of a caries detector dye during cavity preparation: a microbiological assessment. Br Dent J 1993;174:245–248.

28 Lager A, Thornqvist E, Ericson D: Cultivatable bacteria in dentine after caries excavation using rose-bur or Carisolv. Caries Res 2003;37:206–211.

29 Bjørndal L, Larsen T, Thylstrup A: A clinical and microbiological study of deep carious lesions during stepwise excavation using long treatment intervals. Caries Res 1997;31:411–417.

30 Brailsford SR, Lynch E, Beighton D: The isolation of *Actinomyces naeslundii* from sound root surfaces and root carious lesions. Caries Res 1998;32:100–106.

31 Paddick JS, Brailsford SR, Kidd EA, Beighton D: Phenotypic and genotypic selection of microbiota surviving under dental restorations. Appl Environ Microbiol 2005;71:2467–2472.

32 Maltz M, de Oliveira EF, Fontanella V, Bianchi R: A clinical, microbiologic, and radiographic study of deep caries lesions after incomplete caries removal. Quintessence Int 2002;33:151–159.

33 Innes NP, Frencken JE, Bjørndal L, Maltz M, Manton DJ, Ricketts D, van Landuyt K, Banerjee A, Campus G, Domejean S, Fontana M, Leal S, Lo E, Machiulskiene V, Schulte A, Splieth C, Zandona A, Schwendicke F: Managing carious lesions: consensus recommendations on terminology. Adv Dent Res 2016;28:49–57.

34 Lynch E, Beighton D: A comparison of primary root caries lesions classified according to colour. Caries Res 1994;28: 233–239.

35 Fukushima S, Shimizu M, Miura J, Matsuda Y, Kubo M, Hashimoto M, Aoki T, Takeshige F, Araki T: Decrease in fluorescence lifetime by glycation of collagen and its application in determining advanced glycation end-products in human dentin. Biomed Opt Express 2015; 6:1844–1856.

36 Kleter GA: Discoloration of dental carious lesions (a review). Arch Oral Biol 1998;43:629–632.

37 Matsuda Y, Miura J, Shimizu M, Aoki T, Kubo M, Fukushima S, Hashimoto M, Takeshige F, Araki T: Influence of non-enzymatic glycation in dentinal collagen on dental caries. J Dent Res 2016;95: 1528–1534.

38 Black GV: A Work on Operative Dentistry in Two Volumes. Vol. II. The Technical Procedure in Filling Teeth, ed 2. Chicago, Medico-Dental Publishing, 1908.

39 Tomes J: A System of Dental Surgery. London, John Churchill, 1859.

40 Heinrich R, Kneist S, Kunzel W: Clinical controlled study on the treatment of deep carious lesions in deciduous molars (in German). Dtsch Zahnarztl Z 1991;46:581–584.

41 Magnusson BO, Sundell SO: Stepwise excavation of deep carious lesions in primary molars. J Int Assoc Dent Child 1977;8:36–40.

42 Leksell E, Ridell K, Cvek M, Mejare I: Pulp exposure after stepwise versus direct complete excavation of deep carious lesions in young posterior permanent teeth. Endod Dent Traumatol 1996;12: 192–196.

43 Orhan AI, Oz FT, Orhan K: Pulp exposure occurrence and outcomes after 1- or 2-visit indirect pulp therapy vs. complete caries removal in primary and permanent molars. Pediatr Dent 2010; 32:347–355.

44 Hoefler V, Nagaoka H, Miller CS: Long-term survival and vitality outcomes of permanent teeth following deep caries treatment with step-wise and partial-caries-removal: a systematic review. J Dent 2016;54:25–32.

45 Ricketts DN, Kidd EA, Innes N, Clarkson J: Complete or ultraconservative removal of decayed tissue in unfilled teeth. Cochrane Database Syst Rev 2006; 3:CD003808.

46 Schwendicke F, Dorfer CE, Paris S: Incomplete caries removal: a systematic review and meta-analysis. J Dent Res 2013;92:306–314.

47 Schwendicke F, Meyer-Lueckel H, Dorfer C, Paris S: Failure of incompletely excavated teeth – a systematic review. J Dent 2013;41:569–580.

48 Carvalho JC, Dige I, Machiulskiene V, Qvist V, Bakhshandeh A, Fatturi-Parolo C, Maltz M: Occlusal caries: biological approach for its diagnosis and management. Caries Res 2016;50:527–542.

49 Franzon R, Casagrande L, Pinto AS, Garcia-Godoy F, Maltz M, de Araujo FB: Clinical and radiographic evaluation of indirect pulp treatment in primary molars: 36 months follow-up. Am J Dent 2007;20:189–192.

50 Franzon R, Guimaraes LF, Magalhaes CE, Haas AN, Araujo FB: Outcomes of one-step incomplete and complete excavation in primary teeth: a 24-month randomized controlled trial. Caries Res 2014;48:376–383.

51 Innes NP, Ricketts D, Chong LY, Keightley AJ, Lamont T, Santamaria RM: Preformed crowns for decayed primary molar teeth. Cochrane Database Syst Rev 2015;12:CD005512.

52 Innes NP, Evans DJ, Bonifacio CC, Geneser M, Hesse D, Heimer M, Kanellis M, Machiulskiene V, Narbutaite J, Olegario IC, Owais A, Araujo MP, Raggio DP, Splieth C, van Amerongen E, Weber-Gasparoni K, Santamaria RM: The Hall technique 10 years on: questions and answers. Br Dent J 2017;222:478–483.

53 Santamaria RM, Innes NP, Machiulskiene V, Evans DJ, Splieth CH: Caries management strategies for primary molars: 1-year randomized control trial results. J Dent Res 2014;93:1062–1069.

54 Maltz M, Garcia R, Jardim JJ, de Paula LM, Yamaguti PM, Moura MS, Garcia F, Nascimento C, Oliveira A, Mestrinho HD: Randomized trial of partial vs. stepwise caries removal: 3-year follow-up. J Dent Res 2012;91:1026–1031.
55 Brok J, Thorlund K, Gluud C, Wetterslev J: Trial sequential analysis reveals insufficient information size and potentially false positive results in many meta-analyses. J Clin Epidemiol 2008;61:763–769.
56 Wetterslev J, Thorlund K, Brok J, Gluud C: Trial sequential analysis may establish when firm evidence is reached in cumulative meta-analysis. J Clin Epidemiol 2008;61:64–75.
57 Mertz-Fairhurst EJ, Curtis JW Jr, Ergle JW, Rueggeberg FA, Adair SM: Ultraconservative and cariostatic sealed restorations: results at year 10. J Am Dent Assoc 1998;129:55–66.
58 Bjørndal L, Darvann T: A light microscopic study of odontoblastic and nonodontoblastic cells involved in tertiary dentinogenesis in well-defined cavitated carious lesions. Caries Res 1999;33:50–60.

Lars Bjørndal
Section of Cariology and Endodontics, Department of Odontology
Faculty of Health and Medical Sciences, University of Copenhagen
Nørre Allé 20
DK–2200 Copenhagen (Denmark)
E-Mail labj@sund.ku.dk

Schwendicke F, Frencken J, Innes N (eds): Caries Excavation: Evolution of Treating Cavitated Carious Lesions.
Monogr Oral Sci. Basel, Karger, 2018, vol 27, pp 82–91 (DOI: 10.1159/000487838)

Selective Removal of Carious Tissue

David Ricketts[a] · Nicola Innes[b] · Falk Schwendicke[c]

[a] Unit of Restorative Dentistry and [b] School of Dentistry, University of Dundee, Dundee, UK; [c] Operative and Preventive Dentistry, Charité – Universitätsmedizin Berlin, Corporate Member of Freie Universität Berlin, Humboldt-Universität zu Berlin, and Berlin Institute of Health, Berlin, Germany

Abstract

Describing and quantifying how much carious tissue should be removed prior to placing a restoration has been a long-debated issue stretching back as far as G.V. Black's "complete caries removal," now known as non-selective carious tissue removal. Originating in the 1960s and 1970s, from the differentiation between different layers of carious dentine, an outer contaminated ("infected") layer and an inner demineralised ("affected") layer, the former of which needed to be removed during cavity preparation and the latter not, selective carious tissue removal was born. Currently, it is termed selective removal to firm dentine. This chapter describes different selective carious tissue removal techniques (to firm, to leathery, to soft dentine) and how they can be achieved appropriately with conventional and novel techniques. Selective removal to firm dentine is recommended for shallow or moderately deep lesions, while for deep lesions (extending close to the pulp) in teeth with vital pulps, selective removal to soft dentine is recommended to avoid pulpal exposure and to preserve the health of the pulp. Leaving soft carious dentine beneath a restoration does, however, raise certain issues regarding how we truly assess pulpal health, what would other dental practitioners think if the patient moved practice, and how do we monitor such sealed residual caries in the future. These issues will all be discussed in this chapter but should at present not preclude dental practitioners from adopting such a minimally invasive evidence-based approach to carious tissue removal.

Evolution of Caries Tissue Removal

Once a decision has been made to manage a carious lesion operatively, one central question is how to remove carious tissue and then how this can be standardised amongst dental practitioners [1–3]. In an attempt to try and rationalise this central issue it is important to look back at the evolution of carious tissue removal when, over a century ago, G.V. Black [4] wrote in his seminal text of the time the famous words: "Generally when the cavity has been cut to form, no carious dentine will remain." This meant that carious tissue was removed until sound physiological dentine was reached and, for deeper lesions, he wrote that "it is better to expose the pulp of a tooth than to leave it covered only with softened dentine."

Black proposed this approach from a clinical experience standpoint and without the backing of research. Little changed until the 1970s when, using the results of research, Fusayama and coworkers [5, 6] identified 2 distinct zones of carious dentine which could be differentiated with the use of dyes: the inner demineralised (formerly known as "affected") zone and the outer bacterially contaminated (formerly known as "infected") zone. It was recognised that only the outer zone needed to be removed during cavity preparation and that the inner zone, which was often stained but minimally contaminated, resisted excavation (it was firm) and had the potential to remineralise, could be left [7]. This strategy was the starting point of removing carious tissue differently in the central parts of the cavity and the periphery. This action was selective carious tissue removal, in this case to firm dentine, but not termed this at that time. Concurrently, selective removal of carious tissue was also being researched by Massler [8] in the USA, who used the words "infected" and "affected" to term the 2 distinct zones of carious dentine. These 2 words, but particularly the histology-originated word "infected," have had a big influence in the current day erroneous concept of dental caries being an infectious disease and, as a consequence, how carious tissue should be removed.

Risk of Pulpal Exposure and Outcome of Non-Selective Carious Tissue Removal

As described, non-selective ("complete") carious tissue removal as suggested by Black [4] and selective caries removal to firm dentine as suggested by Fusayama and co-workers [5, 6] and Massler [8] both run the risk of pulpal damage or even pulpal exposure in moderate to deep carious lesions which are cavitated (Fig. 1) [9]. The risk of pulpal exposure in deeper lesions was estimated at between 40% (permanent teeth) [10] and 53% (primary teeth) [11]. Once pulpal exposure has occurred, the dental practitioner is faced with the dilemma of how to manage the pulp. Treatment varies between a direct pulp cap, pulpotomy, pulpectomy no, and root canal filling, or even extraction of the tooth, with most preferring the direct pulp cap with calcium hydroxide in symptomless teeth with vital pulps [12]. The reasoning given for this decision is usually ease of use, familiarity, and expected good outcomes. The perceived predictability of the direct pulp cap has mainly been extrapolated from studies which have looked at traumatically exposed teeth where high success rates have been reported [13]. However, following a carious exposure the results are less predictable, with success rates after 3–5 years being as low as 33–37% [13, 14] and after 10 years only 13% [14]. Success rates have been shown to be better in younger patients in teeth with open apices [15] but these will account for only a small proportion of teeth with carious exposures bearing in mind the size of the adult population and caries prevalence. Consequently, we argue for using less invasive alternatives when managing deep lesions. These have been presented as an overview in previous chapters. In this chapter, we will discuss in detail the concept of selective removal of carious tissue.

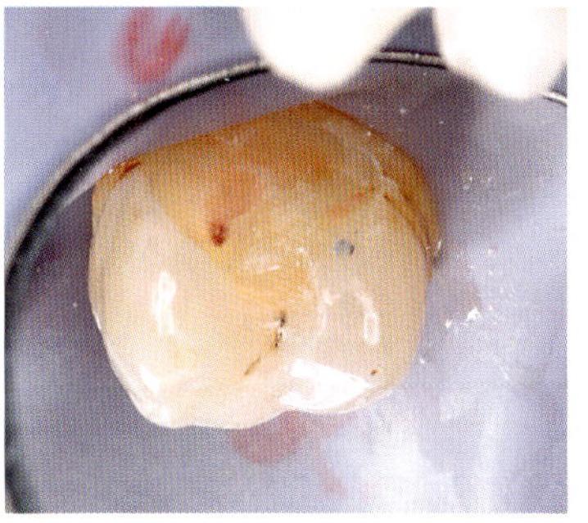

Fig. 1. Non-selective ("complete") carious tissue removal in this deep carious lesion has led to pulpal exposure and a poor long-term prognosis.

Selective Removal to Firm Dentine

Removal of carious tissue in a base of the cavity (overlying the dental pulp) to firm dentine that gives some resistance to an excavator and is more often than not discoloured has been referred to as "selective removal to firm dentine" [3]. This is consistent with the approach advocated by Fusayama and coworkers [5, 6]; removing the outer contaminated dentine and leaving the inner partially demineralised dentine behind (Fig. 2). This approach to carious tissue removal is recommended for central parts of the cavity, while at the cavity periphery carious tissue removal to hard dentine should be performed. Hard dentine feels "scratchy" using a sharp probe. Selective removal to firm dentine is in line with the principles described in the first chapters of this book: to not remove sound or remineralisable tissue, to ensure a good cavity peripheral seal to the restoration, and to achieve optimal restoration longevity. This approach has been advocated for all but deep lesions where pulpal exposure could still occur. Figure 3 shows selective removal to firm dentine, with carious tissue removal to hard (stain free) dentine in the periphery and carious tissue to firm dentine (resistant to a hand excavator) pulpally.

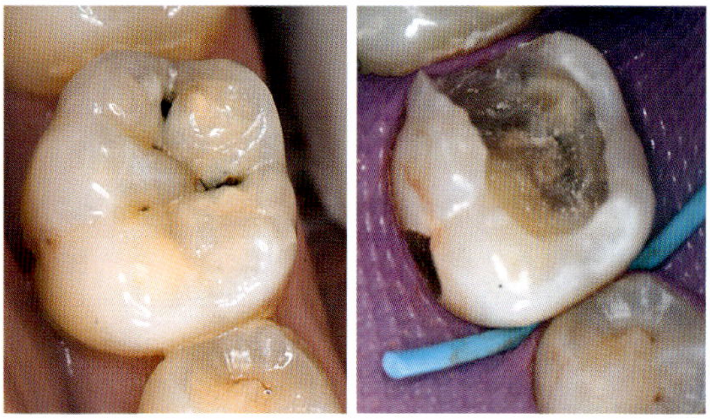

Fig. 2. Tooth 46 shows a deep carious lesion occlusally and distally (left). Carious tissue removal at the periphery of the cavity has been performed until hard dentine remained to achieve a good peripheral seal to the restoration but pulpally there has been selective carious tissue removal to firm dentine (right), i.e., resistant to a hand excavator.

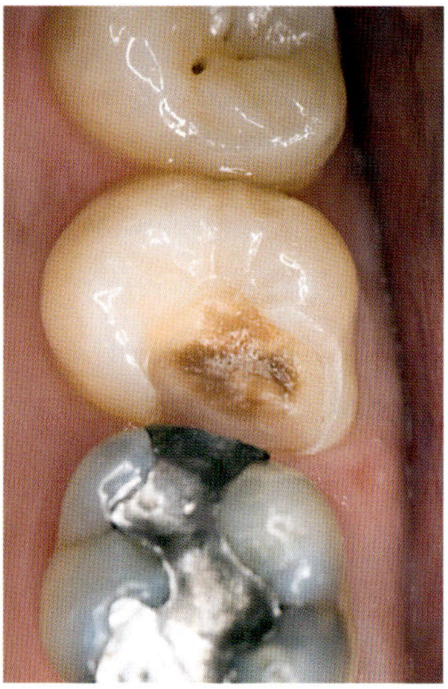

Fig. 3. The upper second molar tooth has undergone peripheral carious tissue removal to hard (stain-free) dentine, whereas pulpally carious tissue removal has been selective to firm, discoloured, and dry dentine caries.

Selective Removal to Soft Dentine

When carious lesions are assessed from a radiograph as penetrating into the pulpal third or quarter of dentine, there is a significant risk of damage or even exposure of the pulp during carious tissue removal, eventually impacting on the long-term prognosis of the entire tooth. In these cases, it is recommended that carious tissue at the periphery of the cavity is, as explained for selective removal to firm dentine, removed to hard, scratchy dentine that will allow a tight hermetic seal to the cavity and restoration, but pulpally soft dentine should be left. This approach is termed selective removal to soft dentine [3]. As described previously, it aims at preserving a healthy pulp whilst allowing a tight seal and a long-lasting restoration.

Figure 4 shows such a case where selective carious tissue removal has been performed, with soft

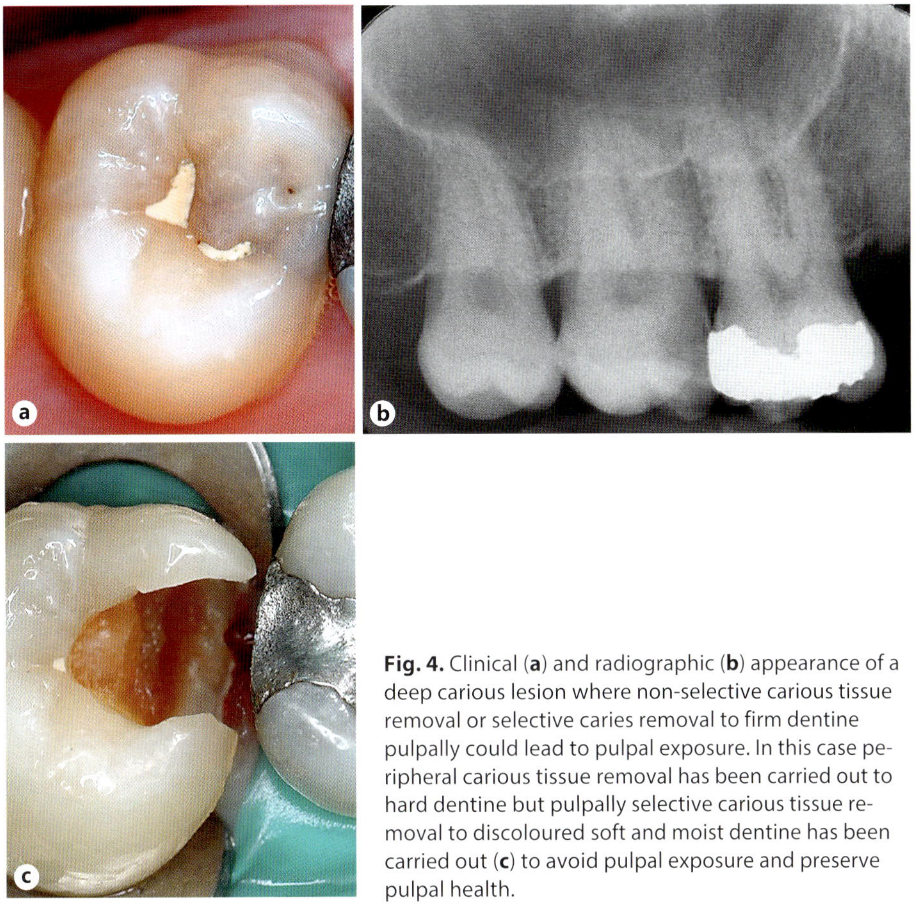

Fig. 4. Clinical (**a**) and radiographic (**b**) appearance of a deep carious lesion where non-selective carious tissue removal or selective caries removal to firm dentine pulpally could lead to pulpal exposure. In this case peripheral carious tissue removal has been carried out to hard dentine but pulpally selective carious tissue removal to discoloured soft and moist dentine has been carried out (**c**) to avoid pulpal exposure and preserve pulpal health.

discoloured dentine remaining pulpally. This dentine is not scratchy or leathery in texture but is soft to the touch with a spoon excavator. It could easily be removed with an excavator and is wet or moist. If pressure were to be applied using a spoon excavator, moisture would ooze from the dentine. Peripherally, the dentine is hard as described.

How to Perform Selective Carious Tissue Removal

Non-selective carious tissue removal to hard, stain, and discolour-free dentine is less subjective than selective removal to firm/soft dentine, where there is little to guide the clinician as to what kind of (histologically characterised) layer of carious dentine is reached. Historically, Sato and Fusayama [5] used a basic fuchsin dye but this liquid fell out of use because of concerns over its carcinogenicity. It has now been replaced with other so-called caries detector dyes, such as 1% acid red in propylene glycol and a range of protein dyes [16]. Dye staining today is rarely used to aid carious tissue removal as it is time consuming with repeated applications and carious tissue removal in gradual stages. In addition, it has subsequently been shown to be neither specific nor sensitive for staining bacterially contaminated dentine in some studies [16]. One study has also shown that when the enamel dentine junction has been clinically rendered to consist of only hard and stain-free dentine, in approximately half of the cases (57%) the dentine will nevertheless stain with a caries detector dye [17]. Subsequent clinical and microbial analysis of such caries detector dye stained and dye stain-free sites at the enamel dentine junction showed that there were only low numbers of recoverable organisms from both sites and that there was no statistically significant difference in the level of organisms at either site [18]. Lastly, and most importantly, caries detector dyes lead to significant risks of pulp exposure and pulp complications. Therefore, caries detector dyes should not be used to dictate carious tissue removal, especially in the pulpal aspect of the cavity: tactile confirmation of the dentine hardness and visual criteria should be used instead.

Other techniques have been investigated to aid in reducing the subjective nature of differentiating the outer contaminated zone of carious dentine from the inner demineralised zone during carious tissue removal. Chemomechanical carious tissue removal with either sodium hypochlorite-based gels (Carisolv) or enzyme-based gels has been described. The sodium hypochlorite-based gels (Carisolv) chlorinate the degraded collagen in the outer zone of caries making removal easier using specifically designed hand instruments, although its specific action is unclear [19, 20]. The enzyme-based gel Papacarie contains papain, chloramine, and toluidine blue, and has antibacterial and anti-inflammatory properties, but its action in facilitating the removal of partially degraded collagen is also unclear [20]. However, both claim to be selective in only removing the outer contaminated zone of carious dentine, leaving the demineralised zone behind. The evidence for the use of chemomechanical carious tissue removal techniques is relatively weak [21], with the main disadvantage being that it can be more time consuming than hand excavation or rotary burrs [7, 21].

In an attempt to make rotary instruments less destructive to tooth tissue, self-limiting polymer burrs have been created. These have been made from medical-grade, glass bead reinforced polymer which are, by the nature of their hardness compared to demineralised dentine, self-limiting in carious tissue removal. They allow removal of the soft carious dentine, but as the demineralised, firm dentine is reached the bur begins to blunt, limiting its destructive nature. The evidence for the use of such burrs is weak and limited; however, preliminary clinical data would suggest that it has potential in being more conservative and selective in carious tissue removal compared to a conventional tungsten carbide burr [22].

Laser fluorescence techniques have long been investigated for the diagnosis of dental carious lesions. One commercially available product, the DIAGNOdent Pen, has been developed based on the detection of bacterial by-products (porphyrins), which fluoresce under a laser light. Whilst primarily developed for caries diagnosis, its use has also been turned to aiding carious tissue removal based on the guiding principle that it will inform the operator whether the carious dentine is heavily bacterially contaminated or not [23]. Compared to carious tissue removal with the aid of a caries detector dye, carious tissue removal aided by the laser fluorescence device may be more conservative and more consistent with tactile evaluation [23]. However, false positive detections (low specificity) are a problem [24, 25] as staining can also lead to fluorescence, which in a carious cavity is an obvious confounding factor. Moreover, the removal of bacteria is not, as described, the most important aim of carious tissue removal and should not be prioritised over maintaining pulp vitality. So far, there is no strong argument to make for fluorescence-aided carious tissue removal.

Attempts at facilitating selective carious tissue removal are commendable. If techniques are to be accepted in clinical practice they have to be efficient (time reducing) as well as effective, and in the future need to be validated against clinically relevant outcomes. It would appear, however, that at present the most efficient and effective way of selectively removing carious dentine would be with the use of a hand excavator [7] or a polymer rotary burr, always comparing against the outlined hardness criteria.

Diagnostic Issues with Selective Carious Tissue Removal to Soft Dentine

When lecturing to dental practitioners on selective carious tissue removal to soft dentine and restoring with a definitive restoration, 3 major themes dominate the discussion. Firstly, how do we truly know that the pulp beneath the sealed carious biomass remains healthy? Secondly, concerns are often expressed over monitoring: what would another dental practitioner think if the patient moved practice and saw residual carious tissue sealed in beneath the restorations placed. Thirdly and finally, what diagnostic techniques are available to monitor the success of sealed soft carious tissue?

Health of Pulp

The guiding principles of carious tissue removal are, as described before, as follows [3]:

- "Preserve non-demineralised and remineralisable tissue;
- Achieve an adequate seal by placing the peripheral restoration onto sound dentine and/or enamel, thus controlling the lesion and inactivating remaining bacteria;
- Avoid discomfort/pain and dental anxiety;
- Maintain pulpal health by preserving residual dentine (avoiding unnecessary pulpal irritation/insult) and preventing pulpal exposure (i.e., leave soft dentine in proximity to the pulp if required)."

Ironically, the concern of dental practitioners is also one of the major guiding principles of appropriate carious tissue management [3]. The problem we have where pulpal health is concerned at the histological level is that it is difficult if not impossible to assess clinically at the chairside for sure. At best, a healthy blood supply to the pulp (pulp vitality) can be assessed through laser Doppler flowmetry and pulse oximetry, and this is often regarded as the "gold standard" against which pulp sensibility tests are compared [26]. As these techniques which assess the blood supply to the tooth are not commercially available for chairside use, the best that can be achieved are surrogates for this, namely assessing neuronal responses in pulp sensibility tests on the assumption that if there is no blood supply, nerves would not survive and respond to such tests. However, sensibility tests are notoriously unreliable alone with false positive and negative responses recognised. Therefore, in clinical practice, it is the overall pain history (or lack of pain) and clinical findings (evidence of peri-radicular pathology, namely tenderness to percussion and/or buccal palpation or presence of a sinus/fistula) together with the sensibility test results which enable the dental practitioner to make a judgement as to the health of the pulp. It is these sequelae to operative procedures in the long term that allow the health of the pulp to be assessed. In studies where selective carious tissue removal to soft dentine has taken place or where carious tissue has been sealed into the tooth with no dentine carious tissue removal, there would appear to be no adverse effects to the pulp based on these assumptions, in the medium to long term [9, 27]. In the absence of a good predictive technology for giving a threshold beyond which a lesion has progressed too far, a radiopaque band of "normal" appearing dentine separating the carious lesion from the dental pulp is often useful as an indicator that it is appropriate to carry out selective carious tissue removal.

Monitoring Carious Lesion Progression

Selective carious tissue removal to soft dentine and placement of a definitive restoration presents the dental practitioner with 2 further dilemmas:

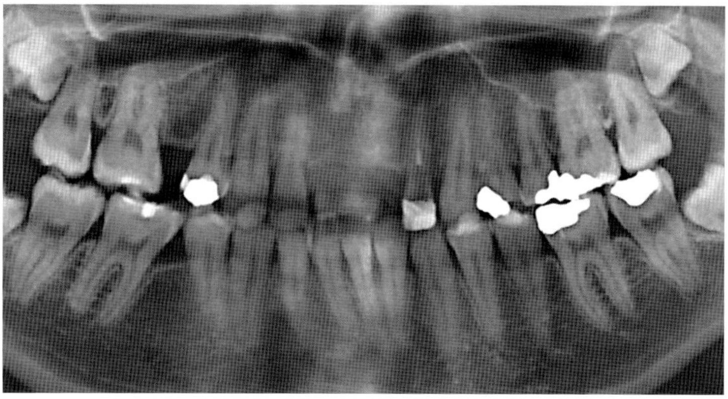

Fig. 5. Dental panoramic tomogram of a young adult patient showing residual sealed soft carious dentine beneath restorations in teeth 14, 24, 25, 26, 36, 37, and 46. Non-selective carious tissue removal to hard dentine or selective carious tissue removal to firm dentine in a number of these teeth would have led to pulpal exposure. Note there is no evidence of peri-radicular pathology in relation to any of these teeth.

from a medico-legal point of view if the patient moves practice, and at recall how to monitor the sealed carious tissue. Figure 5 shows a dental panoramic tomogram of a young adult patient where carious tissue removal to soft dentine has taken place in a number of teeth subsequently restored with amalgam restorations. Whilst the evidence to suggest that the residual carious lesion is unlikely to progress beneath the restorations is strong, surveys of dental practitioners suggest that this sits uncomfortably with them [28–30]. This may be due to various factors, such as when the dental practitioner was trained, with older practitioners sticking to their more traditional education and implementation, local environmental incentives such as remuneration (government-funded schemes or private health insurance schemes sanctioning and restricting many items of treatment), regulatory governance bodies, and fear of litigation for not performing traditional caries removal [31]. In an era when there is great emphasis on clinical governance and the practice of "evidence-based dentistry," involving some of these stakeholders, including educators, may be the first step in breaking down the barriers between the evidence base and implementation [32].

Figure 6 also demonstrates the problem of how such sealed-in carious lesions can be monitored over time. The integrity of the restoration can be assessed clinically with traditional visual and tactile examination and, because carious tissue is excavated to hard dentine at the periphery of the cavity, the marginal integrity of the restoration should not be different to any other restoration placed irrespective of how much carious tissue is removed pulpally [33]. At this juncture, it is important to differentiate between monitoring residual carious lesions sealed in beneath the restoration and new carious lesions developing adjacent to the restoration (traditionally called secondary lesions or recurrent lesions). Whilst traditional and novel diagnostic techniques may perform well in detecting carious lesions adjacent to restorations [34], once sealed, monitoring whether sealed carious lesions have truly arrested and are not progressing is not possible. The only technique available is conventional bitewing radiography and this requires a standardised radiographic technique. However, even this is not straightforward as it relies on the subjective interpretation of consecutive images viewed side by side. One novel technique which may overcome this in the future is subtraction radiography, which has been shown to improve the certitude with which dentists can say whether demineralisation is continuing or not on occlusal and proximal surfaces and beneath restorations [35–37].

Take the series of bitewing radiographs in Figure 6, which were taken of the same child between

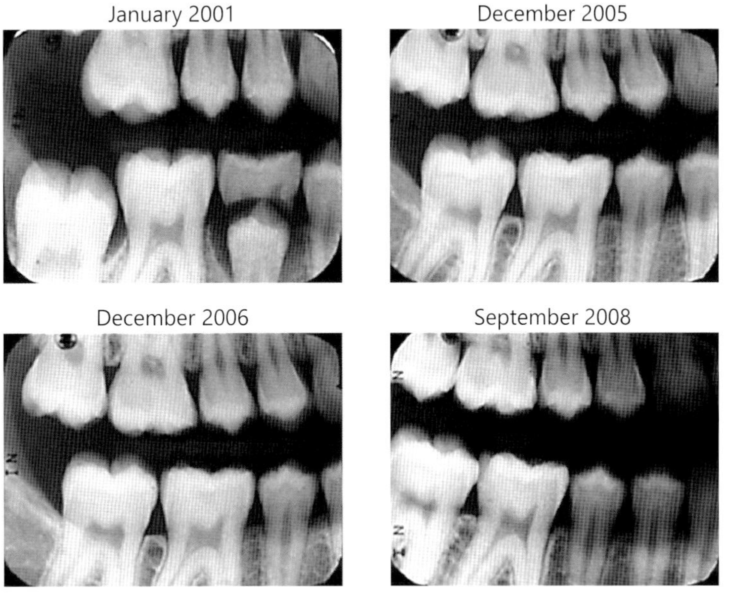

Fig. 6. Series of bitewing radiographs taken of a child showing an occlusal carious lesion in the lower right first molar tooth (tooth 46) between 2001 and 2008.

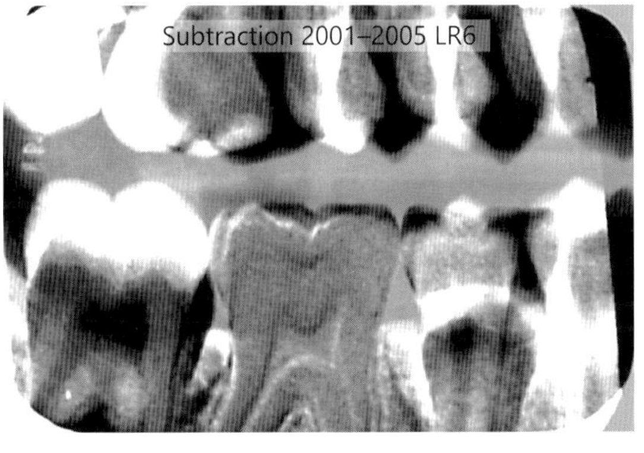

Fig. 7. Subtraction image of tooth 46 comparing 2001 and 2005 images clearly shows net mineral loss and a dark shadow (the lesion has progressed).

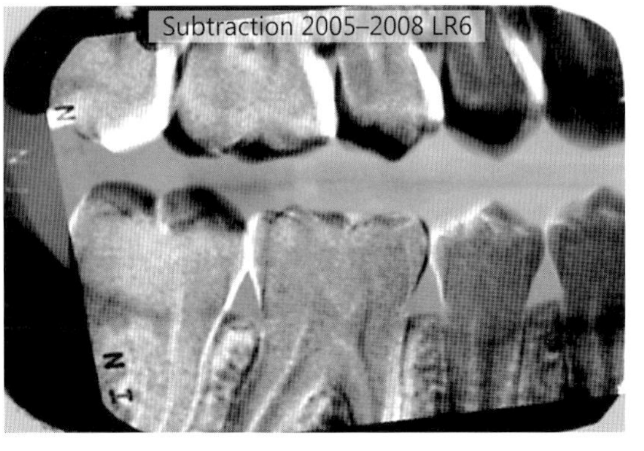

Fig. 8. Subtraction image of tooth 46 comparing 2005 and 2008 images clearly shows no net mineral loss and no dark shadow (the lesion has not progressed).

2001 and 2008. In 2001, there was a suggestion of an occlusal radiolucency in relation to tooth 46, however, it is difficult for sure to know whether it is getting worse in the 2005, 2006, and 2008 images. Between 2001 and 2005 a subtraction image (Fig. 7) clearly shows net mineral loss as a dark shadow and without doubt the lesion was progressing. Tooth 46 was fissure sealed in 2005. Subsequent follow-up in 2006 and 2008 was perhaps more difficult to interpret and determine with a degree of certitude whether the sealed lesion was progressing or not. The subtraction image that resulted from comparing the 2005 and 2008 image (Fig. 8) shows no shadow on the occlusal surface and demonstrated with a degree of certainty that the lesion has now arrested beneath the sealant.

Improvement in monitoring sealed soft carious tissue in the future with radiographs and perhaps techniques such as subtraction radiography may further break down the barriers in implementing the evidence base presented throughout this chapter. Issues related to restoring a cavity that has been cleaned to firm or soft dentine are presented in the chapter by Göstemeyer et al. [this vol., pp. 42–55].

Conclusion

During carious tissue removal, dental practitioners should "preserve non-demineralised and remineralisable tissue," "achieve an adequate seal by placing the peripheral restoration onto sound dentine and/or enamel," "avoid discomfort/pain and dental anxiety," and "maintain pulpal health by preserving residual dentine and preventing pulp exposure." This can be achieved through the evidence-based selective carious tissue removal approaches described in this chapter. For shallow to moderately deep lesions, dentists should perform selective carious tissue removal to firm dentine, while for deep lesions in teeth with vital pulps, selective removal to soft dentine should be performed. Whilst it is acknowledged that there are opponents to such strategies and that there are potential issues on monitoring pulpal health, carious lesion activity beneath a restoration, and restoration integrity, the need to preserve a vital pulp and the long-term health and prognosis of the tooth are of greater concern. These latter arguments should lead dental practitioners to implement more selective and conservative evidence-based carious tissue removal techniques.

References

1 Kidd EA: How "clean" must a cavity be before restoration? Caries Res 2004;38:305–313.

2 Innes NP, Frencken JE, Bjørndal L, Maltz M, Manton DJ, Ricketts D, Van Landuyt K, Banerjee A, Campus G, Doméjean S, Fontana M, Leal S, Lo E, Machiulskiene V, Schulte A, Splieth C, Zandona A, Schwendicke F: Managing carious lesions: consensus recommendations on terminology. Adv Dent Res 2016;28:49–57.

3 Schwendicke F, Frencken JE, Bjørndal L, Maltz M, Manton DJ, Ricketts D, van Landuyt K, Banerjee A, Campus G, Doméjean S, Fontana M, Leal S, Lo E, Machiulskiene V, Schulte A, Splieth C, Zandona AF, Innes NP: Managing carious lesions: consensus recommendations on carious tissue removal. Adv Dent Res 2016;28:58–67.

4 Black GV: The Technical Procedures in Filling Teeth. A Work on Operative Dentistry. Chicago, Medico-Dental Publishing, 1908, vol 2.

5 Sato Y, Fusayama T: Removal of dentin by fuchsin staining. J Dent Res 1976;55:678–683.

6 Kuboki Y, Liu CF, Fusayama T: Mechanism of differential staining in carious dentin. J Dent Res 1983;62:713–714.

7 Banerjee A, Kidd EA, Watson TF: In vitro evaluation of five alternative methods of carious dentine excavation. Caries Res 2000;34:144–150.

8 Massler M: Pulpal reactions to dental caries. Int Dent J 1967;17:441–460.

9 Ricketts D, Lamont T, Innes NP, Kidd E, Clarkson JE: Operative caries management in adults and children. Cochrane Database Syst Rev 2013;3:CD003808.

10 Leksell E, Ridell K, Cvek M, Mejàre I: Pulp exposure after stepwise versus direct complete excavation of deep carious lesions in young posterior permanent teeth. Endod Dent Traumatol 1996;12:192–196.

11 Magnusson BO, Sundell SO: Stepwise excavation of deep carious lesions in primary molars. J Int Assoc Dent Child 1977;8:36–40.

12 Stangvaltaite L, Schwendicke F, Holmgren C, Finet M, Maltz M, Elhennawy K, Kerosuo E, Doméjean S: Management of pulps exposed during carious tissue removal in adults: a multi-national questionnaire-based survey. Clin Oral Investig 2017;21:2303–2309.

13 Al-Hiyasat AS, Barrieshi-Nusair KM, Al-Omari MA: The radiographic outcomes of direct pulp-capping procedures performed by dental students: a retrospective study. J Am Dent Assoc 2006;137:1699–1705.

14 Barthel CR, Rosenkranz B, Leuenberg A, Roulet JF: Pulp capping of carious exposures: treatment outcome after 5 and 10 years: a retrospective study. J Endod 2000;26:525–528.

15 Aguilar P, Linsuwanont P: Vital pulp therapy in vital permanent teeth with cariously exposed pulp: a systematic review. J Endod 2011;37:581–587.

16 McComb D: Caries-detector dyes – how accurate and useful are they? J Can Dent Assoc 2000;66:195–198.

17 Kidd EA, Joyston-Bechal S, Smith MM, Allan R, Howe L, Smith SR: The use of a caries detector dye in cavity preparation. Br Dent J 1989;167:132–134.
18 Kidd EA, Joyston-Bechal S, Beighton D: The use of a caries detector dye during cavity preparation: a microbiological assessment. Br Dent J 1993;174:245–248.
19 Kathuria V, Ankola AV, Hebbal M, Mocherla M: Carisolv – an innovative method of caries removal. J Clin Diagn Res 2013;7:3111–3115.
20 Hamama H, Yiu C, Burrow M: Current update of chemomechanical caries removal methods. Aust Dent J 2014;59: 446–456.
21 Hamama HH, Yiu CK, Burrow MF, King NM: Systematic review and meta-analysis of randomized clinical trials on chemomechanical caries removal. Oper Dent 2015;40:E167–E178.
22 Prabhakar A, Kiran NK: Clinical evaluation of polyamide polymer burs for selective carious dentin removal. J Contemp Dent Pract 2009;10:26–34.
23 Akbari M, Ahrari F, Jafari M: A comparative evaluation of DIAGNOdent and caries detector dye in detection of residual caries in prepared cavities. J Contemp Dent Pract 2012;13:515–520.
24 Bader JD, Shugars DA: A systematic review of the performance of a laser fluorescence device for detecting caries. J Am Dent Assoc 2004;135:1413–1426.
25 Gimenez T, Braga MM, Raggio DP, Deery C, Ricketts DN, Mendes FM: Fluorescence-based methods for detecting caries lesions: systematic review, meta-analysis and sources of heterogeneity. PLoS One 2013;8:e60421.
26 Alghaithy RA, Qualtrough AJ: Pulp sensibility and vitality tests for diagnosing pulpal health in permanent teeth: a critical review. Int Endod J 2017;50:135–142.
27 Schwendicke F, Dörfer CE, Paris S: Incomplete caries removal: a systematic review and meta-analysis. J Dent Res 2013;92:306–314.
28 Oen KT, Thompson VP, Vena D, Caufield PW, Curro F, Dasanayake A, Ship JA, Lindblad A: Attitudes and expectations of treating deep caries: a PEARL Network survey. Gen Dent 2007;55:197–203.
29 Weber CM, Alves LS, Maltz M: Treatment decisions for deep carious lesions in the Public Health Service in Southern Brazil. J Public Health Dent 2011;71: 265–270.
30 Schwendicke F, Meyer-Lueckel H, Dörfer C, Paris S: Attitudes and behaviour regarding deep dentin caries removal: a survey among German dentists. Caries Res 2013;47:566–573.
31 Schwendicke F, Göstemeyer G: Understanding dentists' management of deep carious lesions in permanent teeth: a systematic review and meta-analysis. Implement Sci 2016;11:142.
32 Schwendicke F, Doméjean S, Ricketts D, Peters M: Managing caries: the need to close the gap between the evidence base and current practice. Br Dent J 2015; 219:433–438.
33 Schwendicke F, Kern M, Blunck U, Dörfer C, Drenck J, Paris S: Marginal integrity and secondary caries of selectively excavated teeth in vitro. J Dent 2014;42: 1261–1268.
34 Brouwer F, Askar H, Paris S, Schwendicke F: Detecting secondary caries lesions: a systematic review and meta-analysis. J Dent Res 2016;95:143–151.
35 Wenzel A, Halse A: Digital subtraction radiography after stannous fluoride treatment for occlusal caries diagnosis. Oral Surg Oral Med Oral Pathol 1992;74: 824–828.
36 Ricketts DN, Ekstrand KR, Martignon S, Ellwood R, Alatsaris M, Nugent Z: Accuracy and reproducibility of conventional radiographic assessment and subtraction radiography in detecting demineralization in occlusal surfaces. Caries Res 2007;41:121–128.
37 Martignon S, Ekstrand KR, Gomez J, Lara JS, Cortes A: Infiltrating/sealing proximal caries lesions: a 3-year randomized clinical trial. J Dent Res 2012; 91:288–292.

David Ricketts
Unit of Restorative Dentistry, Dundee Dental Hospital and School
University of Dundee
2 Park Place
Dundee DD1 4HR (UK)
E-Mail d.n.j.ricketts@dundee.ac.uk

Schwendicke F, Frencken J, Innes N (eds): Caries Excavation: Evolution of Treating Cavitated Carious Lesions.
Monogr Oral Sci. Basel, Karger, 2018, vol 27, pp 92–102 (DOI: 10.1159/000487836)

Atraumatic Restorative Treatment: Restorative Component

Soraya Leal[a] · Clarissa Bonifacio[c] · Daniela Raggio[b] · Jo Frencken[d]

[a]Department of Dentistry, Faculty of Health Sciences, Universidade de Brasília, Brasília, [b]Department of Orthodontics and Pediatric Dentistry, School of Dentistry, University of São Paulo, São Paulo, Brazil; [c]Department of Conservative Dentistry, Academic Centre for Dentistry Amsterdam – ACTA, Amsterdam, [d]Department of Oral Function and Prosthetic Dentistry, College of Dental Sciences, Radboud University Medical Center, Nijmegen, The Netherlands

Abstract

Atraumatic restorative treatment (ART) is a method of managing dental caries based on 2 pillars: sealants for preventing carious lesions in pits and fissures, and restorations for cavitated dentine carious lesions. ART uses only hand instruments for opening/enlarging the cavity and for removing carious tissue. The amount of carious tissue that should be removed depends mainly on the cavity depth. In cavities of shallow and medium depth, carious tissue is removed up to firm dentine. In deep/very deep cavities, in which there is no sign of pulp exposure, pulp inflammation and/or history of spontaneous pain, some soft dentine can be left in the pulpal floor/wall with the aim of avoiding pulp exposure. The ART restorative method is indicated for treating single-surface cavities in primary and permanent teeth, and in multiple-surface cavities in primary teeth. Insufficient information is available to conclude on its use for treating multiple-surface cavities in permanent teeth.

The aim of this chapter is to present how the atraumatic restorative treatment (ART) method came into existence, how carious tissue removal is performed using it, and its indications, contraindications, and limitations for restoring tooth cavities. Finally, survival results of ART restorations are provided.

ART was developed in the mid-1980s in response to the unavailability of restorative care for populations with limited resources, where the presence of cavitated lesions frequently led to tooth extractions [1]. On the basis of the principles of the minimum intervention dentistry (MID) concept, the ART method has evolved into a caries management concept for global use. The main goal of ART is to prevent carious lesion development through fissure sealing and to stop its progression through restoring cavitated lesions. The restorative care is performed using hand instruments only and the cavity is filled with an adhesive material, usually a high-viscosity glass-ionomer cement (HVGIC) [1].

Treatment according to ART is always combined with a caries preventive program. The aim of this program is to teach patients the importance of disorganising biofilm from the tooth surfaces regularly and help them in choosing healthy food habits with the intention to shift them from a potentially high risk of caries to a low-risk level. This shift will reduce the number of tooth extractions and increases the number of sound and restored teeth. Although the focus in this chapter is directed towards the restorative part of the ART method, the importance of ART sealants should be highlighted. According to the ART method, fissures that are at high risk of developing a carious lesion and those that have already developed an enamel carious lesion are indications for placing a sealant [2].

The ART method was developed by Dr. Jo Frencken when he was employed at the Dental School in Dar-es-Salaam, Tanzania. In the rural and (sub-) urban areas of Tanzania, decayed teeth were mostly extracted. It was a challenge to provide conventional dental care in the country due to the lack of resources such as electricity, piped water, and finances. The available dental equipment was limited and unreliable. In contrast, hand instruments were available in sufficient numbers. Many cavities were large enough to be cleaned with excavators, which made the need for drilling machines not always necessary. In such underserved communities, the efforts of using mobile dental units with mobile drilling and suction equipment, portable dental chairs, and generators were too expensive, impractical, difficult to maintain, and economically unsustainable [3–5]. Conceived for use in underserved communities, the ART method has widened its indications over the years. These days, the ART method is standard practice in modern dental clinics in many countries and is especially indicative for uncooperative patients, the elderly, and special needs patients [6–9].

In 1986, the results of a pilot study on ART restorations were presented for the first time in a scientific meeting of the Tanzanian Dental Association. In the early 1990s, a randomised control trial comparing ART restorations using a medium-viscosity glass-ionomer cement (GIC) as the filling material with the conventional treatment using amalgam was conducted in permanent and primary teeth. The better than expected survival percentage of 93 for single-surface medium-viscosity ART restorations in permanent teeth at 1 year caught the attention of many public oral health individuals [10]. In 1994, ART was adopted by the World Health Organisation (WHO) and in 2002 by the Word Dental Federation (FDI).

The introduction of ART also challenged some cariology concepts, such as the need for complete removal of affected dentine and that of stepwise excavation [11], and the exclusive use of hand instruments [12]. Studies have shown hand instruments to be more effective and efficient for removing carious tissue in dentine cavitated lesions than rotary instruments. Another advantage is that its use is less likely to lead to over-preparation of the cavity [13–15]. Therefore, ART-prepared cavities are kept as small as necessary [15]. The procedure follows the principles of the MID concept. Because only the "infected" (soft) carious tissue is removed, local anesthesia is seldom required and dental anxiety in children is reduced [16–19]. In this way, ART is not only less traumatic to the patient [16], but also to the tooth structures [13, 14], and is therefore considered a patient-friendly approach [2, 3].

Overall, ART restorations are placed into cavities that are cleaned with hand instruments and restored with a HVGIC that not only fills the cavities, but also seals the pits and fissures adjacent to it. Similarly, ART sealants are placed by pushing HVGIC into the pits and fissures under finger pressure [2].

Indications and Contra-Indications of ART Restorations

In this section, the indications and contra-indications for producing ART restorations are presented in relation to the setting where the dental professional is working, the patients' age and profile, and type of cavities.

Setting

At the beginning of the development of the ART method, the indication for placing an ART restoration was restricted to teeth with dentine cavities in communities where other treatment was unavailable. A few years later, after results of the first clinical studies had been published, the indication for using ART changed. The ART method was considered an "alternative" treatment that could be used in populations not receiving preventive and restorative care [20].

Following the demonstrated success of ART sealants and ART restorations over the years, strong evidence of its quality exists, which has been derived from well-designed randomised control trials, extending the indication for ART to more economically prosperous countries with no shortages in terms of equipment, materials, and related resources. The extension of the indications for ART was a result of research that showed it to be a high-quality treatment option that can be applied, regardless of an individual's economic or social situation, and which showed its effectiveness to be no different to comparable conventional treatments (see Survival of ART Restorations, below).

Patient Age and Profile

As mentioned before, one extremely important aspect related to the ART method is its patient-friendly nature, which positively impacts on preventing children from becoming dentally anxious and on treating already anxious children and adults.

ART allows the treatment of children, even the very young (under 3 years old) [21, 22], adolescents, adults, and the elderly [23]. In addition, special needs patients (physically or mentally impaired) and institutionalised people can benefit from ART [24]. Information is emerging that ART may reduce the need for restorative treatment under general anaesthesia and that the method is cost-effective [25, 26].

Cavities

The correct choice of cavities to be restored using only hand instruments for opening and removing carious dentine can be a challenge. The lesion depth and pulp condition will be discussed in more details in the next section. These conditions are as essential for the success of ART restorations as they are for conventionally placed restorations.

ART restorations are indicated for single-surface cavities in primary and permanent teeth [27–29] and, in our opinion on the basis of solid evidence, should be considered the first choice of treatment for this type of cavity. The performance of ART restorations in multiple-surface cavities in primary teeth is no different from that of comparable conventionally produced amalgam and resin composite restorations, and ART is therefore also indicated for this type of cavity [27, 30]. Insufficient information exists on the level of quality of multiple-surface ART restorations in permanent teeth. Survival results of ART restorations are presented at the end of this chapter.

Caries Tissue Removal in the ART Method

The ART method differs from the traditional way of managing dentine carious lesions as both cavity opening and carious tissue removal are performed exclusively by hand instruments. The non-use of burrs, undoubtedly, represented a paradigm shift in the 1980s, just as the advent of mechanical rotary instruments in the 1880s was, at that time, a revolution in cavity preparation [31]. The use of a burr became essential in dentistry because adequate cavity design and preparation were mandatory requirements for performing high-quality amalgam restorations, the most common direct restorative material for posterior teeth prior to the appearance of composites [32]. However, with the onset and development of adhesive restorative materials, "cavity preparation" has acquired a new meaning. The creation of retention grooves was no longer needed, which meant that a cavity did not need to be prepared, but, instead, properly cleaned before restoration.

Understanding this concept, in combination with better understanding of the dental caries process itself, was crucial for the development of the ART method. Two other important aspects related to this development need to be discussed:

- the amount of carious tissue that needs to be removed before a cavity is ready for the placement of an ART restoration, and
- whether hand instruments are effective at removing carious tissue before placing an ART restoration.

In discussing the first aspect, 2 variables should be considered: "the restorative material" and "the cavity depth." With respect to the second aspect, it is important to understand what happens with bacteria that are left behind in the carious dentine tissue that remains. This is an important aspect in cariology and restorative dentistry as many dentists are not convinced that a tooth cavity in which not all carious tissue is removed can be restored [33]. However, the literature has shown that bacteria become inactivated when properly sealed in the cavity even when no dentine carious tissue removal is performed [34]. This has also been observed for the ART method. The reduction in total volume count per milligram of anaerobic and aerobic microorganisms in "affected" dentine in ART-prepared cavities was 22 and 24%, respectively, in an in vivo experiment of 7 days [35]. The overall conclusion about leaving bacteria inside a cavity is that selective carious removal prior to a well-sealed restoration will always arrest the carious lesion [36]. Ensuring an adequate seal increases the likelihood that the arrestment of the carious lesion will remain in the long term.

Restorative Material in the ART Approach: GICs

Originally, all adhesive restorative materials, including resin composites, were considered appropriate for use with the ART method. However, almost all studies in which the ART approach was tested opted to use chemically activated GIC for both ART sealants and ART restorations.

The choice for this category of GIC was based on some material advantages at the time ART was developed. The absence of the need to use electricity for curing GIC was an important reason for its use as there was no electricity power in the rural areas where ART was pioneered. Since then, conventional GICs have evolved greatly, mainly with respect to their mechanical properties. The emerging HVGIC led to excellent survival percentages of single-surface ART restorations (as discussed below).

Basically, conventional/high-viscosity GICs chemically bind to dentine and enamel, forming an acid-resistant interface [37]. This process involves ionic bonds between the carboxylate groups on the polyacid molecules and calcium ions in the tooth structure [38]. Therefore, it is essential that when carrying out ART and cleaning a cavity for the restoration, a sound margin of dentine and enamel is created to guarantee an excellent bond between the cavity and the GIC, ensuring a proper sealing of the restoration margins (Fig. 1).

Cavity Depth

Cavitated dentine carious lesions and those lesions that can be accessed by means of hand instruments without a history of spontaneous pain and/or pulp involvement are, potentially, cavities suitable to receive an ART restoration. In terms of carious tissue removal, the amount of tissue that needs to be excavated is directly related to the cavity depth, varying from selective carious removal to firm dentine pulpally (shallow/medium-sized cavities) to selective to soft dentine (deep cavities).

An overview paper on ART published more than 20 years ago reported that the process of

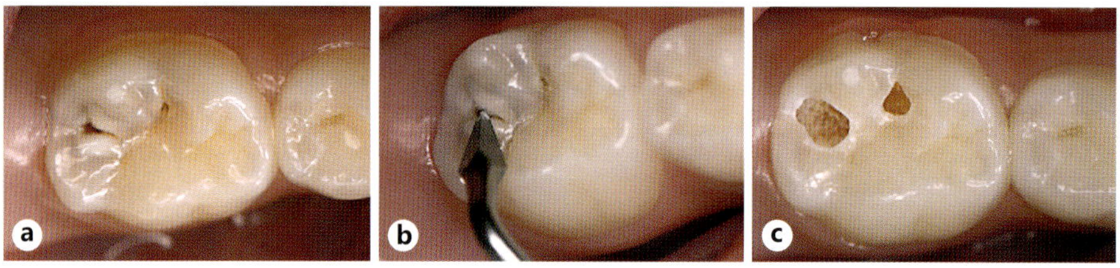

Fig. 1. a Primary molar with a cavitated dentine lesion with a small opening. **b** The opener being used to enlarge the cavity access. **c** The same cavity after being cleaned with hand excavators.

cleaning the cavity entailed the removal of decalcified (infected) dentine while the affected dentine was to be preserved (at that time called partial caries removal) [1]. This strategy was already proposed by Massler [39] and Fusayama et al. [40], who suggested that the soft infected dentine needed to be removed and the harder, affected dentine be retained as it could be remineralised [41]. The innovative aspect of the ART method is related to the fact that all procedures were to be performed using hand instruments only.

The main problem with this concept is the impossibility of clinically defining whether all infected dentine is removed. Therefore, a link between the histological aspects of carious dentine lesions and their clinical features was made, which determined necrotic and contaminated zones as clinically soft dentine and the demineralised tissue as leathery to firm dentine [42]. Thus, using hand instruments, practitioners are able to feel the level of hardness of the dentine and select what needs to be removed and what should remain. This procedure makes the term selective caries tissue removal more appropriate than partial caries removal that was used in the past.

Considering these points, 3 situations can be expected when cleaning a cavity that is indicated to receive an ART restoration:

(a) Shallow to medium deep cavities – in such cavities, the aim is to selectively remove carious tissue to firm dentine pulpally and to firm/hard dentine coronally (Fig. 2). This procedure facilitates a sufficiently large bonding area and does not cause a risk of pulp exposure. However, to be able to achieve this goal it is mandatory to work with sharp excavators as a blunt excavator will leave too much soft dentine behind which may negatively affect the adhesion of the HVGIC to the cavity walls, compromising a good seal at the restoration's margins.

(b) Deep cavities – in order to avoid pulp exposure in vital and symptomless teeth, soft tissue is left on the floor of the cavity (Fig. 3). This approach has been shown to significantly reduce the need for endodontic treatment [43]. However, it is important to highlight that, independently of the restorative procedure (ART or conventional), a very careful tooth history should be elicited, which must collect information about the history of pain/fistula/abscess. Whenever possible, the clinical examination should be accompanied with a radiograph of the tooth. However, this is not always possible, especially when ART is being applied in field conditions. Therefore, the patient should be informed about the risks of a misdiagnosis. Another aspect that merits consideration is that the soft dentine should remain at the floor of the cavity and certainly in the area where there is a risk of exposure, meaning that all the surrounding walls need to be cleaned to firm/hard dentine, which will ensure a proper cavity sealing that is crucial to the success of the treatment.

(c) Cavities with a small opening – it is necessary to widen the entrance of a lesion in which the smallest excavator cannot get inside the cavity.

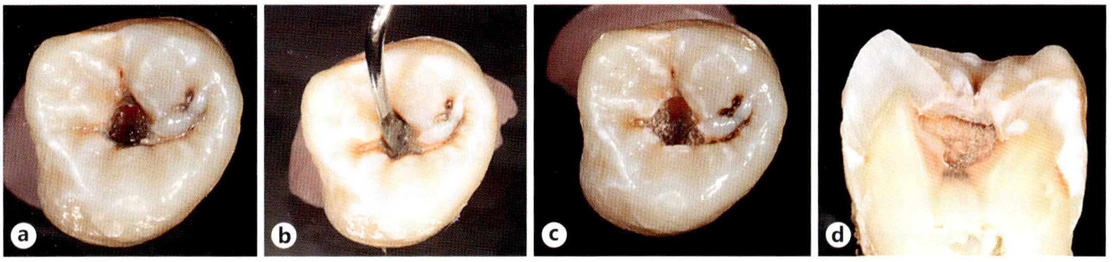

Fig. 2. a Cavitated carious lesion of medium depth in a second permanent molar. **b** The excavator is inserted into the cavity. **c** The cavity after being cleaned with hand instruments only. **d** The tooth was sectioned to show the walls after carious removal up to firm dentine.

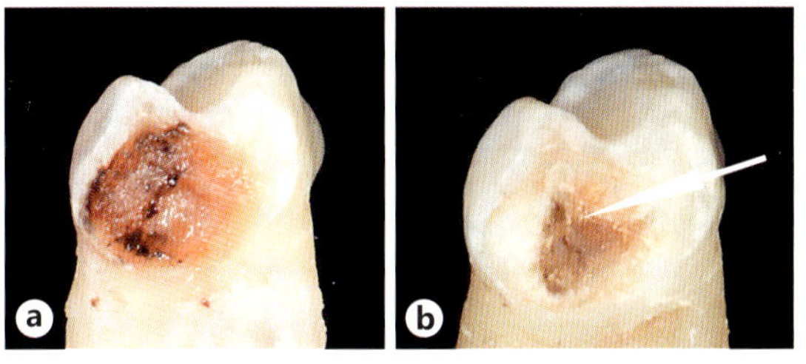

Fig. 3. a A primary tooth presenting a very deep cavitated dentine carious lesion. **b** The same tooth after carious tissue removal performed exclusively with hand excavators. It should be noted that the surrounding walls and the enamel-dentine junction was cleaned up to hard dentine, however, some soft tissue was left at the pulp wall to avoid pulp exposure (arrow).

Small is determined by the working end of a small excavator (Ø = 0.9 mm). If the excavator can enter the cavity, then it is likely that the cavity opening can be widened. If it is not possible, a treatment other than the ART method needs to be employed. Two studies have investigated the effect of using the small excavator as a measuring stick. In an adolescent population in Zimbabwe, with a dentine carious lesion prevalence of 41% and a mean DMFT score of 1.1, it was possible to treat 84% of the dentine carious lesions using hand instruments [44]. A similar result was reported for a group of adolescents from Egypt that had a dentine carious lesion prevalence of 38%. In total, 78% of the dentine carious lesions detected in this study could be treated according to the ART method [45]. An in vitro study concluded that the cavity opening needs to have a diameter of 1.6 mm to facilitate the proper removal of decomposed dentine [46].

In cases where a small excavator cannot enter the cavity, either the practitioner uses the burr to access the cavity or, in field conditions, the cavity can be sealed. If the burr is used, the procedure is no longer ART. Although consensus on sealing such smaller cavities has not been reached, there are some studies that show that this approach can arrest those lesions [47, 48]. In order to attempt widening the cavity entrance, a sharp instrument (hatchet or an ART opener) should be placed in the small cavity opening and rotated backwards and forwards (Fig. 4) to break unsupported enamel and/or crumbling demineralised enamel. When the cavity opening is wide enough, the excavator can be placed into the cavity to properly remove carious tissue to firm/leathery or soft dentine at the pulp wall depending on the cavity depth.

The Use of Hand Instruments

MID is a philosophy that aims to keep the teeth healthy and functional for life [49]. In terms of dental caries, the preservation of sound tooth structure is essential within the MID concept, meaning that over-preparation of cavities by removing sound enamel and remineralisable dentine should be avoided.

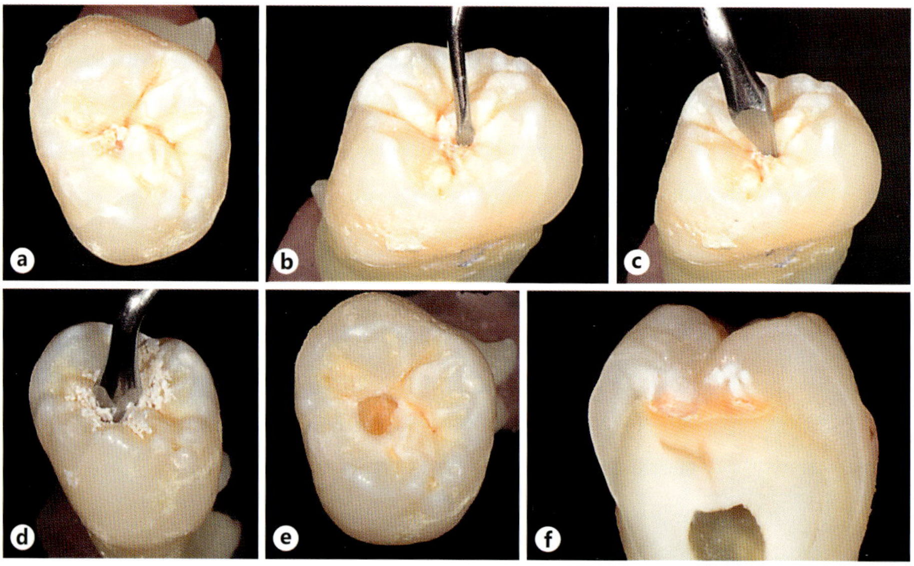

Fig. 4. a Small cavitated dentine carious lesion on the occlusal surface. **b** The smallest excavator is not able to penetrate into the cavity. **c** The opener in position to enlarge the cavity opening. **d** The opener is rotated backwards and forwards. Observe the crumbled enamel on the cavity borders. **e** The cavity after being cleaned. **f** The tooth was sectioned and it is possible to observe a very conservative cavity in which carious dentine was removed up to hard dentine (most likely because the dentine tissue was dry). In future, such a lesion may just be sealed.

In vitro studies using extracted permanent and primary teeth in which different methods for dentine carious removal were compared showed that hand excavation was the best combination of efficiency and effectiveness for carious dentine tissue removal [13, 50]. This shows that the ART approach is a good example of current day cariology in line with the most conservative methods for cleaning a cavity.

Survival of ART Restorations

Criteria to Evaluate ART Restorations

ART restorations have been assessed using the modified Ryge criteria (United States Public Health Services; USPHS), World Dental Association (FDI) criteria [51], and ART restoration criteria. Table 1 presents the ART restoration criteria that have been in use since the start of the ART study in Syria in 1996 [52]. The main difference between the USPHS and the ART restoration criteria concerns the depth of the marginal gap at the interface of the restoration and the tooth. The USPHS criteria have a code that fails a restoration only when a marginal gap exposes dentine, while the comparable ART restoration criteria code considers even a marginal gap of 0.5 mm to have failed. This difference in interpretation of a marginal gap can lead to substantial differences in survival percentages. It is, therefore, likely that the ART restoration criteria are more stringent than the USPHS criteria in long-term studies and lead to lower survival percentages.

Survival of Single- and Multiple-Surface ART/HVGIC Restorations in Primary and Permanent Posterior Teeth by Year of Survival

A meta-analysis that included study data up to February 1, 2017, has calculated the survival

Table 1. ART restoration criteria

Code	Description
0	Present, satisfactory
1	Present, slight deficiency at cavity margin of less than 0.5 mm[1]
2	Present, deficiency at cavity margin of 0.5 mm or more[1]
3	Present, fracture in restoration
4	Present, fracture in tooth
5	Present, overextension of approximal margin of 0.5 mm or more[1]
6	Not present, most or all of restoration missing
7	Not present, other restorative treatment performed
8	Not present, tooth is not present
9	Unable to diagnose
C	Caries present

Using this scoring system, restorations that have survived are indicated by codes 1 and 2. Restoration failure was indicated by codes 3–7 and C in the early years, and more recently by codes 2–6 and C. Code 7 is censored in the latter survival calculations. The codes remaining were censored.
[1] As assessed using the 0.5-mm ball-end of a metal CPI probe.

Table 2. Survival percentages and standard errors of single- and multiple-surface ART/HVGIC restorations in primary and permanent posterior teeth by year of survival [53]

	Year of survival				
	1	2	3	4	5
Primary dentition					
Single	95.2 (1.0)	93.0 (1.2)	85.0 (5.7)		
Multiple	79.7 (2.8)	65.4 (3.9)	49.0 (12.4)		
Permanent dentition					
Single	95.9 (0.9)	92.6 (1.4)	87.1 (3.2)	85.7 (3.2)	79.6 (1.7)
Multiple	92.7 (2.8)	78.2 (11.7)	90.3 (5.5)	–	77.0 (9.0)

Data are presented as % (SE). ART, atraumatic restorative treatment; HVGIC, high-viscosity glass-ionomer cement.

percentages of ART/HVGIC restorations in primary and permanent teeth [53]. The survival percentages for single- and multiple-surface ART/HVGIC restorations in primary posterior teeth were based on 19 and 18 studies, respectively. The weighted mean annual failure rates of single- and multiple-surface ART/HVGIC restorations in primary molars over the first 3 years were 5 and 17%, respectively (Table 2).

A total of 23 and 5 studies were included in the meta-analysis on ART/HVGIC single- and multiple-surface restorations in permanent posterior teeth, respectively (Table 2). The weighted mean annual failure rate of single-surface ART/HVGIC restorations in permanent posterior teeth over the first 5 years was 4.1%. The weighted mean annual failure rate of multi-surface ART/HVGIC restorations in permanent posterior teeth was 2.4% over the first year and 3.2% over the first 3 years. It can be concluded that ART/HVGIC restorations perform very well in single-surface cavities in both primary and permanent posterior teeth, and that their performance to treat multi-surface cavities in posterior teeth in both dentitions need further improvement.

ART/HVGIC and Conventionally Produced Restorations

Primary Dentition

A few meta-analyses have compared ART/HVGIC and amalgam restorations in primary teeth. Mickenautsch et al. [54] concluded that there was no significant difference in the survival percentages of single-surface ART/HVGIC and amalgam restorations after 2 years. A more recent meta-analysis [30] concluded that ART/HVGIC restorations have similar survival percentages compared to conventional techniques (amalgam and resin composite) in occlusoproximal cavities in posterior primary teeth.

Permanent Dentition

A 2004 meta-analysis that compared ART and amalgam restorations concluded that there was no difference in survival percentages between single-surface ART and amalgam restorations after 3 years [55]. The follow-up meta-analysis concluded that the longevity of various types of ART restorations in posterior permanent teeth is equal to, or greater than, that of equivalent amalgam restorations up to 6.3 years [54]. The latest meta-analysis on posterior tooth restorations concluded that: "controlled clinical trials with high-viscosity glass-ionomer restorations placed using ART provided the bulk of the available evidence and suggests that the failure rate of direct posterior high-viscosity glass-ionomer in permanent teeth are comparable to that of dental amalgam restorations" [29].

It is fair to conclude that the published meta-analyses show that ART/HVGIC restorations of various types do not differ statistically in their survival percentages compared to conventional, mainly amalgam restorations over a relatively short period of 6 years. Survival data of longer duration are scarce, just as they are for restorations in anterior teeth in both primary and permanent teeth. ART/HVGIC restorations have a place alongside conventionally placed restorations and are often the first choice.

Final Remarks

On the basis of the information presented, we can conclude that the ART principles of carious removal are in accordance with the MID philosophy of preserving sound tooth structure and follow recommendations of the International Caries Consensus Collaboration. Moreover, the ART method can be applied in different settings and benefit people with different profiles by providing restorations of good quality that present acceptable to excellent survival rates.

References

1 Frencken JE, Pilot T, Songpaisan Y, Phantumvanit P: Atraumatic restorative treatment (ART): rationale, technique, and development. J Publ Health Dent 1996;56:135–140.

2 Frencken JE, Leal SC, Navarro MF: Twenty-five year atraumatic restorative treatment (ART) approach: a comprehensive overview. Clin Oral Investig 2012;16:1337–1346.

3 Mickenautsch S, Rudolpf MJ, Ogunbodede EO, Frencken JE: The impact of the ART approach on the treatment profile in a mobile dental system (MDS) in South Africa. Int Dent J 1999;49:132–138.

4 Smales RJ, Yip HK: The atraumatic restorative treatment (ART) approach for primary teeth: review of literature. Pediatr Dent 2000;22:294–298.

5 Frencken JE: Evolution of the ART approach: highlights and achievements. J Appl Oral Sci 2009;17:78–83.

6 Pilot T: Introduction – ART from a global perspective. Community Dent Oral Epidemiol 1999;27:421–422.

7 Honkala E, Behbehani J, Ibricevic H, Kerosuo E, Al-Jame G: The atraumatic restorative treatment (ART) approach to restoring primary teeth in a standard dental clinic. Int J Paediatr Dent 2003; 13:172–179.
8 da Mata C, Allen PF, McKenna G, Cronin M, O'Mahony D, Woods N: Two-year survival of ART restorations placed in elderly patients: a randomised controlled clinical trial. J Dent 2015;43:405–411.
9 Molina GF, Faulks D, Mazzola I, Cabral RJ, Mulder J, Frencken JE: Three-year survival of ART high-viscosity glass-ionomer and resin composite restorations in people with disability. Clin Oral Investig 2018;22:461–467.
10 Frencken JE, Songpaisan Y, Phantumvanit P, Pilot T: An atraumatic restorative treatment (ART) technique: evaluation after one year. Int Dent J 1994;44:460–464.
11 Massara ML, Alves JB, Brandão PRG: Atraumatic restorative treatment: clinical, ultrastructural and chemical analysis. Caries Res 2002;36:430–436.
12 Molina GF, Cabral RJ, Frencken JE: The ART approach: clinical aspects reviewed. J Appl Oral Sci 2009;17:89–98.
13 Celiberti P, Francescut P, Lussi A: Performance of four dentine excavation methods in deciduous teeth. Caries Res 2006;40:117–123.
14 Lenters M, van Amerongen WE, Mandari GJ: Iatrogenic damage to the adjacent surface of primary molars, in three different ways of cavity preparation. Eur Arch Paediatr Dent 2006;7:6–10.
15 Rahimtoola S, van Amerongen E: Comparison of two tooth-saving preparation techniques for one-surface cavities. ASDC J Dent Child 2002;69:16–26.
16 Schriks MC, van Amerongen WE: Atraumatic perspectives of ART: psychological and physiological aspects of treatment with and without rotary instruments. Community Dent Oral Epidemiol 2003;31:15–20.
17 van Bochove JA, van Amerongen WE: The influence of restorative treatment approaches and the use of local analgesia on the children's discomfort. Eur Arch Paediatr Dent 2006;7:11–16.
18 Rahimtoola S, van Amerongen E, Maher R, Groen H: Pain related to different ways of minimal intervention in the treatment of small caries lesions. ASDC J Dent Child 2000;67:123–127.
19 de Menezes Abreu DM, Leal SC, Mulder J, Frencken JE: Patterns of dental anxiety in children after sequential dental visits. Eur Arch Paediatr Dent 2011;12: 298–302.
20 Frencken JE, Makoni F, Sithole WD, Hackenitz E: Three-year survival of one-surface ART restorations and glass-ionomer sealants in a school oral health programme in Zimbabwe. Caries Res 1998;32:119–126.
21 Camargo LB, Olegário IC, Aldrigui JM, Calvo AFB, Carvalho C, Mendes FM, Raggio DP: Atraumatic restorative treatment vs conventional treatment for early childhood caries – randomized clinical trial for survival analysis and physiological discomfort assessment. Dent Health Curr Res 2016;2:3.
22 Tonmukayakul U, Arrow P: Cost-effectiveness analysis of the atraumatic restorative treatment-based approach to managing early childhood caries. Community Dent Oral Epidemiol 2016;45: 92–100.
23 Hayes M, Allen E, da Mata C, McKenna G, Burke F: Minimal intervention dentistry and older patients part 2: minimally invasive operative interventions. Dent Update 2014;41:500–502, 504–505.
24 Molina GF, Faulks D, Frencken J: Acceptability, feasibility and perceived satisfaction of the use of the atraumatic restorative treatment approach for people with disability. Braz Oral Res 2015; 29:1–9.
25 Estupiñan-Day S, Tellez M, Kaur S, Millner T, Solari A: Mananging dental caries with atraumatic restorative treatment in children: successful experience in three Latin America countries. Rev Panam Salud Publica 2013;33:237–243.
26 da Mata C, Allen PF, Cronin M, O'Mahony D, McKenna G, Woods N: Cost-effectiveness of ART restorations in elderly adults: a randomizaed clinical trial. Community Dent Oral Epidemiol 2014;42:79–87.
27 de Amorim RG, Leal SC, Frencken JE: Survival of atraumatic restorative treatment (ART) sealants and restorations – a meta-analysis. Clin Oral Invest 2012; 16:429–441.
28 Mickenautsch S: Are high-viscosity glass-ionomer cements inferior to silver amalgam as restorative materials for permanent posterior teeth? A Bayesian analysis. BMC Oral Health 2015;8:118.
29 Mickenautsch S: High-viscosity glass-ionomer cements for direct posterior tooth restorations in permanent teeth: the evidence in brief. J Dent 2016;55: 121–123.
30 Tedesco TK, Calvo AF, Lenzi TL, Hesse D, Guglielmi CA, Camargo LB, Gimenez T, Braga MM, Raggio DP: ART is an alternative for restoring occlusoproximal cavities in primary teeth – evidence from an updated systematic review and meta-analysis. Int J Paediatr Dent 2017; 27:201–209.
31 Yip HK, Samaranayake LP: Caries removal techniques and instrumentation: a review. Clin Oral invest 1998;2:148–154.
32 Easton GS: Causes and prevention of amalgam failures. JADA 1941;28:392–400.
33 Quock RL, Patel SA, Falcão FA, Barros JA: Is a drill-less dental filling possible? Medical Hypothesis 2011;77:315–317.
34 Paddick JS, Brailsford SR, Kidd EA, Beighton D: Phenotypic and genotypic selection of microbiota surviving under dental restorations. Appl Environ Microbiol 2005;71:2467–2472.
35 Frencken JE, Imazato S, Toi C, Mulder J, Mickenautsch S, Takahashi Y, Ebisu S: Antibacterial effect of chlorhexidine-containing glass ionomer cement in vivo: a pilot study. Caries Res 2007;41: 102–107.
36 Kidd E, Fejerskov O, Nyvad B: Infected dentine revised. Dent Update 2015;42: 802–806, 808–809.
37 Ngo H, Mount D, Peters MC: A study of glass-ionomer cement and its interface with enamel and dentin using a low-temperature, high-resolution scanning electron microscopic technique. Quintessence Int 1997;28:63–69.
38 Fukada R, Yoshida Y, Nakayama Y, Okazaki M, Inoue S, Sano H, Shintani H, Snauwaert J, van Meerbeek B: Bonding efficacy of polyakenoic acids to hydroxyapatite, enamel and dentin. Biomaterials 2003;24:1861–1867.
39 Massler M: Control of dental caries: a new concept. New Zeland Dent J 1962; 58:1–6.
40 Fusayama T, Okuse K, Hosoda H: Relationship between hardness, discoloration, and microbial invasion in carious dentin. J Dent Res 1967;45:1033–1046.
41 Fusayama T: A Simple Pain-Free Adhesive Restorative System by Minimal Reduction and Total Etching. Tokyo, Ishiyaku EuroAmerica, 1993, p 11.

42 Innes N, Frencken JE, Bjorndal L, Maltz M, Manton D, et al: Managing carious lesions: consensus recommendations on terminology. Adv Dent Res 2016;28: 49–57.
43 Ricketts D, Lamont T, Innes NP, Kidd E, Clarkson JE: Operative caries management in adults and children. Cochrane Database Syst Rev 2013;3:CD003808.
44 Makoni F, Frencken JE, Sithole WD: Oral health status among secondary school students in Harare, Zimbabwe. J Dent Assoc S Afr 1997;52:491–494.
45 Mobarak EH, Shabayek MM, Mulder J, Reda AH, Frencken JE: Caries experience of Egyptian adolescents: does the atraumatic restorative treatment approach offer a solution? Med Princ Pract 2011;20:545–549.
46 Navarro MF, Rigolon CJ, Barata TJ, Bresciane E, Fagundes TC, Peters MC: Influence of occlusal access on demineralized dentin removal in the atraumatic restorative treatment (ART) approach. Am J Dent 2008;21:251–254.
47 Bakhshandeh A, Qvist V, Ekstrand R: Sealing occlusal caries lesions in adults referred for restorative treatment: 2–3 years of follow-up. Clin Oral Invest 2012;16:521–529.
48 Hesse D, Bonifácio CC, Mendes FF, Braga MM, Imparato JC, Raggio DP: Sealing versus partial caries removal in primary molars: a randomized clinical trial. BMC Oral Health 2014;28:14:58.
49 Tyas MJ, Anusavice KJ, Frencken JE, Mount GJ: Minimal intervention dentistry – a review. FDI Comission Project 1–97. Int Dent J 2000;50:1–12.
50 Banerjee A, Kidd EA, Watson TF: In vitro evaluation of five alternative methods of carious dentine excavation. Caries Res 2000;34:144–150.
51 Hickel R, Roulet JF, Bayne S, Heintze SD, Mjör IA, Peters M, Rousson V, Randall R, Schmalz G, Tyas M, Vanherle G: Recommendations for conducting controlled clinical studies of dental restorative materials. J Adhes Dent 2007;9: 121–147.
52 Frencken JE, van't Hof MA, Taifour D, Al-Zaher I: Effectiveness of ART and traditional amalgam approach in restoring single-surface cavities in posterior teeth of permanent dentitions in school children after 6.3 years. Community Dent Oral Epidemiol 2007;35:207–214.
53 de Amorim RG, Frencken JE, Raggio DP, Chen X, Hu X, Leal SC: Survival percentages of Atraumatic Restorative Treatment (ART) restorations and sealants in posterior teeth: an updated systematic review and meta-analysis. Clin Oral Invest 2017, submitted.
54 Mickenautsch S, Yengopal V, Banerjee A: Atraumatic restorative treatment versus amalgam restoration longevity: a systematic review. Clin Oral Investig 2010;14:233–240.
55 Frencken JE, van 't Hof MA, van Amerongen WE, Holmgren CJ: Effectiveness of single-surface ART restorations in the permanent dentition: a meta-analysis. J Dent Res 2004;83:120–123.

Soraya Leal
Campus Darcy Ribeiro, Faculdade de Ciências da Saúde
Departamento de Odontologia, Universitdade de Brasília
Brasília, DF 70670-410 (Brazil)
E-Mail sorayaodt@yahoo.com

Schwendicke F, Frencken J, Innes N (eds): Caries Excavation: Evolution of Treating Cavitated Carious Lesions.
Monogr Oral Sci. Basel, Karger, 2018, vol 27, pp 103–112 (DOI: 10.1159/000487837)

Sealing Carious Tissue Using Resin and Glass-Ionomer Cements

Margherita Fontana[a] • Nicola Innes[b]

[a]Cariology, Restorative Sciences and Endodontics, School of Dentistry, University of Michigan, Ann Arbor, MI, USA; [b]School of Dentistry, University of Dundee, Dundee, UK

Abstract

One of the most conservative ways to retain tooth structure, preserve pulpal health, and avoid invasive treatment is to simply completely seal established carious lesions. A tight seal to isolate the biofilm and arrest the lesion can be successfully achieved using a sealant material such as resin or glass-ionomer for non-cavitated lesions, a restorative material for cavitated lesions, or, for primary teeth, preformed stainless-steel crowns. This chapter focuses on sealants and restorative materials. Sealant materials are a viable treatment option for controlling non-cavitated lesions in occlusal and proximal surfaces where there is no significant breach in the surface integrity of the tooth, even if the lesion extends into dentine. Resin infiltration can also be used to manage proximal non-cavitated lesions. Even when the exact depth of lesion that can be sealed has not been established, evidence supports sealing shallow and moderate deep lesions into dentine. For cavitated lesions, sealing lesions without carious tissue removal might be an option when removal of tooth tissue is not required to provide a hard periphery around the lesion/cavity margin (to enhance bonding or to increase cavity depth for enough restorative material to be placed to last). There is little evidence for placing a restorative material over cavitated carious lesions without tissue removal or preparation. However, where there is a significant breach in the surface integrity of the tooth but there is still enough sound tooth tissue to provide bonding for an adhesive restoration, sealing in carious tissue might still be an option.

The aims and principles for managing dentine carious lesions, as described in the chapter by Schwendicke [this vol., pp. 56–67], are to arrest the caries disease process (i.e., demineralisation), promoting lesion remineralisation and/or arrest, while maintaining dental pulp vitality and retaining tooth structure, which can be achieved by avoiding unnecessarily invasive treatment. One of the most conservative ways to retain

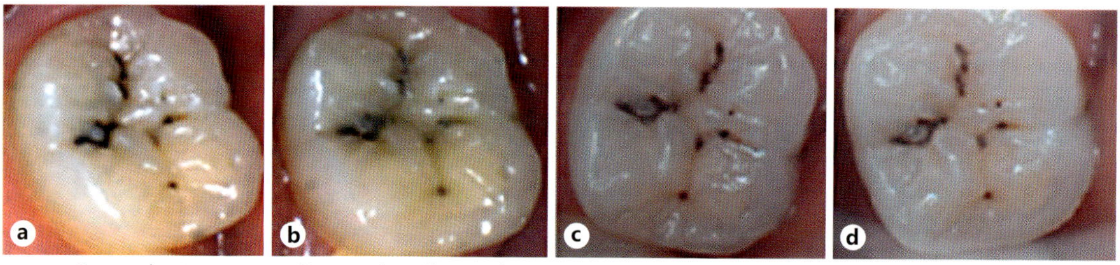

Fig. 1. The photographs show a lower permanent molar where a carious lesion has been sealed with a clear resin sealant to arrest its progress. **a** Before any sealant has been placed. There is shadowing indicating a dentinal lesion. **b** The tooth 1 month following clear resin sealant placement. **c** One year after sealant placement. **d** Two years after sealant placement [1].

tooth structure and avoid invasive treatment, where there is an established carious lesion, is to simply seal the lesion completely into the tooth, without any carious lesion/tissue removal at all. This treatment option works most successfully when a hermetic seal is achieved, isolating the carious lesion from the oral environment (Fig. 1) [1]. This can be accomplished using adhesive materials through a number of methods: completely sealing non-cavitated carious lesions using resin or glass-ionomer sealant materials, sealing cavitated carious lesions using resin-based restorative materials or, for primary teeth, preformed stainless-steel crowns (use of the Hall Technique is covered in the chapter by Santamaria et al. [this vol., pp. 113–123]. The choice of method depends on the overall clinical situation: characteristics of the carious lesion (location, extent, cavitation) and the tooth, as well as the patient's choice, as all decision-making should be carried out in a partnership between the clinician and the patient. This chapter deals with sealing over established lesions to manage them. It includes fissure sealing over lesions, proximal sealing, resin infiltration, restorations placed over dentinal lesions in permanent teeth with no carious tissue removal, and it deals with both cavitated and non-cavitated lesions.

No Excavation of Any Carious Tooth Tissue/Lesion: Effects of Sealing on Bacteria in Lesions

The principles behind carious tissue removal are clearly described in other chapters; however, a brief summary is that tooth tissue removal is sometimes necessary to manage cavitated carious lesions to allow a high-quality restoration to be placed. For example, tissue removal is necessary where there is not a hard periphery at the margins surrounding the lesion for bonding a restoration (this would compromise the seal). Another example is that tissue removal is sometimes required to give more depth to the cavity. This is sometimes necessary to allow placement of an adequate amount of material to ensure a sound restoration (to maximise material/restoration longevity). However, the most minimally destructive approach should always be taken and this should also avoid compromising the health of the dental pulp [2]. The main reason behind aiming to remove all carious tissue used to be because the carious tissue was considered to be "infectious" and as such, to "cure" the disease, the "infected" tissue should be removed. As has been previously discussed in the chapter by Conrads and About [this vol., pp. 1–10], it is now understood that dental carious lesions result from an imbalance in de- and remineralisation resulting from a dysbiosis in the oral microbiome, which changes the proportions of normal constituents of oral biofilms, causing a proliferation of cariogenic bacteria over time. By sealing in lesions, without the need for any tissue removal, the bacterial proliferation can be stopped, and the carious lesions can be arrested.

In 1976, Handelman et al. [3] found that the numbers of viable bacteria were significantly reduced during the first 2 weeks after sealing them under a restoration, and the numbers continued to reduce over time, although to a lesser extent. These results have been replicated many times since [4–7], with a systematic review of the effects of sealants on bacteria levels in carious lesions [8] finding no significant increases in overall bacterial numbers under sealants, and lower numbers of viable bacteria, including *Streptococcus mutans* and lactobacilli, by at least 100-fold. In addition, the number of lesions with any viable bacteria was reduced by about 50%. The effect of restorative materials on bacterial numbers has been recently investigated and, similarly, has been found to be successful in reducing bacterial numbers [6, 7].

Current State of the Evidence

Fissure sealants are known to be highly effective for the prevention of dental carious lesions [9]. However, there have been difficulties with clinicians adhering to clinical guidelines and applying them. One of the most often quoted barriers to the use of preventive fissure sealants is concern over what happens to carious lesions that are sealed in [5]. This concern, together with the evidence from the 1970s and 1980s that lesions seem to arrest when sealed, has stimulated investigations of sealing established carious lesions. In fact, even though sealing over lesions has been shown to be a successful treatment option in arresting the lesion and controlling bacteria within the lesion since the late 1970s, it has remained a contentious issue.

Non-Cavitated Occlusal Lesions Managed Using Sealants

Carious lesions sealed in the studies from the 1970s and 1980s [3, 10, 11] provide the beginnings of an, albeit limited, evidence base to support the sealing of non-cavitated lesions. These sealants were mainly placed over shallow lesions, usually less than half way through dentine [10], and used materials that had inferior properties to those available today. More recently, there have been 3 large clinical trials [1, 12–14] with follow-up periods of 24–44 months that have set out to look at what happens when occlusal carious lesions are sealed under fissure sealants. The lesions included in all studies were non-cavitated, apart from one study that included some cavitated lesions [12, 14]. However, the extent to which these lesions had penetrated dentine varied in each of the studies: the Borges study [13] examined lesions that ranged in depth from the enamel dentine junction to the middle third of dentine; in the Bakshandeh study [12, 14] sealed lesions ranged from enamel lesions to cavitated lesions in the middle third of the dentine; and in the Fontana study [1], using ICDAS as a clinical measure, ICDAS 0–4 lesions were included, which extended no more than half way through the dentine radiographically, as long there was no "frank cavitation." All of the studies showed that sealing over lesions was a successful strategy for arresting carious lesions, although there are 2 factors that should be taken into consideration when applying this evidence to clinical care. The first is that 2 of the studies placed fissure sealants under rubber dams [13, 14], and the second is that, although there was variety in the lesions' depths in these studies, it is still not possible to establish a clear threshold for how deep a lesion has to be before it is "too deep" to be successfully sealed.

A 10-year-old review where progression rates of non-cavitated carious lesions for sealed surfaces were compared to unsealed surfaces found a median annual percentage of 2.6% for sealed versus 12.6% for unsealed carious teeth [8]. A recent comprehensive systematic review [15] had similar findings, with sealants effective in arresting the progression of non-cavitated lesions when compared to no sealants being used or fluoride varnishes. This information has been used by the American Dental Association (ADA) and American Academy of Pediatric Dentistry (AAPD) to recommend that "sealants are effective in preventing and arresting pit-and-fissure occlusal carious lesions of primary and permanent molars in children and adolescents compared with the non-use of sealants or use of fluoride varnishes" [16]. They also concluded that sealants could minimise the progression of non-cavitated occlusal carious lesions that received a sealant.

Although there is also evidence to support glass-ionomer sealants to prevent dental carious lesions becoming established [9], they tend to be used primarily in specific circumstances (e.g., when there are difficulties with isolation for moisture control). Furthermore, because there is limited clinical trial evidence on the use of glass-ionomer sealants over existing lesions, it is difficult to draw conclusions as to what would happen when these lesions are sealed under a glass-ionomer. A study in which small enamel and dentine lesions were sealed over with a hand-mixed medium-viscosity glass-ionomer found that, after 3-years, dentine carious lesions reappeared (i.e., the sealant was lost), were seen as cavities, or a new dentine carious lesion developed in 12.6% of the dentinal lesions sealed. For early enamel carious lesions that were sealed, dentine carious lesions developed in 9.1% of the cases, with no significant difference between the progression seen whether it was enamel or dentine lesions sealed.

The recent systematic review [15] and recommendations by the ADA and AAPD [16] focused on papers that included sealant materials available at the time of publication (2016) in the USA, and concluded that there was no evidence of a difference for the preventive effects of any one material over another. Therefore, the guidance provided was that clinicians should take into account the likelihood of experiencing lack of retention (extremely important especially for resin-based sealants, with some questions around the importance of this for glass-ionomer materials [17–19]). A further consideration should be the ability to obtain a dry field during application when choosing the type of material. It is certain that if dry isolation is difficult, such as a tooth that is not fully erupted, and where the operculum still covers part of the tooth (Fig. 2), then a material that is more hydrophilic (e.g., glass-ionomer) would be preferable.

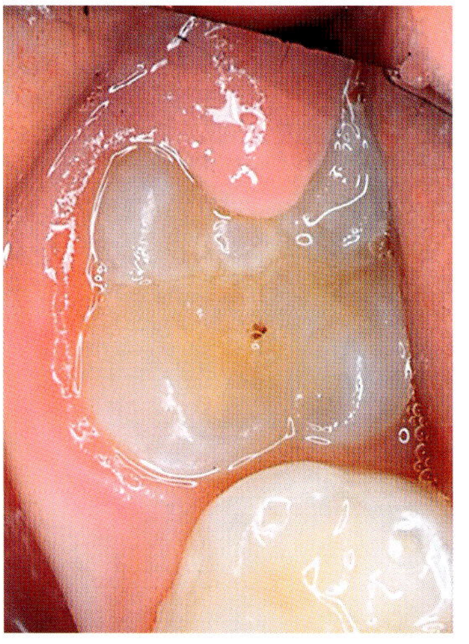

Fig. 2. A lower first permanent molar at high risk of developing a carious lesion, but where adequate moisture control to provide a resin sealant would be difficult to achieve because of the operculum over the distal part of the tooth as it erupts. A glass-ionomer sealant should be placed.

If the tooth can be isolated to ensure a dry site and long-term clinical retention is desired, then the ADA and AAPD recommendations suggest that a resin-based sealant is preferable. Otherwise, the choice of sealant material depends also on the dentist's preference, and the outcome is dependent on the sealant being applied following the highest standard. In all cases, it is important to monitor sealants over time, especially sealants showing a higher risk of experiencing clinical retention loss (i.e., glass-ionomer).

Non-Cavitated Proximal Lesions Sealed Using Sealants and Resin Infiltration

Although this book primarily deals with cavitated dentine lesion management, it is pertinent to include evidence that encompasses both dentine carious lesions and those limited to enamel, as studies have often been carried out on both types of lesions and methods developed for both. Proximal sealing is one such method although its application seems best limited to non-cavitated lesions.

Placing a sealant on a proximal surface can be challenging compared to placing a sealant on the occlusal surface (Fig. 3). Thus, even though this strategy is not common, it is still an effective method for preventing the progress of established non-cavitated lesions [17, 18].

More recently, resin infiltration has been investigated as a method for providing a barrier on the proximal surface but within the demineralised tissue itself, to prevent the progression of lesions (Fig. 4). A Cochrane review supports sealing lesions proximally using sealants or infiltration [18]. Eight trials were included in this review, of which 4 investigated resin sealants, 3 investigated resin infiltration, 1 studied glass-ionomer fissure sealants, and 1 investigated adhesive patches. The conclusion of the review was that sealants, infiltration, and patches placed on non-cavitated proximal lesions were effective for arresting enamel and dentinal lesions. These strategies significantly reduced the likelihood of carious lesion progression compared with non-invasive professional or home care. None of the studies investigated these treatments compared to traditional invasive management options.

Cavitated Lesions Managed Using Adhesive Restorations

The option of no carious tissue removal and sealing frank cavitated lesions using an adhesive restorative material has been investigated in a single clinical trial. As such, the level of evidence is not

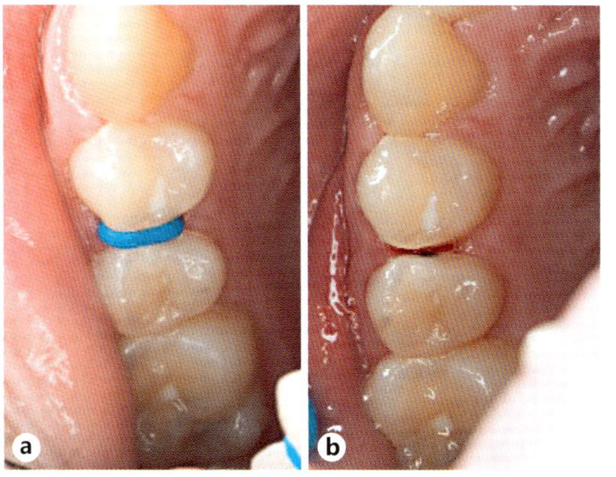

Fig. 3. There is a mesial carious lesion (non-cavitated) on the upper second premolar where a sealant using a conventional acid-etch technique and resin material is going to be placed. **a** An orthodontic separator is placed between the upper first and second premolars for 5 days to create space. **b** The resulting space achieved.

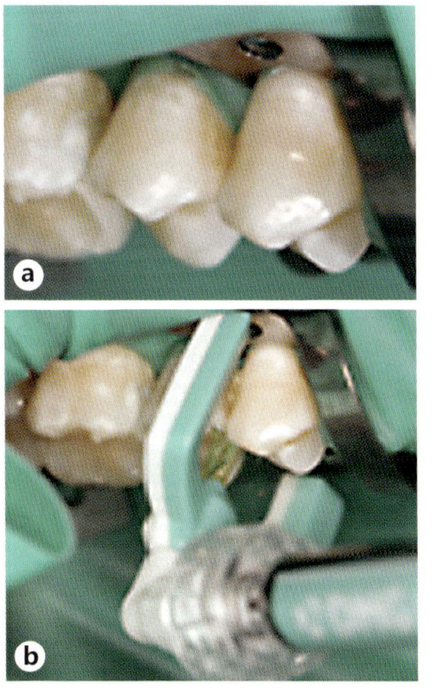

Fig. 4. A carious lesion (non-cavitated) on the upper premolar is having resin infiltration carried out. **a** The teeth with rubber dams placed prior to the infiltration taking place. There is no prior separation as the kit is designed to separate the teeth, creating space during the procedure. **b** The surface of the tooth is etched and will then have infiltrant placed using the application equipment shown.

strong and the limits of the technique have not yet been well established. This single seminal clinical trial [19] assessed bonded and sealed composite restorations placed directly over frank cavitated lesions (i.e., sealed lesions with no dentine caries removal) compared with 2 groups in which complete caries removal was carried out and then restored with either a sealed conservative amalgam restoration or a conventional unsealed amalgam restoration. These materials were applied to permanent teeth with cavitated occlusal carious lesions extending up to half way into dentine. Even though the main aim of the study was to assess restoration longevity, other outcomes such as pulpal pain were also recorded. The participants were followed up over 10 years (the follow-up rate was 54%), with both types of sealed restorations showing better clinical performance and longevity compared with the unsealed amalgam group, although sealed amalgam performed best. The authors also noted that, over the 10 years of the study, the bonded and sealed composite restorations arrested the clinical progress of these lesions.

Effects of Sealing

As stated previously, when carious lesions are sealed under restorations, the microbial biofilm is deprived of its nutrient source. This "starvation" affects the microbes and causes them to enter a dormant state or to die. By reducing the amount and/or activity of the biofilm, the lesion's progress slows down and even stops. Clinical trials support this effect through indirect but clinically relevant evidence on lack of progression of lesions where sealants and restorations remain intact [1, 12, 13, 19]. However, studies investigating the properties of the biofilm sealed under restorations have directly shown that there are fewer bacteria [3, 5, 6] and those present tend to be less diverse and less virulent [4, 6, 7, 20].

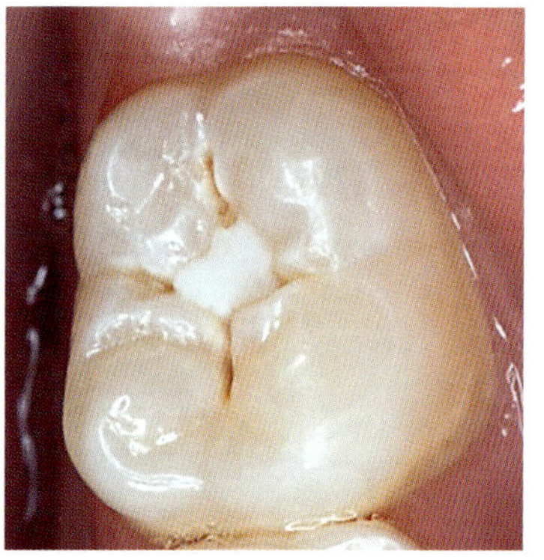

Fig. 5. A second permanent molar where a fissure sealant has worn/failed and there is development of carious lesions in the exposed fissure system. There is evidence of breakdown in the fissures and white areas of demineralisation can be seen around the edges of the fissures. Sealants often need to be topped up and maintained to preserve their seal.

Advantages and Disadvantages, Pulpal and Restorative Issues, Limitations of the Material to Seal

Fissure sealing has long been accepted as a successful method for prevention. As has been shown, there is also a growing body of evidence to support its use, where carious lesions have become established, to prevent their progression (both for proximal and occlusal lesions) [1, 15, 18, 21]. However, evidence for sealants over, and infiltration of, carious lesions has mainly been obtained from studies of shallow or moderately deep lesions where there is no cavitation of the lesion and the materials used to seal have certain limiting properties. Fissure sealant materials are either low filled resins or high-viscosity glass-ionomer materials. Each material has its advantages and disadvantages. Low filled resins, when taken in thin section, are very brittle. Glass ionomer fissue sealant materials have no inherent strength and can wear (Fig. 5).

Therefore, sealants need to be monitored (Fig. 6) and topped up periodically to maintain their integrity, especially when they have been used to seal over lesions, and the conditions in the

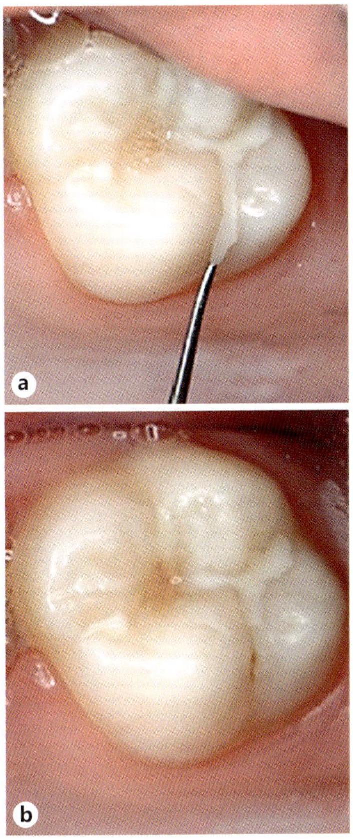

Fig. 6. The adherence of the sealant should be checked around the full circumference of the material at each oral health assessment appointment ("check-up"). **a** The sealant has been extended to the palatal fissure to protect it but is not sticking to the tooth. A probe can be inserted beneath the loose edge and can lift it off. **b** After the sealant is removed, the fissure can be seen to be developing a carious lesion underneath it that had not been there originally.

mouth/around the tooth might still allow the progression of the lesion.

In one long-term study of occlusal sealants placed over carious lesions [1], 11% of sealants needed to be repaired after 1 year, 22% by 2 years, and 30% by 44 months. There seemed to be an increased need for repair linked to higher baseline ICDAS scores, but not to radiographic depth.

As stated previously, glass-ionomer materials have not been widely studied over carious lesions and the evidence supporting their long-term performance is limited. Furthermore, in general glass-ionomer sealants have the disadvantage of having a significantly higher wear over time than resin materials, but they have the advantage of being a more hydrophilic material, thus allowing for placement in clinical circumstances where humidity control may not allow for consideration of a more retentive resin sealant [15, 22].

Slowing down the repeat restorative cycle is one of the aims of modern dentistry [23] and the most minimal approach to managing the dentinal carious lesion would be to remove no tooth tissue, carious or sound. This has been shown to be successful in clinical trials of the Hall Technique where a preformed metal crown is simply pushed over a tooth without any tissue removal to provide a seal. These trials show success rates that are much higher (over 90% at 5 years and higher in shorter timeframes) than in other trials where restorative materials are used to seal lesions [24, 25], and this is probably related to the quality of the seal that can be achieved predictably with the crown, and does not rely heavily on clinician skill, in restoration material placement or on material properties. The difficulties with providing a sealant with the same highly predictable results are that the material has more limited physical properties. In the seminal Mertz-Fairhurst study [19] where cavitated carious lesions were not removed in one of the groups and a resin was placed over it, additional means of sealing over traditional amalgam restorations were used in one of the other groups using resin fissure sealant materials to ensure that as good a seal as possible was achieved.

Diagnostic Challenges

The evidence that has been produced has variable definitions and there is no agreed terminology. Most of the evidence has been produced on lesions that were described as non-cavitated and assessment of the extent of "shallow" or "moderately deep" lesions varied depending on the method used – radiographic or clinical (e.g., ICDAS recording). However, using good standard diagnostic methods to visualise the surface of the tooth (clean, dry) should ensure that there is no significant frank cavitation prior to placing a resin sealant. Radiographs can be used to give some assessment of the depth of the dentinal lesion and supplement any clinical diagnosis.

When and When Not to Seal Carious Tissue

Although the evidence to support sealants over lesions is compelling, coming from different settings and showing results all in the same direction (that sealants can prevent the progression of lesions), there are variable failure rates in available studies. A systematic review on the extent of the carious lesion that can be successfully sealed (as assessed by its depth in dentine radiographically), compared 3 different groups of treatment options for pit and fissure caries: (1) where there is no hard tissue management, for example non-invasive treatments such as fluoride/anti-bacterial medicament applications and diet change; (2) those where etching of hard tissues is used, such as sealing, and (3) techniques that involve removing carious dentine. The study concluded that shallow or moderately deep lesions are likely to be successfully managed by sealants, but that there is not enough evidence to make recommendations for deeper lesions [26].

The properties of sealants suggest that they may have limited suitability for use with carious lesions where demineralisation of enamel and dentine has taken place to such an extent that the ability of the tooth to withstand biting forces has been compromised (i.e., large or deep cavitations). This is because in these cases sealants will provide protection from the ingress of bacteria but will not add much to the strength of the tooth. In cases where the lesion is very deep, the sealant may not prevent the lesion surface from breaking down if the forces are too great. In fact, clinical evidence is still limited for sealing deep lesions, and the exact extent of the carious lesion that can be sealed using currently existing materials has not been measured in any great detail. Clinically, in the case of a deep lesion, even where there is very little cavitation clinically visible (usually because the breach in enamel is at the base of a fissure and cannot be seen), the dentinal lesion has demineralised the dentine. Healthy dentine has around 70% mineralisation, but this is greatly reduced after the dentine is affected by the acids from the biofilm and proteolytic enzymes denaturing the collagen. A further consideration is that one of the features noticeable when carrying out stepwise caries removal is that, on re-entry to the dentinal lesion for the second step of the process, there tends to be a gap beneath the temporary restoration and what was a moist and soft carious tissue is seen to become hard and dry. This shrinkage and drying of dentine has not been quantified but could result in the restoration sitting on a base that is not sound, possibly compromising the quality of the restoration. Thus, for fissure sealants over deep dentinal lesions, there could still be drying and shrinking of the dentinal tissues that could compromise the tooth structural strength.

Even though the lack of clarity in the studies around definitions of non-cavitated or micro-cavitated lesions make it difficult to recommend exactly what kind of carious lesion can be sealed, most studies on shallow to moderately deep non-cavitated lesions agree these lesions can be successfully managed using dental sealants. As mentioned, a recent systematic review could not recommend which material would perform best [15], and 2 of the studies included in the review used rubber dams when placing sealants [12–14], although the necessity of this, or the extent to which it improved outcomes, if at all, remains unknown. Finally, there is too high a degree of clinical heterogeneity between these studies to allow a network meta-analysis to help provide this information.

Summary of Clinical Recommendations

Even when sealing caries lesions has proven to be an effective non-invasive caries management strategy, especially for non-cavitated lesions, there are still many areas in need of further research – the most important seem to be: (1) which type of material is most suited for specific situations; (2) how deep a dentine carious lesion can be sealed with predictably successful results; (3) how extensive can cavitation be and still allow a carious lesion to be sealed, while still providing a predictable and good outcome; (4) how do sealants compare with restorations when managing deep dentine lesions, and (5) what factors should influence the decision to keep repairing sealants that have been placed over non-cavitated carious lesions? Despite this lacking information, taking the evidence presented in this chapter in full, some recommendations can be made:

- Where there is no significant breach in the surface integrity of the tooth, but the lesion still extends into dentine, sealing the tooth/lesion without any tissue being removed is an effective treatment option that should be considered.
- Where there is a significant breach in the surface integrity of the tooth but there is still enough sound tooth tissue to provide bonding for an adhesive restoration, sealing in the existing carious tissue might be a possibility.

References

1 Fontana M, Platt JA, Eckert GJ, González-Cabezas C, Yoder K, Zero DT, Ando M, Soto-Rojas AE, Peters MC: Monitoring of sound and carious surfaces under sealants over 44 months. J Dent Res 2014;93:1070–1075.

2 Schwendicke F, Frencken JE, Bjørndal L, Maltz M, Manton DJ, Ricketts D, van Landuyt K, Banerjee A, Campus G, Doméjean S, Fontana M, Leal S, Lo E, Machiulskiene V, Schulte A, Splieth C, Zandona AF, Innes NP: Managing carious lesions: consensus recommendations on carious tissue removal. Adv Dent Res 2016;28:58–67.

3 Handelman SL, Washburn F, Wopperer P: Two-year report of sealant effect on bacteria in dental caries. J Am Dent Assoc 1976;93:967–970.

4 Jeronimus DJ Jr, Till MJ, Sveen OB: Reduced viability of microorganisms under dental sealants. ASDC J Dent Child 1975;42:275–280.

5 Oong EM, Griffin SO, Kohn WG, Gooch BF, Caufield PW: The effect of dental sealants on bacteria levels in caries lesions: a review of the evidence. J Am Dent Assoc 2008;139:271–278.

6 Orhan AI, Oz FT, Ozcelik B, Orhan K: A clinical and microbiological comparative study of deep carious lesion treatment in deciduous and young permanent molars. Clin Oral Investig 2008;12: 369–378.

7 Paddick JS, Brailsford SR, Kidd EA, Beighton D: Phenotypic and genotypic selection of microbiota surviving under dental restorations. App Environ Microbiol 2005;71:2467–2472.

8 Griffin SO, Oong E, Kohn W, Vidakovic B, Gooch BF: The effectiveness of sealants in managing caries lesions. J Dent Res 2008;87:169–174.

9 Ahovuo-Saloranta A, Forss H, Walsh T, Nordblad A, Mäkelä M, Worthington HV: Pit and fissure sealants for preventing dental decay in permanent teeth. Cochrane Database Syst Rev 2017; 7:CD001830.

10 Handelman SL, Stege PM, Baric JM, Espeland MA, Saunders RH: Clinical radiographic evaluation of sealed carious and sound tooth surfaces. J Am Dent Assoc 1986;113:751–754.

11 Handelman SL, Leverett DH, Solomon ES, Brenner CM: Use of adhesive sealants over occlusal carious lesions: radiographic evaluation. Community Dent Oral Epidemiol 1981;9:256–259.

12 Bakhshandeh A, Qvist V, Ekstrand K: Sealing occlusal caries lesions in adults referred for restorative treatment: 2–3 years of follow-up. Clin Oral Investig 2012;16:521–529.

13 Borges BC, de Souza Borges J, Braz R, Montes MA, de Assunção Pinheiro IV: Arrest of non-cavitated dentinal occlusal caries by sealing pits and fissures: a 36-month, randomised controlled clinical trial. Int Dent J 2012;62:251–255.

14 Qvist V, Borum MK, Moller KD, Andersen TR, Blanche P, Bakhshandeh A: Sealing occlusal dentin caries in permanent molars. JDR Clin Trans Res 2017;2: 73–86.

15 Wright JT, Crall JJ, Fontana M, Gillette E J, Nový BB, Dhar V, Donly K, Hewlett ER, Quinonez RB, Chaffin J, Crespin M, Iafolla T, Siegal MD, Tampi MP, Graham L, Estrich C, Carrasco-Labra A: Sealants for preventing and arresting pit-and-fissure occlusal caries in primary and permanent molars: a systematic review of randomized controlled trials – a report of the American Dental Association and the American Academy of Pediatric Dentistry. J Am Dent Assoc 2016;147:631–645.e18.

16 Wright JT Tampi MP, Graham L, Cameron E, Crall JJ, Fontana M, Gillette EJ, Nový BB, Dhar V, Donly K, Hewlett ER, Quinonez RB, Chaffin J, Crespin M, Iafolla T, Siegal M, Carrasco-Labra A: Evidence-based clinical practice guideline for the use of pit-and-fissure sealants: a report of the American Dental Association and the American Academy of Pediatric Dentistry. J Am Dent Assoc 2016; 147:672–682.e12.
17 Basili C.P, Emilson CG, Corvalan GC, Moran MP, Torres C, Quiroz MD, Gomez SS: Preventive and therapeutic proximal sealing: a 3.5-year randomized controlled clinical trial follow-up. Caries Res 2017;51:387–393.
18 Dorri M, Dunne SM, Walsh T, Schwendicke F: Micro-invasive interventions for managing proximal dental decay in primary and permanent teeth. Cochrane Database Syst Rev 2015;11:CD010431.
19 Mertz-Fairhurst, E.J., Curtis JW Jr, Ergle JW, Rueggeberg FA, Adair SM: Ultraconservative and cariostatic sealed restorations: results at year 10. J Am Dent Assoc 1998;129:55–66.
20 Going RE, Loesche WJ, Grainger DA, Syed SA: The viability of microorganisms in carious lesions five years after covering with a fissure sealant. J Am Dent Assoc 1978;97:455–462.
21 Ricketts D, Lamont T, Innes NP, Kidd E, Clarkson JE: Operative caries management in adults and children. Cochrane Database Syst Rev 2013;3:CD003808.
22 Kuhnisch J, Mansmann U, Heinrich-Weltzien R, Hickel R. Longevity of materials for pit and fissure sealing – results from a meta-analysis. Dental Mat 2012;28:298 303.
23 Elderton RJ: Overtreatment with restorative dentistry: when to intervene? Int Dent J 1993;43:17–24.
24 Innes NP, Evans DJ, Stirrups DR: Sealing caries in primary molars: randomized control trial, 5-year results. J Dent Res 2011;90:1405–1410.
25 Santamaria RM, Innes NPT, Machiulskiene V, Schmoeckel J, Alkilzy M, Splieth CH: Alternative caries management options for primary molars: 2.5-year outcomes of a randomised clinical trial. Caries Res 2017;51:605–614.
26 Schwendicke F, Jäger AM, Paris S, Hsu LY, Tu YK: Treating pit-and-fissure caries: a systematic review and network meta-analysis. J Dent Res 2015;94:522–533.

Margherita Fontana
Cariology, Restorative Sciences and Endodontics
School of Dentistry, Room 2393, University of Michigan
1011 N University Avenue
Ann Arbor, MI 48109-1078 (USA)
E-Mail mfontan@umich.edu

Schwendicke F, Frencken J, Innes N (eds): Caries Excavation: Evolution of Treating Cavitated Carious Lesions.
Monogr Oral Sci. Basel, Karger, 2018, vol 27, pp 113–123 (DOI: 10.1159/000487835)

Sealing Carious Tissue in Primary Teeth Using Crowns: The Hall Technique

Ruth M. Santamaría[a] · Nicola Innes[b]

[a]Department of Preventive and Pediatric Dentistry, Ernst-Moritz-Arndt University of Greifswald, Greifswald, Germany;
[b]School of Dentistry, University of Dundee, Dundee, UK

Abstract

In line with reducing the invasiveness of interventions in permanent teeth and changes towards more biological approaches, there have also been moves away from traditional restorative approaches to managing primary teeth where carious dentine/lesions were completely excised and a restoration placed. The Hall Technique is a method for managing carious primary molar teeth where a preformed stainless-steel crown, also known as a preformed metal crown, is seated over a tooth, sealing in, and not removing carious tissue. This chapter discusses the rationale behind the Hall Technique, an outline of the clinical procedure to carry it out, its indications and contraindications, together with the evidence supporting its use. The Hall Technique has been found to be acceptable to children and preferred to more invasive treatment options. Like all dental treatment options, it requires careful case selection, precise carious lesion and pulpal status diagnosis (clinically and radiographically), good patient management, and excellent parental cooperation. The Hall Technique has been shown to be a durable (being likely to last the lifespan of the primary molar) and economical management option for primary molars with carious lesions, which in addition offers the benefit of full coronal coverage, reducing the risk of future carious lesion development. As part of our everyday armamentarium in paediatric dentistry, the Hall Technique is an effective management option for controlling carious lesions in primary molars.

The contemporary view of carious lesion management focuses on treating the lesions using less invasive treatment options, where the emphasis is on biofilm alteration to arrest carious lesions, preserving as much as possible of the affected dental hard tissue [1, 2]. Traditionally, complete removal of the carious tissues with placement of a restoration was the standard treatment for carious primary teeth worldwide; however, in the past few decades the understanding of caries has significantly changed. It is now recognised that the process, originating from the plaque biofilm, leading to demineralisation of the dental hard tissues, and ultimately breakdown of the dentine matrix, can be stopped at virtually any stage if the biofilm is disturbed and fluorides delivered at the lesion [3, 4]. Thus, the central goal of carious lesion management now focuses on correcting this chronic imbalance by reducing demineralisation factors and maximising remineralisation of the carious hard tissues [5, 6]. This concept has led to the development of innovative biologically based techniques such as the selective or stepwise carious tissue removal, which are discussed in detail in the chapter by Bjørndal [this vol., pp. 68–81]. In addition, other techniques advocate the inactivation of lesions without carious tissue removal such as non-restorative cavity control, presented in the chapter by van Strijp and van Loveren [this vol., pp. 124–136], or sealing techniques with no carious tissue removal using preformed stainless-steel crowns (SSCs), such as with the Hall Technique.

Overview

In addition to considerations associated with treating carious lesions in children, such as age-related ability to cope, procedure duration, increased requirements for patient cooperation when placing resin-based restorations, etc., it is a priority to provide high-quality treatment, ensuring that the tooth remains symptomless until it sheds naturally [7]. The Hall Technique offers an approach to manage carious primary molars, which significantly reduces some of these treatment barriers. Like all treatment options, it will not be suitable for every tooth, child, or parent. The main characteristics of the Hall Technique are that:

- no carious tissue is removed;
- no local anaesthesia is required;
- no tooth preparation is carried out;
- all carious tissue is sealed under a preformed SSC using glass-ionomer cement.

This biologically based concept aims to control the carious lesion through influencing the biofilm's environment. By sealing it into the tooth, separating the lesion from the oral environment and its substrate, this isolates the carious lesion from the oral environment and the biofilm composition alters to a less cariogenic microflora, slowing the caries process, or even arresting the activity and progress of the carious lesion [8, 9]. In addition, SSCs fitted using the Hall Technique have been proven to be extremely durable, usually for the lifespan of the restored primary molar, well-retained, subject to low technique sensitivity, and the crowned molars benefit from complete coronal coverage, minimising the risk of further carious lesion development or structural weakening [10, 11].

History of the Hall Technique

The first study on the Hall Technique was published in 2006 [12]. It was a retrospective study which analysed the practice records of a general dental practitioner from Scotland, Dr. Norna Hall. Dr. Hall simplified the standard technique to restore primary teeth using preformed SSCs and used it with her patients. This retrospective study involved a total of 978 crowns fitted in 259 children using her novel technique (today known as the Hall Technique). Most crowns were placed when there was clinical evidence of a proximal carious lesion into dentine and marginal ridge breakdown. This study showed the Hall Technique to have comparable outcomes to those achieved with other more conventional restorations. Further evaluation of the Hall Technique

Table 1. Overall success rates for 4 randomised control trials of the Hall Technique and their comparator interventions

Study	Country and Study details	Age group, years	Sample	Intervention	Overall success[1], years (%)
Innes et al. [13], 2007, [16], 2011	UK General dentists in NHS practice *Lesions:* occlusal and proximal	3–10 mean 6.8 SD 1.58	66 children/132 teeth (split-mouth design) HT = 132; CR = 132	HT	2 (93) 5 (92)
				Complete and selective removal and restoration according to GDP preference	2 (39) 5 (41.5)
Santamaria et al. [14], 2014, [15], 2017	Germany Specialists in hospital *Lesions:* cavitated proxymal	3–8 mean 5.6 SD 1.5	169 children/teeth HT = 52 NRCC = 52 CR = 65	HT	1 (98) 2.5 (92.5)
				Complete caries removal and Compomer restoration	1 (71) 2.5 (67)
				Non-restorative cavity control	1 (75) 2.5 (70)
Narbutait et al. [17], 2017	Lithuania Specialists in hospital *Lesions:* cavitated proxymal	3–8 mean 5.69 SD 1.23	122 children/teeth HT = 35 NRCC = 35 CR = 52	HT	1 (94)
				Caries removal and restoration according to GDP preference	1 (73)
				Non-restorative cavity control	1 (47)
Araujo et al. [18], 2017	Brazil Specialists and undergraduate students in field school setting *Lesions:* cavitated proxymal	5–10 mean 8.08 SD 1.11	131 children/teeth HT = 66 ART = 65	HT	1 (98.5)
				Atraumatic restorative treatment	1 (58.5)

HT, Hall Technique; NRCC, non-restorative cavity control; CR, conventional restoration; ART, atraumatic restorative treatment; GDP, general dental practitioner.
[1] Overall success: none of the following; signs or symptoms of reversible or irreversible pulpitis, restoration loss, fracture/wear requiring intervention, dental abscess requiring pulpotomy or extraction, unrestorable tooth.

was carried out in a split-mouth randomised clinical trial [13] in general dental practices in Scotland. This study compared the clinical effectiveness and acceptance of the Hall Technique compared to traditional restorative techniques used by the general dentists (mainly glass-ionomer cement fillings) in 132 children. Annual clinical and radiographic follow-up checks were conducted. Failures were recorded as either "major" (signs and/or symptoms of irreversible pulpal disease) or "minor" (loss of restoration, restoration requiring repair, and caries progression). Two-year results showed that the Hall Technique was clinically more effective than conventional restorations with success rates (no major or minor failures) of 93%. Similar results were reported from a parallel-arm randomised clinical trial performed in a University setting in Germany [14, 15]. This study, of 169 children, compared the 2.5-year clinical efficacy and survival rates of 3 caries treatment approaches: the Hall Technique; non-restorative caries control (NRCC; opening the cavity without caries removal and with fluoride application), and conventional restorations (compomer fillings), for the management of occlusoproximal carious lesions in primary molars. The Hall Technique performed better than NRCC and conventional restorations, with success rates of 92.5% (no major or minor failures) as compared to 70% in the NRCC group and 67% in the conventional restorations arm.

Further supporting the evidence from randomised control trials (Table 1), retrospective and prospective observational studies [19–21] assessing the Hall Technique over a 1.5- to 5-year time span have shown high success rates (>95%), similar to conventional crowns. The consistently high success rates of the Hall Technique independent of the type of study (retrospective or prospective/observational or randomised control), setting (primary or secondary care), practitioner (undergraduate, general practitioner, specialist), or country where it has been used (Australia, Belgium, Brazil, Chile, Germany, India, the Netherlands, New Zealand, the UAE, the UK and the USA) speak for themselves. These wide-ranging success rates have likely influenced the dissemination of the Hall Technique, increasing its use as a caries management option for carious primary molars [22].

Summary

The success rates of the Hall Technique have been consistently high independent of practitioner, the setting (delivery of care), country where it was performed, or the comparator used (material/technique). This has influenced the dissemination of the Hall Technique and its increasing use as a management option for carious primary molars in many countries in the world, e.g., Australia, Belgium, Brazil, Chile, Germany, India, the Netherlands, New Zealand, the UAE, the UK, and the USA amongst others [22].

Technique Acceptance

Pain and discomfort directly influence the behaviour of child patients during treatment [23–25]. In paediatric dentistry, the ideal "child friendly" caries therapies manage the lesion without causing the child any stress or discomfort.

Innes et al. [13] reported that 77% of children, 83% of parents, and 81% of clinicians preferred the Hall Technique over conventional fillings. Similarly, Santamaria et al. [7] showed that clinicians reported significantly more negative behaviour in children when using conventional fillings compared to the Hall Technique (37 vs. 13%). In addition, around three quarters of clinicians (77%) rated the Hall Technique as a very simple procedure to perform compared to 50% in the conventional filling arm. The Hall Technique offers a simple to use option with a low level of challenge for children to cooperate with. This may reduce treatment-induced anxiety and encourage future patient cooperation.

Summary

Reduction of pain and discomfort during treatment with the Hall Technique compared to more invasive techniques may support the relationship between the clinician and the child, build confidence, reduce anxiety, and encourage positive dental attitudes for future visits.

Cost-Effectiveness

The cost-effectiveness of the Hall Technique has been compared to other options (conventional filling and pulpotomy) for treating asymptomatic carious primary teeth [26]. Simulation modelling was performed using a carious molar in a 5-year-old child followed until exfoliation (maximum follow-up of 7 years) to calculate treatment cost (in Euros). The Hall Technique proved to be the most cost-effective option within a German healthcare setting, with yearly costs of EUR 9.77 compared to EUR 13.31 for conventional fillings and EUR 11.75 for an immediate pulpotomy.

Summary

The Hall Technique has the potential to avoid negative child health impacts and costs of treatment (including of repeated treatment). This technique can be considered as a behavioural management technique as it improves compliance in young children and reduces anxiety associated with dental treatment.

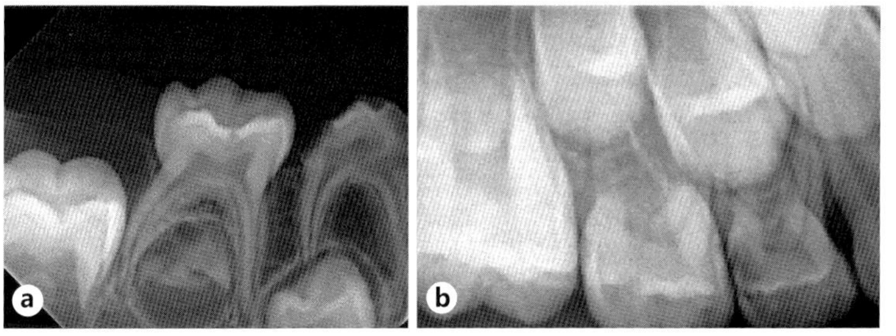

Fig. 1. a This mandibular first primary molar (84) has a large disto-occlusal cavity. It is symptomless, and no inter-radicular pathology is visible. There is a band of "normal" appearing dentine between the carious lesion and the pulp chamber. **b** This maxillary first primary molar (54) has a moderately advanced proximal lesion where the position and extent of the cavity make it difficult to achieve a good seal using an adhesive restorative material.

The Hall Technique Step by Step

Although the Hall Technique is technically a simple procedure to perform in terms of clinical skills, like all dental procedures it will not be a solution to treat carious primary molars for uncooperative children. For success, the Hall Technique requires careful case selection, precise caries and pulpal diagnosis, good patient management, and parental cooperation.

The steps for carrying out the Hall Technique are given below. For further information a manual on the Hall Technique is available for free download at https://en.wikipedia.org/wiki/Hall_Technique.

Step 1: Case Selection

Analyse the suitability of the Hall Technique for each specific patient, and evaluate the extent of the lesion and pulp involvement both clinically and radiographically.

For Which Teeth Is the Hall Technique Indicated?

At the tooth level, the Hall Technique is effective treatment for the management of asymptomatic carious primary molars where the lesion has extended into dentine. The following aspects should be considered:

- extent of the carious lesion: there must be sufficient sound coronal tissue to retain the crown;
- depth of the carious lesion: a dentine bridge (i.e., a band of dentine that appears "normal") must be present between the advancing edge of the carious lesion and the pulp (Fig. 1) on a radiograph. There should be no evidence of peri-radicular pathology of the surrounding bone;
- tooth vitality and dental pulp involvement: assessing pulp status involves a combination of history (past and existing symptoms and main complaint), clinical extra-oral and intra-oral examination of the soft and hard tissues including palpation, percussion, and testing tooth mobility.

Teeth presenting with provoked pain of short duration and diagnosed as a reversible pulpitis might be candidates for treatment with the Hall Technique. Where a reversible pulpitis is present, it is common in both primary and permanent teeth to remove some of the carious lesion (as this is provoking the pain) and place a dressing to allow the dental pulp the chance to lay down reactionary dentine and wall itself from the lesion, relieving the pain. This also encourages the lesion to arrest as it is isolated from nutrients. Usually none of the carious tissue is removed, but in the case of a reversible pulpitis removing some of the lesion might help reduce enough stimuli from the lesion to allow the dental pulp to settle and lay down reparative dentine. However, if there is unprovoked pain, or other signs or symp-

Table 2. Indications and contraindications for the Hall Technique at the tooth and patient level

Indications	Contraindications
Tooth level/lesion Asymptomatic proximal and multi-surface carious primary molars (cavitated or non-cavitated, active or inactive[1]) Asymptomatic occlusal lesions (class I; cavitated or non-cavitated, active or inactive[1]), if the patient is unable to accept a conventional restoration Hypoplastic primary molars Asymptomatic carious lesions in primary molars, regardless of the surfaces involved, where the patient has a high caries risk	*Tooth level/lesion* Signs or symptoms of irreversible pulpitis, or dental abscess/fistula Radiographic signs of pulpal involvement, or peri-radicular pathology Lack of a clear band of dentine between the lesion and the dental pulp on a radiograph Lack of sufficient sound tissue to retain the crown Atypical tooth shape, so that a crown cannot be easily fitted
Patient level Anxious children (e.g., fear of injections, drilling) Behavioural disorders (e.g., attention deficit hyperactivity disorder) or young children with limited attention spans As a potential treatment for improving cooperation and building confidence	*Patient level* Where there is no cooperation as there is a risk of crown aspiration or swallowing Patients at risk of infective endocarditis Immunocompromised children

[1] The decision to place a Hall crown on an inactive and/or non-cavitated carious lesion should be based on the individual caries risk, lesion activity, child's attendance pattern, and on the overall likely benefit to the patient.

toms of irreversible pulpitis, these teeth are not candidates to be treated with the Hall Technique and need pulp therapy or to be extracted.

For Which Patients Is the Hall Technique Indicated?

Besides being indicated generally for children with carious lesions (see below for the type of teeth and lesions), the Hall Technique is particularly appropriate for carious lesions in anxious children, especially where the specific anxieties are around injections and the use of air rotor instruments. It is also well accepted by young children with short attention spans (because the treatment times are short) or where there is some ability to cooperate, although this might be limited. It is also useful as a therapy option for cooperation improvement and building a child's confidence in their ability to cope with treatment. As already stated though, if the child is unable to cooperate with treatment, this option should not be considered. Indications and contraindications of the Hall Technique are presented in Table 2.

Step 2: Child and Parent Preparation and the Materials Needed

Child and parental cooperation are crucial for procedure success. The use of the "tell, show, do" technique is recommended to introduce the child to the procedure, giving clear and specific instructions with the right level of physical interaction (e.g., show the child the crown and allow them to handle a spare one), accompanied by verbal reassurance. Using an empathetic communication style, children can be introduced to the idea of the Hall crown being "a shiny helmet, just like soldiers wear to protect their heads," "an iron man," "pirate" or "twinkle" tooth, or "a precious, shiny, princess crown." Parents should be in-

Table 3. Instruments and materials used to perform the Hall Technique

Material	Comment
Dental mirror	
Straight probe	Can be used to remove orthodontic separators, though care must be taken not to injure the tissues when the separator is loosened
Tooth brush or a bristle brush	To clean the tooth preceding crown cementation
Excavator	Can also be used to remove orthodontic separators To remove the crown if this becomes necessary To remove excess glass-ionomer cement
Heidemann spatula or flat plastic	To load the crown with glass-ionomer cement
Preformed stainless steel crowns (Fig. 2)	All sizes (1–7), although sizes 4, 5, and 6 are the most commonly used
Cotton wool rolls	For child to bite down on and push crown over tooth, and to wipe away residual cement
Glass-ionomer cement	Luting cement for crown cementation
Orthodontic elastic separators and dental floss (Fig. 3)	To gain some space mesially/distally where there are tight contact areas
Band forming pliers	To adjust the crown, mainly if the primary molars have lost mesio-distal length due to cavitated proximal carious lesions
Sticking plaster	To stick the crown to the finger, aiding airway protection

formed about the specifics of the technique, such as there being no carious tissue removal and the associated increase of the occlusal vertical dimension (OVD).

The instruments used for the Hall Technique are all commonly found in a dental practice. The essential dental instruments and consumable materials needed are presented in Table 3 and Figures 2 and 3.

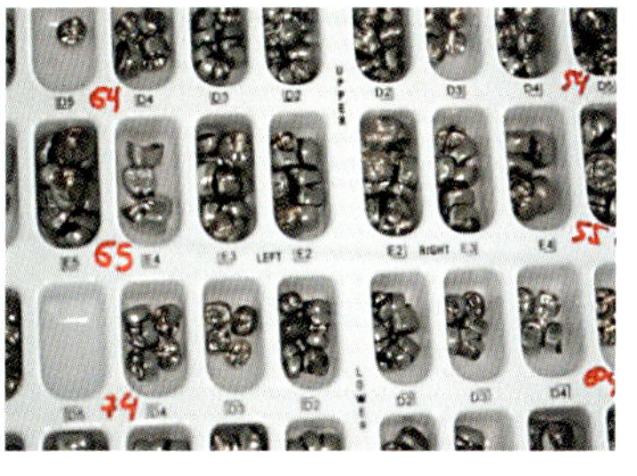

Fig. 2. Various sizes of preformed SSCs used for the Hall Technique: sizes 4, 5, and 6 are the most commonly used.

Step 3: Assessment of Crown Morphology, Contact Areas and Occlusion

- Crown morphology: aberrations in tooth shape can make placing a Hall crown more challenging. This can also become a problem when there is a proximal carious lesion with marginal ridge breakdown in the first or second primary molars. In this case, there can be a migration of the adjacent molar into the cavitated area leaving a narrower mesiodistal space to place the crown. To solve this problem, the crown margins can be adjusted using band-forming pliers, making a concavity to adapt the intruding marginal ridge of the adjacent tooth.
- Contact areas: Hall crowns can be easily fitted successfully to primary molars where the marginal ridge is still intact. Primary teeth often have broad contact areas, which can make placing the crown easier. However, for closed contacts it can be necessary to create a small amount of space for the crown by using orthodontic separators. These should be placed 2–3 days before fitting the Hall crown and removed immediately prior to crown placement (Fig. 4).
- Occlusion: it is to be expected that placing a Hall crown will cause a premature contact and

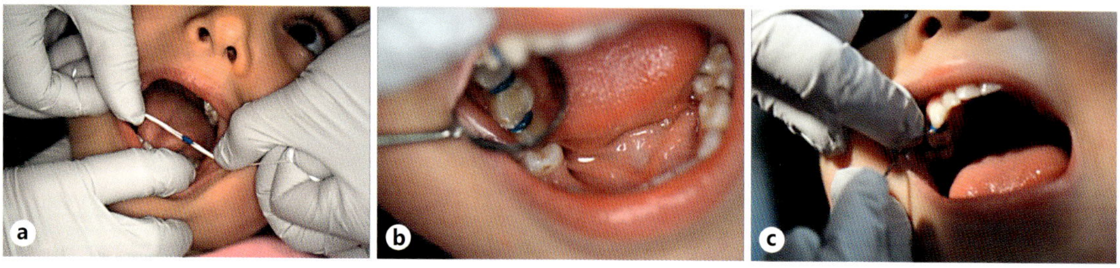

Fig. 3. a, **b** Placing of orthodontic elastic separators with dental floss to create space for fitting an SSC using the Hall Technique. **c** Careful removal of the orthodontic separators using a straight probe.

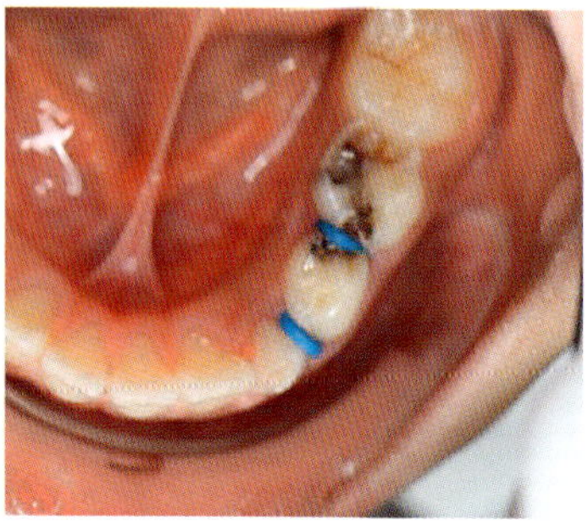

Fig. 4. Orthodontic elastic separators placed mesial and distal to create space for fitting a Hall crown on this mandibular first primary molar (74).

an increase in the OVD as there is no occlusal tooth reduction (Fig. 5). Patients and parents should be advised that the child may notice the crown as being "high in the bite," although reassured that this does not cause pain. Many children even do not consider the increase in OVD as something uncomfortable or even notice it.

- In a controlled clinical trial (performed in Surinam) the changes in the OVD after placing a Hall crown were assessed. Immediately after crown placement, the overbite decreased significantly compared to baseline (mean from 2.45 to 0.54; $p = 0.026$). Two weeks after treatment, the overbite had significantly increased (mean 1.96). Thirty days after placing the crown, the overbite did not show significant differences as compared to baseline (mean 2.75; $p = 0.317$) [27]. This study showed the primary dentition's ability to adjust to a slightly opened bite over a few days, with full re-establishment within a few weeks with no evidence of adverse effects [27]. Similar results were found in a study that examined serial photos and study models of teeth following the placement of crowns using the Hall Technique [28].

Step 4: Size of the Hall Crown

Care must be taken to protect the airway and the child should be seated upright so that if the crown falls into the mouth it lands on the floor of the mouth rather than the throat. This can also be done by using a small piece of sticking plaster on the finger to hold the crown.

The aim is to select the smallest crown size that will seat over and cover the whole tooth. The clinician should feel a slight "spring back" when trying on the crown (Fig. 6). The crown is not fully seated through the contact points before cementation; it can be very hard to remove. As described above, orthodontic separators may be placed in the proximal spaces 2–3 days before fitting the Hall crown to create space and facilitate crown placement.

When fitting a crown for a second primary molar and where the first permanent molar has not yet erupted, care must be taken not to fit an oversized crown as this may interfere with the eruption path of the first permanent molar, in-

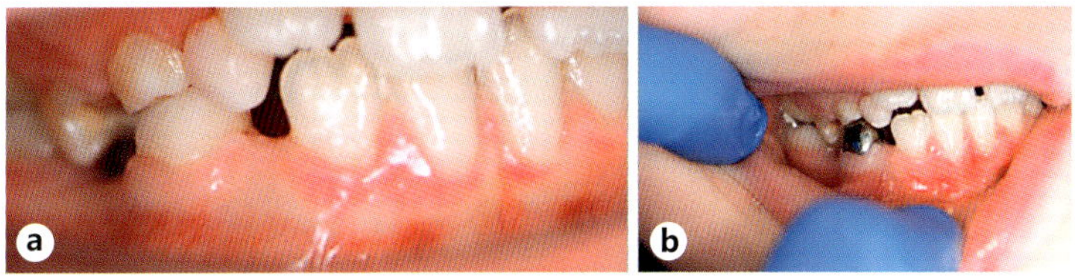

Fig. 5. Anterior view of the dentition before fitting a crown on a mandibular first primary molar (84; **a**) and immediately after crown cementation (**b**). An increase of around 1.5 mm can be observed.

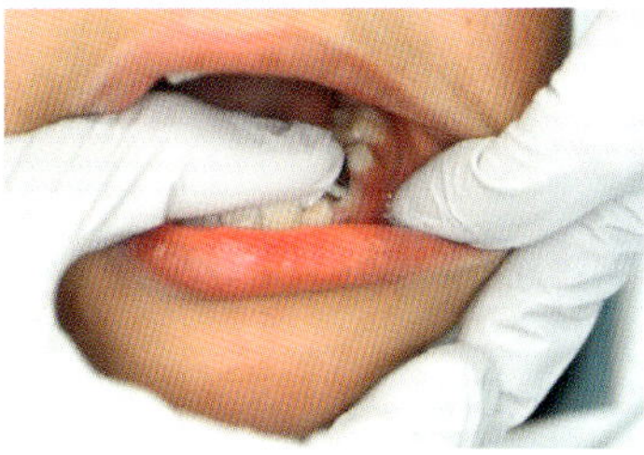

Fig. 6. Selecting the correct crown size to fit a Hall crown on a mandibular first primary molar (74).

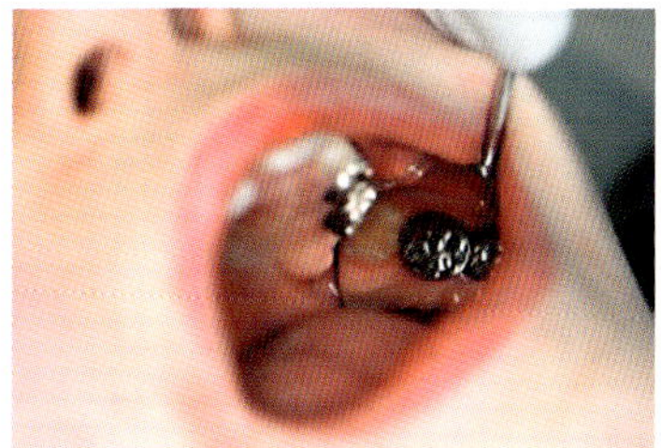

Fig. 7. Situation after 2 years. An oversize Hall crown was fitted on a maxillary second primary molar (65) interfering with the eruption path of the maxillary first permanent molar (26).

creasing its risk of impaction (Fig. 7). Before placing the crown residual bacterial plaque over the tooth can be removed with a rotary bristle brush or a toothbrush (Fig. 8).

Step 5: Fill the Crown

Clean and dry the crown using the triple syringe or cotton wool rolls. Load the crown generously with glass-ionomer luting cement from the base upwards and ensure that the cement covers the walls (Fig. 9). Be careful to avoid air blows and gaps.

Step 6: Fit and Seat the Crown

The Hall crown should be placed evenly on top of the tooth. The clinician should seat the crown by finger pressure ensuring the crown seats evenly over the tooth. As the crown is seated over the tooth excess cement should be seen to flow out from the margins. Then the child is asked to bite down on the crown. If they do not want to do this or do not bite hard enough, the crown can be pushed on by the clinician. As soon as the crown is seated, the patient should be asked to open their mouth to allow the crown position to be checked and to remove the excess of cement. If the crown fails to fully seat, it should be removed rapidly, using a spoon excavator.

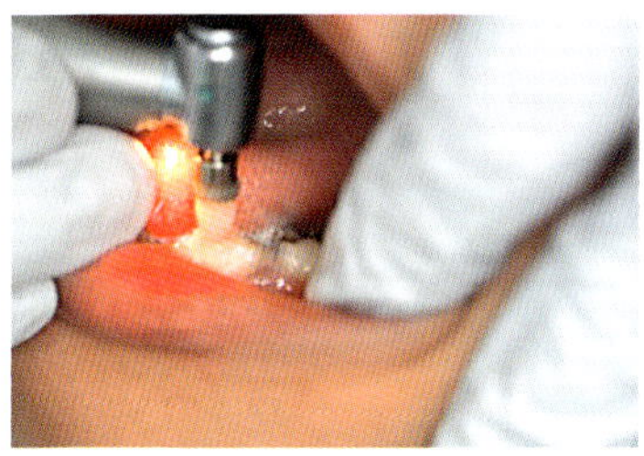

Fig. 8. Cleaning a mandibular first primary molar (74) with a rotary bristle brush before crown fitting.

Step 7: Further Seating

Having checked that the crown is in the ideal position, the child should be instructed to bite down firmly again on the crown (or cotton wool) for 2–3 min until the cement has set (Fig. 10). Alternatively, the clinician should hold

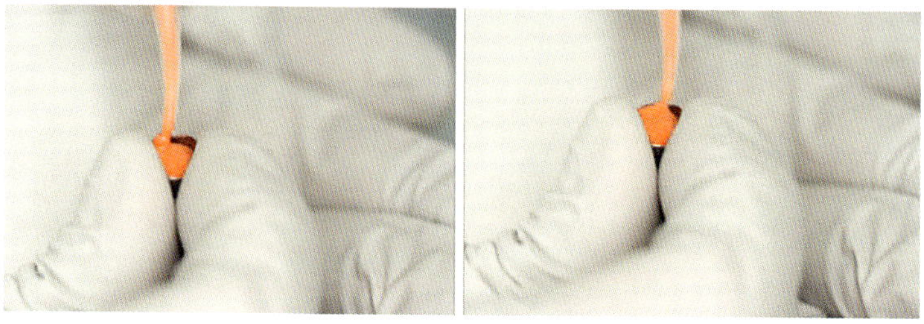

Fig. 9. Loading the Hall crown with a glass-ionomer luting cement (at least two thirds full).

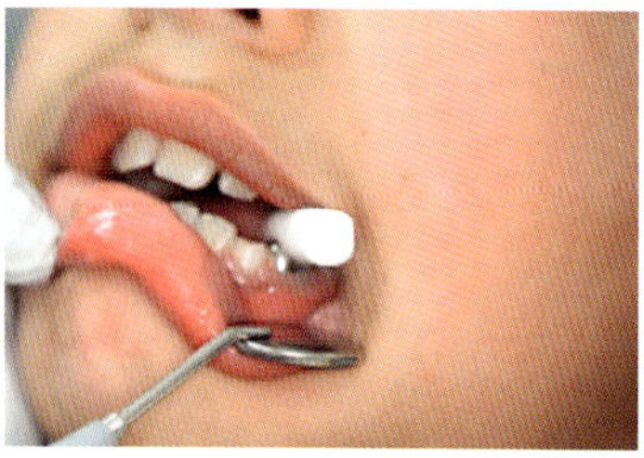

Fig. 10. Fitting the crown on a mandibular first primary molar (74). The child seats the crown by biting firmly on it.

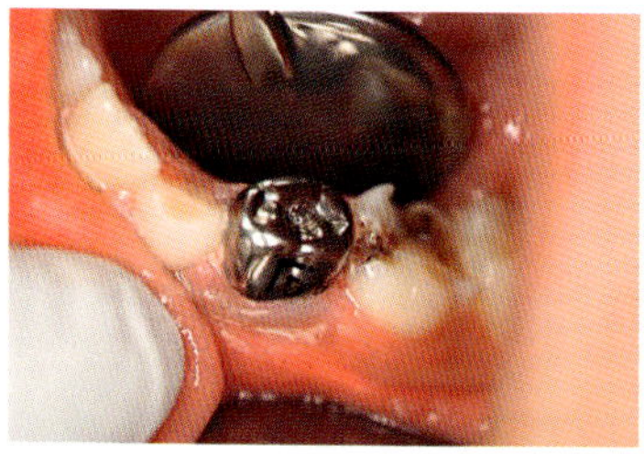

Fig. 11. Cement should be removed and the occlusion checked before discharging the patient.

down the crown with firm finger pressure to prevent it from springing back up and compromising the seal.

Step 8: Final Cement Clearance and Occlusion Check

The next step is to go around the teeth with a hand excavator to remove any excess cement and floss between the contacts (Fig. 11). It is important to inform parents that the child will notice the crown as being high in the bite, which should resolve within 1 day, with the occlusion fully re-establishing within a few weeks.

Conclusion

The Hall Technique is a low invasive, biologically based, simple procedure to perform, which is clinically effective and well accepted by patients, their carers, and clinicians [13–18, 19, 21, 29, 30]. The Hall Technique is an extremely durable (likely to last the lifespan of the primary molar) [14–18] and economical caries management option for primary molars, which in addition offers the benefit of full coronal coverage, reducing the risk of future caries development [26].

References

1 Schwendicke F, Frencken JE, Bjørndal L, Maltz M, Manton DJ, Ricketts D, van Landuyt K, Banerjee A, Campus G, Doméjean S, Fontana M, Leal S, Lo E, Machiulskiene V, Schulte A, Splieth C, Zandona AF, Innes NP: Managing carious lesions: consensus recommendations on carious tissue removal. Adv Dent Res 2016;28:58–67.

2 Kidd EA. How "clean" must a cavity be before restoration? Caries Res 2004;38:305–313.

3 Fejerskov O, Nyvad B, Kidd EA: Pathology of dental caries; in Fejerskov O, Nyvad B, Kidd EAM (eds): Dental Caries: The Disease and Its Clinical Management, ed 3. Oxford, Wiley Blackwell, 2005.

4 Kidd E: Should deciduous teeth be restored? Reflections of a cariologist. Dent Update 2012;39:159–162, 165–166.

5 Innes NPT, Frencken JE, Bjørndal L, Maltz M, Manton DJ, Ricketts D, van Landuyt K, Banerjee A, Campus G, Doméjean S, Fontana M, Leal S, Lo E, Machiulskiene V, Schulte A, Splieth C, Zandona AF, Schwendicke F: Managing carious lesions: consensus recommendations on terminology. Adv Dent Res 2016;28:49–57.
6 Innes NP, Evans DJ: Modern approaches to caries management of the primary dentition. Br Dent J 2013;214:559–566.
7 Santamaria RM, Innes NP, Machiulskiene V, Evans DJ, Alkilzy M, Splieth CH: Acceptability of different caries management methods for primary molars in a RCT. Int J Paediatr Dent 2015; 25:9–17.
8 Innes N, Evans D, Hall N: The Hall technique for managing carious primary molars. Dent Update 2009;36:472–474, 477–478.
9 Innes N, Evans D, Stirrups D: The Hall technique. Br Dent J 2008;205:167–168.
10 Innes NP, Ricketts D, Chong LY, Keightley AJ, Lamont T, Santamaria RM: Preformed crowns for decayed primary molar teeth. Cochrane Database Syst Rev 2015;12:CD005512.
11 Seale NS, Randall R: The use of stainless steel crowns: a systematic literature review. Pediatr Dent 2015;37:145–160.
12 Innes NP, Stirrups DR, Evans DJ, Hall N, Leggate M: A novel technique using preformed metal crowns for managing carious primary molars in general practice – a retrospective analysis. Br Dent J 2006;200:451–454, discussion 444.
13 Innes NP, Evans DJ, Stirrups DR: The Hall technique; a randomized controlled clinical trial of a novel method of managing carious primary molars in general dental practice: acceptability of the technique and outcomes at 23 months. BMC Oral Health 2007;7:18.
14 Santamaria RM, Innes NP, Machiulskiene V, Evans DJ, Splieth CH: Caries management strategies for primary molars: 1-yr randomized control trial results. J Dent Res 2014;93:1062–1069.
15 Santamaría RM, Innes NPT, Machiulskiene V, Schmoeckel J, Alkilzy M, Splieth CH: Alternative caries management options for primary molars: 2.5-year outcomes of a randomised clinical trial. Caries Res 2017;51:605–614.
16 Innes NP, Evans DJ, Stirrups DR: Sealing caries in primary molars: randomized control trial, 5-year results. J Dent Res 2011;90:1405–1410.
17 Narbutait J, Innes NPT, Santamaria RM, Splieth CH, Machiulskiene V: One-year outcomes of dental caries management using different approaches in primary molars of Lithuanian children. Caries Res 2016;50:323.
18 Araujo MP, Olegario IC, Hesse D, Innes NP, Bonifacio CC, Raggio DP: ART versus Hall technique in primary molars: 1-year survival and cost analysis of a RCT. Caries Res 2016;50:330.
19 Ludwig KH, Fontana M, Vinson LA, Platt JA, Dean JA: The success of stainless steel crowns placed with the Hall technique. J Am Dent Assoc 2014;145: 1248–1253.
20 BaniHani A, Duggal M, Toumba J, Deery C: Outcomes of the conventional and biological treatment approaches for the management of caries in the primary dentition. Int J Paediatr Dent 2018; 28:12–22.
21 Clark W, Geneser M, Owais A, Kanellis M, Qian F: Success rates of Hall technique crowns in primary molars: a retrospective pilot study. Gen Dent 2017; 65:32–35.
22 Innes NP, Evans DJ, Bonifacio CC, Geneser M, Hesse D, Heimer M, Kanellis M, Machiulskiene V, Narbutaité J, Olegário IC, Owais A, Araujo MP, Raggio DP, Splieth C, van Amerongen E, Weber-Gasparoni K, Santamaria RM: The Hall technique 10 years on: questions and answers. Br Dent J 2017;222:478–483.
23 van Bochove JA, van Amerongen WE: The influence of restorative treatment approaches and the use of local analgesia, on the children's discomfort. Eur Arch Paediatr Dent 2006;7:11–16.
24 American Academy on Pediatric Dentistry Clinical Affairs Committee – Behavior Management Subcommittee: Guideline on behavior guidance for the pediatric dental patient. Pediatr Dent 2009;30:125–133.
25 Goumans C, Veerkamp JS, Aartman IH: Dental anxiety and behavioural problems: what is their influence on the treatment plan? Eur J Paediatr Dent 2004;5:15–18.
26 Schwendicke F, Stolpe M, Innes N: Conventional treatment, Hall technique or immediate pulpotomy for carious primary molars: a cost-effectiveness analysis. Int Endod J 2016;49:817–826.
27 van der Zee V, van Amerongen WE: Short communication: influence of preformed metal crowns (Hall technique) on the occlusal vertical dimension in the primary dentition. Eur Arch Paediatr Dent 2010;11:225–227.
28 So D, Evans DJ, Borrie F, Roughley M, Lamont T, Keightley A, Innes NPT: Measurement of occlusal equilibration following Hall crown placement – a pilot study (abstract). J Dent Res 2015; 94(spec. issue A):0080.
29 Innes NPT, Ricketts D, Chong LY, Keightley AJ, Lamont T, Santamaria RM: Preformed crowns for decayed primary molar teeth. Cochrane Database Syst Rev 2015;12:CD005512.
30 Boyd DH, Page LF, Thomson WM: The Hall technique and conventional restorative treatment in New Zealand children's primary oral health care – clinical outcomes at two years. Int J Paediatr Dent 2018;28:180–188.

Ruth M. Santamaría
Department of Preventive and Pediatric Dentistry
Ernst-Moritz-Arndt University of Greifswald
Rotgerbergstrasse 8
DE–17487 Greifswald (Germany)
E-Mail ruth.santamaria@uni-greifswald.de

Schwendicke F, Frencken J, Innes N (eds): Caries Excavation: Evolution of Treating Cavitated Carious Lesions.
Monogr Oral Sci. Basel, Karger, 2018, vol 27, pp 124–136 (DOI: 10.1159/000487839)

No Removal and Inactivation of Carious Tissue: Non-Restorative Cavity Control

Guus van Strijp · Cor van Loveren
Academic Centre for Dentistry (ACTA), Amsterdam, The Netherlands

Abstract

Non-restorative cavity control (NRCC) is a 3-part treatment option for dentine cavities in the primary dentition, for root carious lesions and cavitated coronal smooth surface lesions. The first part is that the patient's oral hygiene procedure/habits improve and involve the exposed dentine. For this, it may be necessary to expose the cavity (second part) so that it is accessible for the toothbrush (the lesion exposure method). As long as the dentine carious lesion is diagnosed as active or there is increased risk that carious lesion activity will recur, it is advisable to support the treatment with a 38% silver diamine fluoride (SDF) or a 5% sodium fluoride (NaF) varnish therapy (third part). NRCC has advantages over traditional restorative therapy as it avoids the stress and fear initiation that often results from invasive restorative therapy. It avoids a futile or detrimental repeat restorative cycle when cavity outlines have to be designed in caries active areas and it increases awareness of people's own responsibility for oral health and the quality of the oral hygiene procedure. NRCC has been advocated, particularly in primary dentitions, for patients or parents/carers who are able to accept responsibility for the disease and commit to remedial action including diet modification and regular, frequent toothbrushing with a fluoride toothpaste. It should not be used when immediate invasive action is required such as in the case of pain, infection, or sepsis. Professionals who choose NRCC commit themselves to being critical regarding their educational qualities and to commence a cycle of quality improvement.

Minimal invasive intervention treatments are based on the paradigm shift that the biofilm overlying the carious lesion is the driving force of the carious process and not the bacteria present in infected dentine. Daily removal or disruption of this biofilm by brushing with a fluoridated toothpaste will slow down the carious process or even bring it to a halt. A prerequisite for adequate removal of the biofilm from within a cavity, however, is the cavity's level of accessibility. A cavity can be made accessible by removing overhanging enamel or, in the case of a cavity in the approximal surface, by slicing that surface. Treating a cavity in this way is termed non-restorative cavity control (NRCC) [1]. NRCC can be defined as a causal therapy, i.e., fighting the cause of the disease and not its symptoms. Examples of NRCC treatment are: (1) daily biofilm removal with toothbrush and fluoride toothpaste, supported by 3-monthly fluoride varnish application or application of a glass-ionomer layer; (2) application of silver diamine fluoride (SDF) followed by daily biofilm removal with toothbrush and fluoride toothpaste.

NRCC in primary teeth aims at preserving the functionality of the tooth until exfoliation without causing pain or inflammation. It is considered a child-friendly treatment as no drilling or anaesthesia is needed. Avoiding or postponing a restorative treatment and a likely retreatment by using this low-threatening treatment avoids or at least reduces fear and anxiety of the child towards oral health and increases his/her confidence in the professional. However, its success depends in a large part on the parent's/caretaker's ability and willingness to take responsibility for their child's oral health in general, and especially for cleaning cavities. Oral hygiene should be performed adequately and daily. For the general dental practitioner NRCC is another tool in guiding a young child and parents in keeping primary teeth functional and pain free [2].

In the permanent dentition, a minimal invasive treatment is applicable for managing root carious lesions or coronal smooth surface lesions. In these cases, the main goal is to avoid a futile repetative restorative cycle, which starts as cavity outlines are prepared in caries-active areas. By first preventing lesion activity, the only reason for any treatment becomes esthetical or functional. The only negative impact concerns the fact that the lesion will frequently darken in colour over time as the mineral content in the surface of the lesion increases and/or because of the Maillard reaction and/or because extrinsic stains are incorporated into the arresting lesion. NRCC has the ability to become one of the most effective ways of managing cavitated dentine lesions and, thus, avoiding placing a restoration. If aesthetics is an issue for the patient, then a minimally invasive tooth-coloured restoration may be placed. The evidence supporting NRCC treatments is presented later on in this chapter.

It is obvious that if a cavity has developed, primary prevention has failed. Just restoring a cavity, without putting emphasis on improving oral hygiene, is not the way forward. To improve patients' oral hygiene habits, a tailor-made approach to communicate with the patient may be necessary. This would be more easily achieved with NRCC treatments than with a restorative approach. During restorative sessions patients are generally not open for preventive counselling [3].

For an NRCC treatment to become successful, a paradigm shift in the mind of dental practitioners is also necessary. An example is reported in the study by Varsio et al. [4]. The authors observed that the treatment strategy used for the 6-year-old high-caries patients was not preventive oriented. High-caries patients had 3–4 times as many visits as all 6-year-old children on average, but the visits mostly served for providing operative treatment. In spite of these operative efforts, only 39% of treatment courses among the non-cooperative and in 63% among the cooperative high-caries patients were completed. Non-cooperative patients (approx. 34% of this population) had more past and present caries in their deciduous teeth, more dental visits, and received more demanding treatment than the cooperative high-caries patients. Caries preventive treatment given to all high-caries patients was rare, the number of preventive interventions per patient and per visit tended to correlate negatively with patient cooperation. In the remainder of this chapter, we discuss NRCC treatments and present the scientific evidence obtained so far.

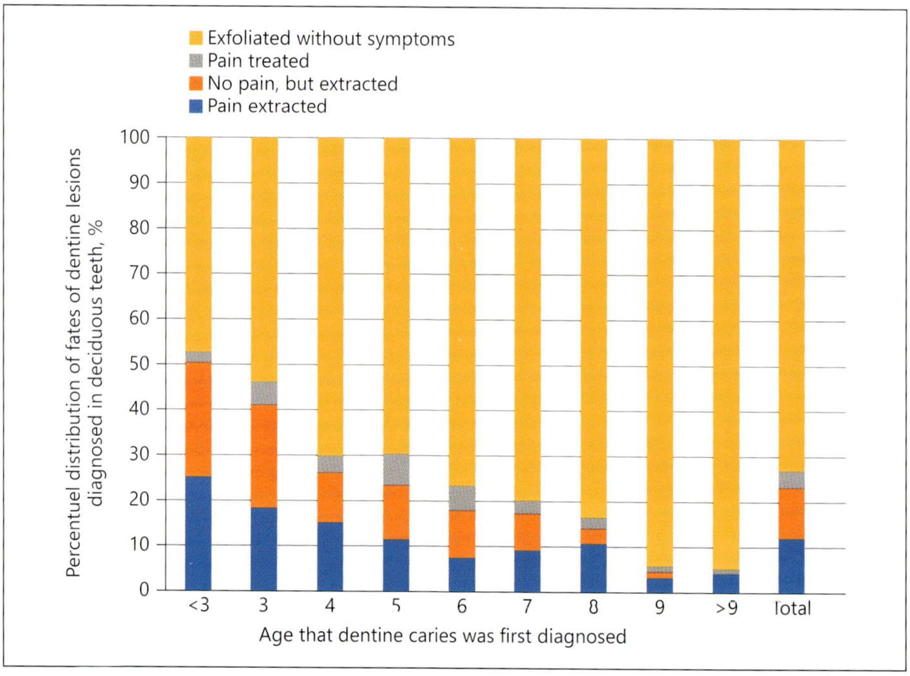

Fig. 1. Fate of diagnosed dentine caries at various ages (adapted from Levine et al. [5]).

Is Restorative Treatment Necessary?

In oral health, we often forget to pose the question of what would happen if we do not interfere at all. This question is of interest as the actual prognosis of the disease may determine the choice of treatment. Mostly, dental practitioners still act based on the idea that the disease will progress if the lesion is not restored. Is this presumption always correct? In a retrospective study, Levine et al. [5] showed that it is not always necessary to restore cavities in primary teeth as most of the not-restored teeth in his study exfoliated without symptoms. This study was performed in 2 general practices in northern England. When the first of these practices was established in 1976, the prevalence of caries was much higher than today and the pressure on the available resources within the newly established practices required priority to be given to pain relief and treatment of carious permanent teeth. Asymptomatic carious primary teeth were frequently seen, but usually left unrestored and this policy continued over the years. Management consisted of regular reinforcement of simple dietary and toothbrushing advice. Where appropriate, fluoride dietary supplements were prescribed. Of 1,587 non-treated cavitated primary teeth in 481 children, 84% showed no clinical symptoms like pain or abscesses after the mean observation time of 1,332 days (Fig. 1). However, even those teeth that were extracted had a median survival time of 490 days.

Non-Restorative Cavity Control: Primary Dentition

For NRCC treatments to be successful, the cooperation of the child and parents/caregivers in keeping the carious lesion(s) clean is a prerequisite. It needs the motivation and long-term cooperation of both. Transfer of knowledge to the par-

Table 1. Examples of words that should not be used when motivating patients

Words to avoid	Reason	Alternative
This session will not take long	Patient may only hear "long" and "not long"	I will use 2 minutes of your time
(active remark), but...	Destructive	(active remark), and.........
Why?	Destructive	Can you tell me the reasons
Can you try...?	Suggestive for answer: off course I can	I see you have some doubts, can you share these with me...?

ents/caregiver about the caries process and the awareness that self-care can stop this process are essential. The professional should have knowledge of behavioural change techniques and apply these systematically with the consequences of recall sessions [6]. Changing the behaviour of the family where the lifestyle and actions have led to initiation of the disease is very challenging and should not be underestimated.

To check if behavioural change techniques have been applied well, it is advisable to occasionally make a voice recording of these sessions. The conversation can be examined and alternative strategies planned if necessary [6]. You can ask yourself: did I create a safe and open atmosphere, did I align with the patient, did I motivate (or did I actually do the opposite), did we reach an action plan? and so. In short, was I active and constructive? As an example, a phrase like "you brushed well but you have to move your brush more to the back" (active, but destructive) stimulates a patient differently compared with the phrase "you brushed well and if you move your brush a little more to the back it is perfect" (active and constructive; Table 1).

Indication of NRCC

In a number of cases in primary teeth, NRCC can be considered an alternative to restorative treatment. From a medical ethical point of view, that tells us that a medical/dental professional should chose the least invasive treatment option available, the use of NRCC treatments as the first choice of treatment can be defendable unless there is an immediate threat of pain, infection, or need for extraction. Restorative treatment may be the first choice if the tooth cavity is small and the dentition, generally speaking, well maintained. In general, NRCC treatments would be the first choice for the following indications [7]:

- young children (4 years or younger) – non-invasive treatments prevent or at least postpone threatening invasive treatments to an older age when the child can better cope with these;
- children who are very afraid of a restorative treatment – this treatment may not be needed (age-dependent) or be postponed;
- children (8–9 years and older) with many active caries lesions in the primary dentition to prevent restorative treatment until exfoliation – in cases of pain and infection extraction is the treatment of choice.

The advantage of this cause-related therapy is that success or failure can be observed (activity of the lesion) in time and discussed with the child and/or parents/caregiver. The effect of the causal therapy can be assessed by the hardness and most often shiny appearance of the demineralised tooth surface. NRCC can "buy" time for a child to develop the cognition to understand and cope with a more invasive treatment should it be necessary. Also, it allows time for them to

Table 2. Treatment protocol of NRCC consists of several steps (adapted from Gruythuysen [7])

Administrative	Contract involving the informed consent, clarifying the purpose of the treatment and the role of the dental professional and patient, parents/caregiver to make the treatment successful
Technical	Make the cavity accessible for (professional) home care cleaning; using a hatchet or diamond burr overhanging enamel can be removed; in the case of an approximal cavity, slicing (in a V-form shape without losing contact with the neighbouring tooth) will enhance accessibility. Teach and check the skills of the patient, parents/caregiver in how to clean the cavity adequately with the preferred toothbrush
Behavioural	Use appropriate behavioural change techniques like motivational interviewing; this includes a step of checking that the information has been understood; make voice recordings of the sessions for educational purposes for yourself
Safety net	Apply fluoride varnish (every 3 months), SDF (once/twice a year), or a remineralisation-promoting liner (glass-ionomer) until the dentine has rehardened
Periodic evaluation	Tailor periodic evaluation to the alleged success for the next period; at most a 3-month period, unless a longer period argued for; Use light photographs and/or a notation system like Ekstrand, Nyvad or ICDAS to monitor caries/lesion activity/size; Decide whether the treatment is still justified; Reinforce of the self-care strategy

become acclimatised to the dental environment. Moreover, it does not need local anaesthesia or rotary instruments.

Treatment Protocol of NRCC

As the success of NRCC depends highly on the collaboration of patients and parents/caregivers, the goals and the obligation of all parties should be clear (Table 2). Therefore, it is advisable to sign a contract involving the informed consent from the patient and/or the parents/caregiver which mentions the purpose of the treatment, the role of the dental professional and that of the patient and/or parents/caregiver to assist in bringing the treatment to a success. The technical protocol implies making the cavity accessible (lesion exposure) for home care cleaning with the preferred toothbrush (removal of the biofilm). It may be necessary to slice (approximally) the tooth surface or to remove overhanging enamel with a hatchet, enamel access cutter, or diamond burr. In cases where slicing is performed, the resulting situation should avoid food impaction and loss of interproximal space. It is essential that patients/parents/caregivers are motivated and instructed to clean the cavity twice daily. Special care should be given to clean approximal surfaces which is comparable to cleaning erupting molars (Fig. 2). Communicate effectively (motivational interviewing techniques), use behavioural change techniques, and keep an adequate patient health record. A safety net support can be given by the application of fluoride varnish at every visit, or application of SDF or a remineralisation-promoting liner (glass-ionomer). Monitor caries activity and the lesion size by taking clinical coloured pictures. Determine a recall period that is dependent on the level of activity of the carious lesion and the cooperation of patient/caregiver. A recall period might initially be very short, but can be en-

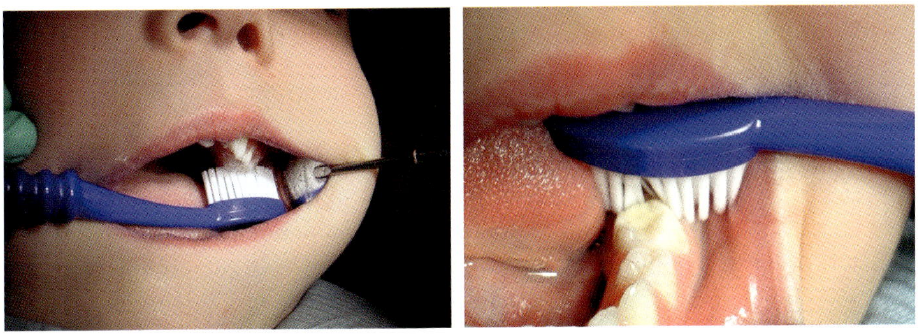

Fig. 2. To reach the occlusal surface of a partially erupted permanent molar in the mixed dentition, it might be necessary to brush perpendicular to the dental arch (also known as lateral brushing). (Photographs: René Gruythuysen, Amsterdam).

Table 3. Clinical criteria for active and inactive dentine carious lesions (adapted from Fejerskov and Nyvad [8])

Active lesion	
Visual appearance	Yellowish or light brownish; dull/matte; typically covered by biofilm
Tactile features	Soft, sticky/leathery on gentle probing; with/without localised/manifest cavitation; margins of cavity are sharply demarcated
Inactive lesion	
Visual appearance	Yellowish, brownish or black; shiny smooth; often not covered by biofilm
Tactile features	Feels hard on gentle probing; cavity formation may be rough/uneven; margins of cavity are smooth

larged depending on the performance of the patient/caregiver and the success obtained.

Active cavitated dentine lesions are lesions that are considered to be progressing at the time of examination. Active dentine lesions are yellowish or light brownish in colour and are typically covered by a microbial deposit. The carious tissue feels soft or leathery on gentle probing (Table 3). Inactive lesions are considered to be arrested and re-activation is controlled by daily toothbrushing with fluoride toothpaste. The inactive (arrested) lesion is typically dark brown – often almost black. The surface of the lesion is usually shiny and smooth, and hard on gentle probing. However, colour per se is not considered a reliable diagnostic criterion [9]. The diagnostic characteristics of these types of lesions are mandatory to apply in daily clinical practice to avoid unnecessary treatments. To monitor caries development notation systems like ICDAS, Nyvad, or Ekstrand can be used [see the chapter by Neuhaus and Lussi; this vol., pp. 24–31].

Scientific Evidence for Success of NRCC in Primary Dentition

NRCC corresponds to a causal approach of caries and is targeted to improve oral health and to keep teeth functional. NRCC in the primary dentition

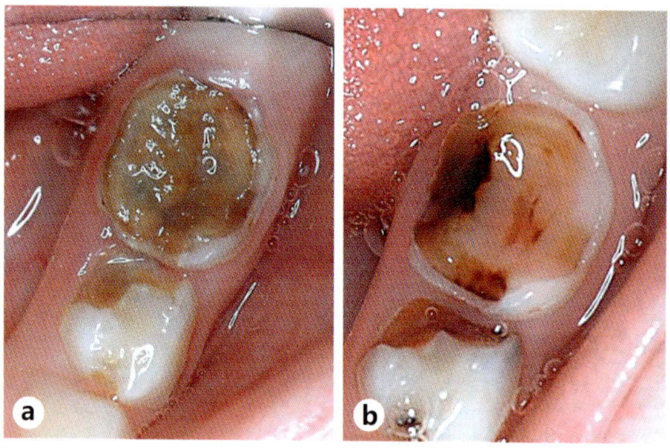

Fig. 3. Successful NRCC treatment of carious lesions in 84 and 85. Active lesions (**a**) were still arrested after 12 months (**b**). (Photographs: Nicola Innes, Dundee).

may even be an alternative for invasive treatments under general anaesthesia. NRCC is successful when the carious lesion has become arrested (Fig. 3).

NRCC is not new. G.V. Black, in his textbook of 1908 [10], wrote: "All buccal and labial cavities in which decay is burrowing should be fully opened by clipping away all the overhanging enamel and left as wide open as possible in order to admit free washing, both in artificial cleaning and in fresh clean saliva." This advice concurs with the observation from Anderson in 1938 [11], who showed that carious lesion progression within a cavity was arrested in primary teeth after making the occlusal cavitated lesion accessible for cleaning. This observation was made in the pre-fluoride era. Since then, a number of population-based studies have been reported, and these are presented below.

An interesting observation was made during a longitudinal school-performed study originally designed to prevent caries in the primary dentition [12, 13]. The prevention program for 168 Chinese children (aged 3–6 years) consisted of tooth brushing with a 1,000-ppm fluoride toothpaste under the supervision of a trained teacher. The teachers also taught the children prevention and oral hygiene procedures. After the evaluation period of 3 years, 28% of the cavitated carious dentine lesions had become inactive, while in the control groups only 12% of such lesions became arrested. A multiple linear regression analysis indicated that the baseline ds score and its interactions with the prevention programme, gender, and the child's oral hygiene all had a significant effect on the number of tooth surfaces with arrested carious lesions at the final examination. It has to be remarked that in this study there was no involvement of the parents.

In an observational clinical study [14] with 30 toddlers who suffered from early childhood caries, the NRCC approach was shown to be successful. Active carious lesions in the proximal surfaces of anterior teeth were made accessible for cleaning by slicing the surface. The children received a fluoride gel (2% sodium fluoride; NaF) treatment every 2 months. The caregivers were instructed how to clean the lesions and were advised regarding a healthy diet and oral health. After 1 year, 90% of these anterior lesions became inactive and did not show any complications.

Several studies compared NRCC with the traditional approach (complete excavation and restoration) and with atraumatic restorative treatment (ART) or the use of a Hall crown (no excavation of carious dentine, sealing in the caries process with a stainless-steel crown filled with glass-ionomer cement).

Mijan et al. [15, 16] compared the survival percentages of cavitated primary molars treated traditionally with amalgam (CRT), the ART method, and the UCT (ultra conservative treatment) method among 6- to 7-year-old Brazilian children. In the UCT group, small cavities were treated according to the ART method and medium- and large-sized cavities were made accessible, if needed, and cleaned with toothbrush and fluoride toothpaste (NRCC). After 3.5 years, no significant differences in survival percentages were observed between the 3 treatment modalities of CRT, ART, and UCT (90.9, 90.4, and 89.0%, respectively). In the UCT group, cavity cleaning was performed every day under the supervision of a trained dental auxiliary during school days (200 days/year). This study showed that the UCT approach showed good results. An investigation of quality of life was also part of this study [17]. After 1 year, no significant difference in quality of life was observed between the treatment groups. The different treatments were equally effective in the decrease of pain sensation, insomnia, and irritability.

In a practice-based randomised clinical trial, Santamaria et al. [18] compared 3 treatment protocols in children with a high caries risk. The investigated treatments were conventional restoration (compomer), Hall Technique, and NRCC. NRCC comprised enhancing the accessibility of approximal cavities in primary teeth and the application of a fluoride varnish. The caregivers of the children (aged 3–8 years) received instruction in how to brush the lesion perpendicular to the dental arch. The fluoride varnish application (5% NaF) and the instructions were repeated every 3 months. After 2.5 years, 142 children could be included for evaluation. The results showed that the Hall Technique was superior (2.5% major failures) compared to conventional restorations (9.0% major failures) and NRCC (9.0% major failures). Comparing the conventional treatment with NRCC, no significant difference was observed in the percentage of failures (abscesses, pulpal complaints, or necessity for a endodontic treatment). Within the NRCC group, most failures were found in children not adhering to the 3-month recall interval. Children treated according to the conventional treatment modality showed less cooperative behaviour compared to children treated according to the Hall Technique or NRCC [19].

In a study evaluating 30 cavities in approximal surfaces of primary molars that had been treated daily through site-specific oral hygiene with a fluoridated toothpaste, supplemented by professional topical fluoride treatment and dietary advice, 50% of the cavitated approximal cavities survived without complaints after an average period of 26 months (9–44 months). Five cavities showed major failures (pulpal/periapical pathology) due to unsuccessful cooperation of mother or child. In 5 cases, failure occurred due to technical imperfections (failure to open up lesions sufficiently or lesions extended too far apically to render the lesion cleansable). Finally, 5 cavities were filled because of sensitivity or lesion progression making the lesion uncleansable. Children and parents were highly satisfied with the NRCC treatment. The authors concluded that this NRCC treatment can be a helpful method to control carious lesion progression in primary teeth and may familiarise the child with dental treatment [20].

In addition to the described clinical studies, well-documented clinical case studies have demonstrated the usefulness of NRCC, supported with fluoride varnish, in arresting carious lesion progression and its beneficial effect for the child in accepting a needed treatment [21]. NRCC requires an accurate monitoring of the activity of the lesion. Lesion activity is the reflection of the cooperation of the parent/caregiver or child. It must be kept in mind that the same parent/caregiver were not able or willing to prevent the present cavities. To persuade them to improve their attitude towards performing a better oral hygiene regime for their child is not an easy task. To allow NRCC to work, it needs parents/carers (or older children) who are able to accept responsibility for the disease and commit to remedial action, including diet modification and regular, frequent toothbrushing with a fluoride toothpaste.

Non-Restorative Cavity Control: Permanent Dentition

In permanent dentition, NRCC can be used in cases of cavitated coronal smooth surface lesions or in root carious lesions. Similarly to the management of cavitated lesions in the primary denti-

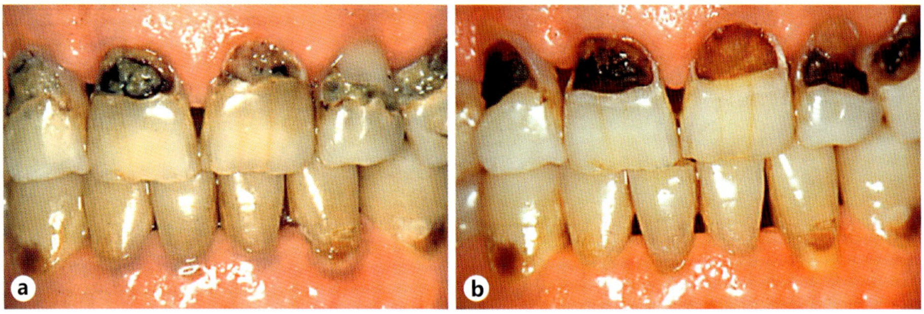

Fig. 4. NRCC of active smooth surface carious lesions in upper anterior teeth. **a** Multiple carious lesions are covered by plaque. **b** Appearance after 14 days. Overhanging enamel has been removed to make the cavities accessible for cleaning and the lesions were brushed with a fluoride toothpaste twice daily. Lesions had turned towards inactivity. (Photographs: Peter van Amerongen, Amsterdam).

tion, accessibility of the lesion for cleansing is a prerequisite for inactivating the caries process. In smooth surface lesions as well as in root carious lesions adjacent to the dentine-enamel junction, smoothening of the cavity border and removing overhanging enamel will improve the cleansability (lesion exposure method). Depending on the activity of the lesion, additional application of a fluoride will enhance remineralisation. An example of the inactivation of active smooth surface lesions by making the lesions accessible for cleaning and an improved cleansing with fluoride toothpaste is shown in Figure 4.

Scientific Evidence for Success of NRCC in Permanent Dentition

The success of a causal approach of cavitated lesions was shown in an 18-month observational study [22] where active cavitated root carious lesions became inactive just by cleaning the surface of the lesions with a fluoride toothpaste twice daily and 2% NaF application at the start of the study and after 8 weeks. Even when the root surface has been severely demineralised, the collagen fibres in the dentine are retained as a scaffold into which redeposition of mineral may take place. Great caution should, therefore, be taken to not remove or damage the softened tissue by probing or scaling before any attempt to reharden the softened tissue has taken place. Enabling mineral deposition into a partly demineralised root surface takes several months. The important factor is to ensure that the patient can perform a proper daily oral hygiene using a fluoridated toothpaste. Furthermore, a topical application of a 2% NaF solution, APF gel (2.7% NaF), fluoride varnish, or SDF is recommended at 3-month intervals as long as lesions show signs of activity [23, 24]. Changing the environmental conditions does not only modify the surface features of the root carious lesion, but also enhances the biological response in the dentine, leading to increased sclerosis deep into the previously demineralised zone. These interventions may therefore have an effect on the experience of pain within weeks.

In recent years, research has focused on high fluoride concentrations in toothpaste for improved control of root caries development. Four short-term clinical trials of 6–8 months [25–28] have concluded that root caries progression might be halved by exchanging a conventional toothpaste (1,100, 1,350, 1,450 ppm F) with a 5,000-ppm-F toothpaste [29].

The Role of Fluoride in Arresting Dentine Caries

In several studies, the topical use of fluoride has been part of the treatment protocol to remineralise dentine carious lesions. There is, however, little evidence on the efficacy of this process, although in situ studies provided evidence that fluoride is essential in root caries control [30]. The basic chemical similarity between dentine and enamel indicates that similar physicochemical processes are responsible for caries development and progression in these tissues. Histological differences between enamel and dentine predict, however, that fluoride is less effective in protecting dentine than in protecting enamel. Knowledge from experiments with enamel cannot be easily translated to dentine. Therefore, more evidence should be collected to show the effectiveness of fluoride on the protection and remineralisation of dentine carious lesions. When comparing coronal and root dentine, the basic histological similarity indicates that fluoride may be equally effective for both tissues.

SDF solution/varnish and NaF varnish are the most often professionally applied products tested for dentine caries control. The mode of action of SDF is based on the antimicrobial effect of silver and the formation of a "sclerotic coating" at the surface of carious dentine. Bacterial killing is, however, not a long-lasting cure for root caries [31]. SDF has again attracted attention in recent decades. A number of clinical studies are presented below.

A prospective controlled clinical trial investigated the effectiveness of topical fluoride applications in arresting dentine caries [32]. Three hundred and seventy-five children, aged 3–5 years, with carious upper anterior teeth were divided into 5 groups. Children received annual applications of SDF solution (44,800 ppm F) or NaF varnish (22,600 ppm F) applications every 3 months. For half of the children, soft carious tissue was removed prior to fluoride application, which was not performed in the other half. After 30 months, the respective mean percentages of arrested carious tooth surfaces in the SDF groups were approximately 50% irrespective of the type of excavation, while in the NaF varnish groups the rate was approximately 30%, the same percentage as in the control group.

In another study [2], children aged 3–4 years who had at least 1 active dentine carious lesion were randomly allocated into 3 intervention groups: group 1, application of 30% SDF solution every 12 months; group 2, 3 applications of 30% SDF solution at weekly intervals at baseline, and group 3, 3 applications of 5% NaF varnish at weekly intervals at baseline. After 18 months, the caries arrest rates at tooth surface level were 40, 35, and 27% for groups 1, 2, and 3, respectively ($p < 0.001$). The presence of plaque on lesion surfaces, tooth type, and tooth surface all had significant effects on caries arrest rates.

In another study [33], annual application of SDF was compared to the semi-annual application and to annual application of high fluoride-releasing glass-ionomer. The caries arrest rates were 79, 91, and 82% for the 3 groups, respectively ($p = 0.007$).

In a prospective randomised clinical trial, Yee et al. [34] showed the caries-arresting effectiveness of a single spot application of: (1) 38% SDF with tannic acid as a reducing agent to accelerate the deposition of silver phosphate; (2) 38% SDF alone; (3) 12% SDF alone, and (4) no SDF application in the primary teeth of 976 Nepalese schoolchildren. The single application of 38% SDF with or without tannic acid was effective in arresting caries, but the 12% application was not. After 6 months, 50–60% of the dentine lesions had arrested, but of those approximately 50% became active again after 24 months. The authors concluded that 38% SDF provides an alternative when restorative treatment for primary teeth is not an option.

An annual application of 38% SDF has been shown to prevent and arrest root carious lesions in elderly people compared to education only, after 24–30 months of follow-up [23, 24]. Li et al. [24] showed that 90% of root carious lesions arrested after the application of SDF against 45% for the control group in a 30-month clinical trial. SDF has also been applied into prepared cavity lesions, reducing secondary root caries development around class V restorations [35].

In summary, SDF seems to be more effective than NaF varnish. Based on single studies it seems that semi-annual applications of 38% SDF are slightly better than annual applications. Removal of soft carious dentine prior to SDF application seems not to be necessary. Lower concentrations of SDF appear to be less effective.

Adverse Effects of SDF

SDF application usually blackens the teeth to an unacceptable level and caution has to be taken when visible areas are treated. Duangthip et al. [36] demonstrated that blackening of carious lesions was common, affecting 36.7 and 49.5% of the lesions when 12% SDF was applied annually or semi-annually, and 65.6 and 76.3% of the lesions when 38% SDF was applied annually or semi-annually, respectively. They did not report significantly high rates of adverse effects, including tooth or gum pain, gum swelling, gum bleaching, and systemic toxicity. Overall, the prevalence of tooth and gum pain as perceived by patients and reported by parents was 6.6%, while gum swelling and gum bleaching were 2.8 and 4.7%, respectively. These adverse effects may last for up to 48 h [37, 38]. Based on parental reporting, SDF did not cause acute systemic illness.

Conclusion

Dentine caries can be arrested. The first option to achieve this is through brushing the surface with a fluoride toothpaste (1,000–1,500 ppm F). For adults, a better result is achieved when the toothpaste contains 5,000 ppm F. Additionally, an annually or semi-annually applied solution of 38% SDF or a 3-monthly 5% NaF varnish may also be useful in arresting dentine caries. If a cavity is not accessible for cleaning its surface, the lesion has to be exposed further. This "lesion exposure method" can be applied in the primary dentition for coronal lesions or in the permanent dentition for root carious and cavitated coronal smooth surface lesions. The concept, exposing the lesion and brushing the surface to reharden it, is designated as an NRCC treatment. This method has advantages for patients and dental professionals. The advantages for the patient is that a cavitated carious lesion can be managed without having to place a restoration and sometimes avoiding restorative care under general anesthesia, and that restorative treatment can be postponed or avoided. A futile or detrimental repetative restorative cycle may also be avoided. For younger children, an additional advantage is that fear-inducing restorative treatments may not be necessary while the child may benefit from the improved self-care over the course of their lifetime, which is the key to success for NRCC and for maintaining a healthy dentition. Cooperation of the parents/caregiver or patient is a prerequisite to implement NRCC successfully. This requires a meticulous monitoring of the activity of the lesion. It also requires a dedicated dentist/oral health worker who constantly improves his/her qualities in personal health education.

References

1 Innes NP, Frencken JE, Bjørndal L, et al: Managing carious lesions: consensus recommendations on terminology. Adv Dent Res 2016;28:49–57.

2 Duangthip D, Chu CH, Lo EC: A randomized clinical trial on arresting dentine caries in preschool children by topical fluorides – 18 month results. J Dent 2016;44:57–63.

3 Duijster D, de Jong-Lenters M, Verrips E, van Loveren C: Establishing oral health promoting behaviours in children – parents' views on barriers, facilitators and professional support: a qualitative study. BMC Oral Health 2015;15:157.

4 Varsio S, Vehkalahti M, Murtomaa B: Dental care of six-year-old high-caries patients in relation to their cooperation. Community Dent Health 1999;16:171–175.

5 Levine RS, Pitts NB, Nugent ZJ: The fate of 1,587 unrestored carious deciduous teeth: a retrospective general dental practice based study from northern England. Br Dent J 2002;193:99–103.

6 Zwart E, Gresnigt-Bekker CO: Preventieve tandheelkunde 2. De macht der gewoonte en verandering naar gezond mondhygiënegedrag. Ned Tijdschr Tandheelk 2017;124:28–33.

7 Gruythuysen RJ: Non-restorative cavity treatment: managing rather than masking caries activity. Ned Tijdschr Tandheelk 2010;117:173–180.

8 Fejerskov O, Nyvad B: Root surface caries – rationale behind good diagnostic practice. Monogr Oral Sci 2017;26:43–54.

9 Lynch E, Beighton D: A comparison of primary root caries lesions classified according to colour. Caries Res 1994;28:233–239.

10 Black GV: A Work on Operative Dentistry. Chicago, Medico-Dental Publishing, 1908.

11 Anderson BG: Clinical study of arresting dental caries. J Dent Res 1938;17:443–452.

12 Lo EC, Schwarz E, Wong MC: Arresting dentine caries in Chinese preschool children. Int J Paediatr Dent 1998;8:253–260.

13 Schwarz E, LO EC, Wong MC: Prevention of early childhood caries – results of a fluoride toothpaste demonstration trial on Chinese preschool children after three years. J Public Health Dent 1998;58:12–18.

14 Peretz B, Gluck G: Early childhood caries (ECC): a preventive-conservative treatment mode during a 12-month period. J Clin Pediatr Dent 2006;30:191–194.

15 Mijan M, de Amorim RG, Leal SC, et al: The 3.5-year survival rates of primary molars treated according to three treatment protocols: a controlled clinical trial. Clin Oral Investig 2014;8:1061–1069.

16 Mijan M, de Amorim RG, Leal SC, et al: Correction to: The 3.5-year survival rates of primary molars treated according to three treatment protocols: a controlled clinical trial. Clin Oral Investig 2018;22:545.

17 Leal SC, Bronkhorst EM, Fan M, Frencken JE: Effect of different protocols for treating cavities in primary molars on the quality of life of children in Brazil – 1 year follow-up. Int Dent J 2013;63:329–335.

18 Santamaria RM, Innes NP, Machiulskiene V, et al: Alternative caries management options for primary molars: 2.5-year outcomes of a randomised clinical trial. Caries Res 2017;51:605–614.

19 Santamaria RM, Innes NP, Machiulskiene V, et al: Acceptability of different caries management methods for primary molars in a RCT. Int J Paediatr Dent 2015;25:9–17.

20 Hansen NV, Nyvad B: Non-operative control of cavitated approximal caries lesions in primary molars: a prospective evaluation of cases. J Oral Rehabil 2017;44:537–544.

21 Gruythuysen RJM: Niet-Restauratieve Caviteitsbehandeling. Houten, Accredidact, 2012.

22 Nyvad B, Fejerskov O: Active root surface caries converted into inactive caries as a response to oral hygiene. Scand J Dent Res 1986;94:281–284.

23 Zhang W, McGrath C, Lo EC, Li JY: Silver diamine fluoride and education to prevent and arrest root caries among community-dwelling elders. Caries Res 2013;47:284–290.

24 Li R, Lo EC, Liu BY, Wong MC, Chu CH: Randomized clinical trial on arresting dental root caries through silver diammine fluoride applications in community-dwelling elders. J Dent 2016;51:15–20.

25 Baysan A, Lynch E, Ellwood R, Davies R, Petersson L, Borsboom P: Reversal of primary root caries using dentifrices containing 5,000 and 1,100 ppm fluoride. Caries Res 2001;35:41–46.

26 Ekstrand K, Martignon S, Holm-Pedersen P: Development and evaluation of two root caries controlling programmes for home-based frail people older than 75 years. Gerodontology 2008;25:67–75.

27 Ekstrand KR, Poulsen JE, Hede B, Twetman S, Qvist V, Ellwood RP: A randomized clinical trial of the anti-caries efficacy of 5,000 compared to 1,450 ppm fluoridated toothpaste on root caries lesions in elderly disabled nursing home residents. Caries Res 2013;47:391–398.

28 Srinivasan M, Schimmel M, Riesen M, et al: High-fluoride toothpaste: a multicenter randomized controlled trial in adults. Community Dent Oral Epidem 2014;42:333–340.

29 Wierichs RJ, Meyer-Lueckel H: Systematic review on noninvasive treatment of root caries lesions. J Dent Res 2015;94:261–271.

30 Nyvad B, ten Cate JM, Fejerskov O: Arrest of root surface caries in situ. J Dent Res 1997;76:1845–1853.

31 Kidd E, Fejerskov O, Nyvad B: Infected dentine revisited. Dental Update 2015;42:808–809.

32 Chu CH, Lo EC, Lin HC: Effectiveness of silver diamine fluoride and sodium fluoride varnish in arresting dentin caries in Chinese pre-school children. J Dent Res 2002;81:767–770.

33 Zhi QH, Lo EC, Lin HC: Randomized clinical trial on effectiveness of silver diamine fluoride and glass ionomer in arresting dentine caries in preschool children. J Dent 2012;40:962–967.

34 Yee R, Holmgren C, Mulder J, et al: Efficacy of silver diamine fluoride for arresting caries treatment. J Dent Res 2009;88:644–647.

35 Zhao IS, Mei ML, Burrow MF, Lo EC, Chu CH: Prevention of secondary caries using silver diamine fluoride treatment and casein phosphopeptide-amorphous calcium phosphate modified glass-ionomer cement. J Dent 2017;57:38–44.

36 Duangthip D, Fung MHT, Wong MCM, Chu CH, Lo ECM: Adverse effects of silver diamine fluoride treatment among preschool children. J Dent Res 2018; 97:395–401.

37 Deutsch A: An alternate technique of care using silver fluoride followed by stannous fluoride in the management of root caries in aged care. Spec Care Dentist 2016;36:85–92.

38 Rosenblatt A, Stamford TC, Niederman R: Silver diamine fluoride: a caries "silver-fluoride bullet." J Dent Res 2009; 88:116–125.

Guus van Strijp
Department of Cariology Endodontology Pedodontology
Academic Centre for Dentistry (ACTA)
University of Amsterdam and VU University Amsterdam
Gustav Mahlerlaan 3004
NL–1081 LA Amsterdam (The Netherlands)
E-Mail a.vstrijp@acta.nl

Schwendicke F, Frencken J, Innes N (eds): Caries Excavation: Evolution of Treating Cavitated Carious Lesions.
Monogr Oral Sci. Basel, Karger, 2018, vol 27, pp 137–145 (DOI: 10.1159/000487840)

Evidence-Based Deep Carious Lesion Management: From Concept to Application in Everyday Clinical Practice

Sophie Doméjean[a–c] · Brigitte Grosgogeat[d–f]

[a]Université Clermont Auvergne, UFR d'Odontologie, [b]CHU Estaing Clermont-Ferrand, Service d'Odontologie, and [c]Centre de Recherche en Odontologie Clinique EA 4847, Clermont-Ferrand, and [d]Université Lyon 1, UFR Odontologie, [e]Laboratoire des Multimatériaux et Interfaces, UMR CNRS 5615, and [f]Hospices Civils de Lyon, Service de Consultations et de Traitements Dentaires, Lyon, France

Abstract

This chapter aims to discuss the way dental practitioners manage deep carious lesions (DCL) in routine practice and the barriers and incentives/facilitators to changes in accepted practice. In concert with the philosophy of minimal intervention dentistry, the concept of quaternary prevention (actions taken to prevent overtreatment and reduce harm to the patient) emerges in dentistry. This can be applied to carious tissue removal (CTR) in DCL given the risks associated with this procedure (high risk of pulp exposure, pulpal complications, tooth substance loss, and unsuccessful invasive, expensive outcomes). Recently conducted questionnaire surveys show that a gap exists between research findings and professional practices in relation to DCL management. It is, therefore, important to identify the barriers to the implementation of evidence-based dentistry into dental practices for the management of DCL in order to create appropriate corrective interventions to encourage practitioners in the use of selective CTR as a procedure.

Primary, secondary, and tertiary prevention apply to medicine, but also to dentistry in general and to cariology in particular. Together with the adequate diagnosis of dental caries and identification of carious lesions, they are cornerstones of minimal intervention dentistry (MID) [1] (Table 1). The concept of quaternary prevention has been more recently defined in medicine [2, 3]. It concerns the need for protecting patients from new unnecessary and/or excessive medical

Table 1. Primary to quaternary preventions in cariology

Type of prevention	Definition in terms of cariology	Examples of strategies (non-exhaustive list)
Primary	Prevention of caries disease occurrence at a population or individual level	Population level: water fluoridation Individual level: – Prevention of early contamination in infants – Fluoride varnish application – Preventive sealant application
Secondary	Detection of early signs of caries disease at a population or individual level Prevention of carious lesion progression	Comprehensive diagnosis (presence of a lesion, severity, activity) Therapeutic sealants Lesion arrest and remineralisation Oral hygiene counselling Diet counselling
Tertiary	Prevention of complications (e.g., restoration failures) Prevention of occurrence of new carious lesions	Fluoride regimen Follow-up at intervals based on the individual caries risk level
Quaternary	Prevention of iatrogenic damage and over-treatment	Avoid unnecessary or excessive intervention

interventions and their consequences. Quaternary prevention is also applicable to dentistry as visiting a dentist does not necessarily improve a patient's oral health and the restorative treatment by itself does not cure the disease [4, 5]. Quaternary prevention is of particular relevance to deep carious lesion (DCL) management. The conventional restorative approach, based on the removal of all soft and coloured dentine ("complete" carious lesion excavation), leads to an increased risk of pulp exposure, pulpal complications, and unsuccessful invasive and expensive outcomes in the long-term that compromises the tooth longevity [6, 7]. Recent consensus papers [8, 9], based on the latest literature on the topic, concluded that bacterially contaminated and/or demineralised tissues close to the pulp do not need to be removed and that preserving pulpal health is the priority in vital teeth with DCLs. This conclusion encompasses the idea of a key aspect of quaternary prevention – the principle of primum non nocere or "first do no harm."

The present chapter aims to report the way dental practitioners manage DCLs in routine dental practice and to discuss ways that would facilitate the integration of current concepts of keeping pulp vitality and preserving dental hard tissues (e.g., selective carious tissue removal; CTR) into everyday clinical dental practice.

What Do Dental Practitioners Do in Practice?

Evidence-based medicine/dentistry (EBM/EBD) is the best method for guiding clinical decisions [10, 11]. EBM/EBD is defined as the judicious integration of systematic assessments of clinically relevant scientific evidence, relating to the patient's oral and medical condition and history, with the dentist's clinical expertise and the patient's treatment needs and preferences [12]. Tremendous scientific evidence underlies the basic sciences and clinical procedures in cariology and in particular for selective CTR in DCL management [13]. Unfortunately, recent papers have shown that a gap exists between the results of studies and adoption of these into professional practice for DCL management. A systematic review and meta-analysis showed that, based on 9 questionnaire studies in various countries (Brazil, France, Germany, Norway, and the USA), dental practitioners rejected evidence-based CTR strategies for DCL in permanent teeth [14]. The review also concluded that wide variations exist between respondents in terms of basic knowledge but also in terms of treatment planning and clinical procedures. For example, an international study showed that most dentists thought that complete CTR was required to avoid lesion progression (France: 68%; Germany: 66%; Norway: 63%) [15]. These results are in line with those regarding the criteria used for assessing CTR. The review showed that most respondents aimed to keep only hard dentine (France 70%; Germany 77%; Norway: 69%). There was also variability between the 3 countries towards the clinical procedures. For a given clinical case (DCL in a permanent tooth with a vital, painless pulp in a 20-year-old female), 84% of the Norwegian respondents would choose stepwise excavation, whereas more than 66% of the French and German respondents opted for complete CTR. Hand-excavation was only recommended by 50% of the German respondents, but by 70 and 75% of the French and the Norwegian respondents, respectively.

Since the publication of that systematic review, a questionnaire survey of US dentists reported similar conclusions [16]. This clearly shows a gap between research evidence from studies and actual clinical practice, with a majority of respondents being in favour of complete CTR until hard dentine is felt. The survey further showed that clinical practice varied between different dental specialties. Paediatric dentists (31%) were more likely to remove carious tissues partially than general dental practitioners (GDPs; 12%) and endodontists (4%). It is very surprising that the variability also applied to diagnosis procedures; 90% of the endodontists reported that they routinely used pulp vitality tests, but only 30% of the GDPs and 4% of the paediatric dentists would use this device. The low percentage recorded among paediatric dentists may be explained by the difficulty in assessing the pulpal status in young children properly. The difference in testing pulp vitality between endodontists and GDPs cannot be explained by this factor. This outcome is a surprise as accurate diagnosis of the status of the pulp is the basis of a rational clinical decision making.

Unfortunately, it is clearly evident that there is lack of implementation of the recently proven concepts toward DCL management and preservation of pulp vitality in clinical practice. This gap is not specific to DCL but concerns various domains of cariology and MID in general, such as restorative decision thresholds [17–21], caries risk assessment [22, 23], repair of defective restorations [24–26], dental sealant placement [27, 28], and use of professional fluoride [29].

The fact that clinical practice does not follow scientific principles strictly and that GDPs predominantly rely on invasive treatment strategies despite a body of evidence in favour of MID is unquestionable. Care provision has been shown to be influenced by a range of cultural, social, and economic resources [30–34].

Facilitators and Barriers to Implementing Science into Practice

It takes time for changes in treatment provision and fundamental philosophies to diffuse to practitioners [18, 35]. Implementing new care concepts and/or changing existing ones in organisations, services, and systems require changes in individual and collective behaviour. Changing behaviour requires an understanding of the influences on behaviour in the context in which they occur [36]. It is thus essential to identify the barriers and to define priority fields to create appropriate corrective interventions such as training, education, environmental restructuring, and coercion, which correspond to the behaviour change wheel system proposed by Michie et al. [37].

The first hypothesis that comes to mind is the potential effect of both under- and post-graduate educations and concurrently the date of graduation – the "don't know" barrier described by Innes et al. [38]. Indeed, from the 9 surveys included in the Schwendicke and Gostemeyer [14] systematic review, it appeared that dental practitioners' age/year of graduation (5 studies out of 9) was the most cited variable related to the decision-making process. This shows the impact of undergraduate education on the implementation of oral health care. Very little is known on the specific topic of DCL management and what is taught in dental schools. Indeed, to our knowledge, only one survey is currently available; it involved 43 dental schools among 65 registered in the USA, and provides us a good overview of the current landscape of dental education toward CTR in the USA [39]. The study reported a wide range of teaching content with marked differences between schools regarding the criteria used for CTR and its assessment, the management of DCL, and the definition of "caries remaining at cavity preparations." It can be hypothesised that such variability might exist worldwide and that teaching harmonisation is essential. Table 2 presents the principal statements/conclusions related to CTR and DCL reported in current cariology curricula/consensus for undergraduate dental education [40–44]. It illustrates the recent evolution of evidence related to partial/selective CTR and the fact that this is not clearly taken into consideration in the development of current curricula content, except in the USA. The latest article relating to a core curriculum in cariology was published by Fontana et al. [44] in 2016; it mentions the term "partial excavation" and the need for a US dentist to be capable, on graduation, of performing and understanding the indications of different excavation techniques. Two years earlier, Martignon et al. [43] reported a more general conclusion (without any clear mention of "partial excavation" or "stepwise excavation"), stating that Colombian dentists must be capable, on graduation, of deciding when, how, and to what extent to remove carious tissue before placing a restoration. Nevertheless, the 2011 conclusions of the first consensus workshop on the development of a European curriculum in cariology were based on the literature available at that time and, thus, are quite evasive toward CTR [40, 41]. It can be stated that: (1) further investigations are needed to present a clear description of the current teaching with respect to DCL across the globe, and that cariology curricula must be regularly redefined, or at least amended, based on the latest evidence, and (2) there is a lack of data regarding post-graduate education and long-life learning in general in relation with DCL.

If the impact of education on clinical decision making is of importance, other factors influence professional practices. Indeed, expected failures are not limited to GDPs who graduated many years ago and/or do not attend continuing education programs [37]. Other paths have been identified to be a key support factor for transferring knowledge, such as external networks of trusted peers and respected practitioners [45]. According to Sbaraini [45], this type of network could be even more important than the established "centrally produced guidelines and academic advice." In the same vein, the fact that investigations are most often performed within academic environments may also create a barrier to new technique adoption, as GDPs do not recognise themselves in that specific clinical setting/environment and perhaps do not see the results as relevant to their setting in general practice. It is essential to provide clear recommendations/clinical guidelines in a variety of languages to be applicable to the greatest number of clinicians, as recently published in English in the special issue of *Advances in Dental Research* [8, 9]. Nevertheless, clinical guidelines, isolated from other actions, have been shown to only moderately impact dental practices [45, 46]. Guidelines are often considered necessary but not sufficient [47, 48].

Table 2. Cariology curriculums/consensus for undergraduate dental education

Location and study	Considerations related to surgical interventions and CTR
Europe Schulte and Pitts [40], 2011; Buchalla et al. [41], 2011	The caries process How to deal with an infection: to date, removal of bacterially softened dental hard tissue is recommended Caries removal Caries removal is part of many restorative therapies for the management of a carious lesion; recently, a discussion has started among cariologists as to what extent dental hard tissue affected by the caries process has to be removed; there is consensus among the experts that the aim of removal of carious dental hard tissue is to preserve tooth vitality and facilitate the long-term success of the restoration being placed; in an environment where evidence in favour of either complete or partial removal of carious tissue is currently lacking, a cariology curriculum should allow for those responsible in establishing the curriculum in individual dental schools to teach this issue according to the best evidence available to them; beyond a specific caries removal approach taught, the dentist upon graduation should be familiar with a range of strategies for surgical caries management comprising both identification of what needs to be removed and the physical act of removal of carious tooth tissue
Brazil Ferreira-Nobilo Nde et al. [42], 2014	Learning cycle: clinical; discipline: dentistry Surgical interventions with the aim of treatment and conservation of dental elements, patients with carious lesions and/or larger structures, preserving the preventive principles inherent to maintaining a good oral health status
Colombia Martignon et al. [43], 2014	Domain IV: operative treatment decision making 4.6. On graduation, a dentist must be capable of deciding when, how, and to what extent to remove carious tissue before the placement of a restoration, considering the restorability of the tooth, preservation of tooth structure and pulp vitality and periodontal viability and the functionality
USA Fontana et al. [44], 2016	Domain IV: surgical therapies and clinical decision making 4.9. On graduation, a dentist must be capable of performing and understanding the indications of different techniques of caries tooth structure removal (e.g., partial vs. complete, stepwise excavation, indirect and direct pulp capping) while preserving tooth structure and pulp vitality

CTR, carious tissue removal.

The complexity of the procedure/care and the potential anxiety arising from a lack of experience may be a hindrance to changes [34]. Nevertheless, in the particular case of DCL management, clinical procedures are easy to carry out and do not need specific skills or devices. Schedule difficulties are also often reported (time constraints, lack of cooperation among the dental team members) as being a barrier to practice changes [31–33, 49]. However, there is no objective reason why selective CTR and restoration within a single visit may impact negatively on the financial viability of the practice compared to traditional complete excavation into 1 or, even more, into 2 steps.

Financial considerations at the health care system level (inappropriate funding system/remuneration, lack of financial support for innovation) and/or at the practitioner level (lack of financial advantage for new practices, risk of income loss/

reduction) also impact clinical practices. For example, methods of remuneration may have a counterproductive effect regarding MID implementation in general as some are still more lucrative for more invasive interventions [50]. Suga et al. [51] evaluated the factors driving GDPs towards, or away from, preventive measures in cariology and concluded that further education and training, coupled with a fairer payment scheme, would be a reasonable approach to change the balance in favour of the provision of preventive measures. Similar conclusions may be hypothesised toward DCL management.

Habits are strong barriers to changing professional practice [32]. There is sparse literature about practitioners' desire for changing their practices, but it seems that GDPs do not feel the need for changing their routine [49]. Monaghan underlined that resistance to change and to authority is part of human nature [52]. It is essential to bring practitioners to an awareness that EBM/EBD is not a limitation to clinical freedom, but that, on the contrary, it offers an opportunity to improve decision making for patient welfare [52].

Over and above these barriers, inherent to the practitioner and his/her professional environment, many studies also present some related to patient's expectations. Well-informed, shared decision making, and patient-centred quality outcomes become an absolute priority [53, 54]. Traditionally, outcome assessment of dental carious lesion management was often limited to restoration longevity and/or tooth vitality. Unfortunately, little is known about patient satisfaction and expectations toward DCL management. Indeed, to our knowledge, only 1 paper has been published on the topic [55]. It described a study aiming to have a better understanding of how patients (qualitative study: 12 focus group members; quantitative study: 150 patients, aged 18–25 years) feel and think regarding CTR and the associated risks. Globally, it showed that patients are lacking knowledge toward recent concepts of DCL management. For example, it appeared that none of the focus group members were aware of the concept of selective CTR. Moreover, the majority of participants in the quantitative study perceived complete CTR as a better option than selective CTR. This was especially true for those with strong dental anxiety, those with a lower level of education, and those who frequently changed their dentist. Similar lack of understanding and reluctance have been described toward non-invasive strategies for non-cavitated carious lesions [56]; indeed, in some cases, restorations were placed at the patient's request for lesions that could have benefited from strictly non-invasive options.

Conclusion and Perspectives

The literature is lacking about the facilitators and barriers to implementing EBD into DCL management. Further investigations, such as theoretical domains framework (TDF)-based studies [57], may help to understand the evolution of dental professional practices and patient thought processes. The TDF, developed in 2012, consists of a theory-informed interview based on 14 different domains (e.g., knowledge, skills, beliefs about capabilities, beliefs about consequences) and it provides a theoretical lens through which to view the cognitive, affective, social, and environmental influences on behaviour [35]. The TDF has been used to describe barriers and facilitators of professional practices toward antibiotic prescription [58], preventive oral healthcare delivery (e.g., risk recording, risk-based recall interval determination, fluoride varnish application, preventive sealant placement) [59, 60] or dental management of patients on bisphosphonates [61]. Using TDF in the context of DCL management may help to address the persisting barriers to changes and to denounce the potential iatrogenesis of current practices.

References

1 Frencken JE, Peters MC, Manton DJ, Leal SC, Gordan VV, Eden E: Minimal intervention dentistry for managing dental caries – a review: report of a FDI task group. Int Dent J 2012;62:223–243.

2 Jamoulle M, Roland M: Quaternary prevention. WICC annual workshop: Wonca congress proceedings. Hong Kong, 1995.

3 Jamoulle M: Quaternary prevention, an answer of family doctors to overmedicalization. Int J Health Policy Manag 2015;4:61–64.

4 Elderton RJ: Iatrogenesis in the treatment of dental caries. Proc Finn Dent Soc1992;88:25–32.

5 Elderton RJ: Overtreatment with restorative dentistry: when to intervene? Int Dent J 1993;43:17–24.

6 Ricketts D, Lamont T, Innes NP, Kidd E, Clarkson JE: Operative caries management in adults and children. Cochrane Database Syst Rev 2013;3:CD003808.

7 Schwendicke F, Stolpe M, Meyer-Lueckel H, Paris S, Dorfer CE: Cost-effectiveness of one- and two-step incomplete and complete excavations. J Dent Res 2013;92:880–887.

8 Schwendicke F, Frencken JE, Bjorndal L, Maltz M, Manton DJ, Ricketts D, van Landuyt K, Banerjee A, Campus G, Domejean S, Fontana M, Leal S, Lo E, Machiulskiene V, Schulte A, Splieth C, Zandona AF, Innes NP: Managing carious lesions: consensus recommendations on carious tissue removal. Adv Dent Res 2016;28:58–67.

9 Innes NP, Frencken JE, Bjorndal L, Maltz M, Manton DJ, Ricketts D, van Landuyt K, Banerjee A, Campus G, Domejean S, Fontana M, Leal S, Lo E, Machiulskiene V, Schulte A, Splieth C, Zandona A, Schwendicke F: Managing carious lesions: consensus recommendations on terminology. Adv Dent Res 2016;28:49–57.

10 Ballini A, Capodiferro S, Toia M, Cantore S, Favia G, De Frenza G, Grassi FR: Evidence-based dentistry: what's new? Int J Med Sci 2007;4:174–178.

11 Innes NP, Schwendicke F, Lamont T: How do we create, and improve, the evidence base? Br Dent J 2016;220:651–655.

12 American Dental Association (ADA): Policy on evidence-based dentistry. http://www.ada.org/en/about-the-ada/ada-positions-policies-and-statements/policy-on-evidence-based-dentistry (accessed December 2017).

13 Banerjee A, Frencken JE, Schwendicke F, Innes NPT: Contemporary operative caries management: consensus recommendations on minimally invasive caries removal. Br Dent J 2017;223:215–222.

14 Schwendicke F, Gostemeyer G: Understanding dentists' management of deep carious lesions in permanent teeth: a systematic review and meta-analysis. Implement Sci 2016;11:142.

15 Schwendicke F, Stangvaltaite L, Holmgren C, Maltz M, Finet M, Elhennawy K, Eriksen I, Kuzmiszyn TC, Kerosuo E, Doméjean S: Dentists' attitudes and behaviour regarding deep carious lesion management: a multi-national survey. Clin Oral Investig 2017;21:191–198.

16 Koopaeei MM, Inglehart MR, McDonald N, Fontana M: General dentists', pediatric dentists', and endodontists' diagnostic assessment and treatment strategies for deep carious lesions: a comparative analysis. J Am Dent Assoc 2017;148: 64–74.

17 Innes NPT, Schwendicke F: Restorative thresholds for carious lesions: systematic review and meta-analysis, J Dent Res 2017;96:501–508.

18 Doméjean S, Maltrait M, Espelid I, Tveit A, Tubert-Jeannin S: Changes in occlusal caries lesion management in France from 2002 to 2012 – a persistent gap between evidence and clinical practice. Caries Res 2015;49:408–416.

19 Rechmann P, Doméjean S, Rechmann BM, Kinsel R, Featherstone JD: Approximal and occlusal caries lesions: restorative treatment decisions by California dentists. J Am Dent Assoc 2016;147: 328–338.

20 Kopperud SE, Tveit AB, Opdam NJ, Espelid I: Occlusal caries management: preferences among dentists in Norway. Caries Res 2016;50:40–47.

21 Bussaneli DG, Boldieri T, Diniz MB, Rivera LM, Santos-Pinto L, Cordeiro Rde C: Influence of professional experience on detection and treatment decision of occlusal caries lesions in primary teeth. Int J Paediatr Dent 2015;25:418–427.

22 Doméjean S, Léger S, Simon A, Boucharel N, Holmgren C: Knowledge, opinions and practices of French general practitioners in the assessment of caries risk: results of a national survey. Clin Oral Investig 2017;21:653–663.

23 Kakudate K, Sumida F, Matsumoto Y, Yokoyama Y, Riley JL 3rd, Gilbert GH, Gordan VV: Dentists' decisions to conduct caries risk assessment in a dental practice-based research network. Community Dent Oral Epidemiol 2015;43: 128–134.

24 Gordan VV, Riley J 3rd, Geraldeli S, Williams OD, Spoto JC 3rd, Gilbert GH; National Dental PBRN Collaborative Group: The decision to repair or replace a defective restoration is affected by who placed the original restoration: findings from the National Dental PBRN. J Dent 2014;42:1528–1534.

25 Staxrud F, Tveit AB, Rukke HV, Kopperud SE: Repair of defective composite restorations: a questionnaire study among dentists in the public dental service in Norway. J Dent 2016;52:50–54.

26 Kanzow P, Dieckmann P, Hausdorfer T, Attin T, Wiegand A, Wegehaupt FJ: Repair restorations: questionnaire survey among dentists in the Canton of Zurich, Switzerland. Swiss Dent J 2017;127:300–311.

27 Yokoyama Y, Kakudate N, Sumida F, Matsumoto Y, Gilbert GH, Gordan VV: Evidence-practice gap for dental sealant application: results from a dental practice-based research network in Japan. Int Dent J 2016;66:330–336.

28 Chin ZW, Chong WS, Mani SA: Practice of sealants and preventive resin restorations among Malaysian dentists. Oral Health Prev Dent 2016;14: 125–135.

29 Yokoyama Y, Kakudate N, Sumida F, Matsumoto Y, Gilbert GH, Gordan VV: Evidence-practice gap for in-office fluoride application in a dental practice-based research network. J Public Health Dent 2016;76:91–97.
30 Sbaraini A, Carter SM, Evans RW, Blinkhorn A: How do dentists and their teams incorporate evidence about preventive care? An empirical study. Community Dent Oral Epidemiol 2013;41: 401–414.
31 McGlone P, Watt R, Sheiham A: Evidence-based dentistry: an overview of the challenges in changing professional practice. Br Dent J 2001;190: 636–639.
32 Forbes G, Rutherford S, Stirling D, Young L, Clarkson J: Current practice and factors influencing the provision of periodontal healthcare in primary dental care in Scotland: an explorative study. Br Dent J 2015;218:387–391.
33 Watt R, McGlone P, Evans D, Boulton S, Jacobs J, Graham S, Appleton T, Perry S, Sheiham A: The facilitating factors and barriers influencing change in dental practice in a sample of English general dental practitioners. Br Dent J 2004;197: 485–489.
34 McColl E, Smith M, Whitworth J, Seccombe G, Steele J: Barriers to improving endodontic care: the views of NHS practitioners. Br Dent J 1999;186:564–568.
35 Haugejorden O: Adoption of fluoride-based caries preventive innovations in a public dental service. Community Dent Oral Epidemiol 1988;16:5–10.
36 Atkins L, Francis J, Islam R, O'Connor D, Patey A, Ivers N, Foy R, Duncan EM, Colquhoun H, Grimshaw JM, Lawton R, Michie S: A guide to using the theoretical domains framework of behaviour change to investigate implementation problems. Implement Sci 2017;12:77.
37 Michie S, van Stralen MM, West R: The behaviour change wheel: a new method for characterising and designing behaviour change interventions. Implement Sci 2011;6:42.
38 Innes NP, Frencken JE, Schwendicke F: Don't know, can't do, won't change: barriers to moving knowledge to action in managing the carious lesion. J Dent Res 2016;95:485–486.
39 Nascimento MM, Behar-Horenstein LS, Feng X, Guzman-Armstrong S, Fontana M: Exploring how US dental schools teach removal of carious tissues during cavity preparations. J Dent Educ 2017; 81:5–13.
40 Schulte AG, Pitts NB: First consensus workshop on the development of a European Curriculum in Cariology. Eur J Dent Educ 2011;15(suppl 1):1–2.
41 Buchalla W, Wiegand A, Hall A: Decision-making and treatment with respect to surgical intervention in the context of a European core curriculum in cariology. Eur J Dent Educ 2011;15(suppl 1): 40–44.
42 Ferreira-Nobilo Nde P, Rosario de Sousa Mda L, Cury JA: Cariology in curriculum of Brazilian dental schools. Braz Dent J 2014;25:265–270.
43 Martignon S, Marin LM, Pitts N, Jacome-Lievano S: Consensus on domains, formation objectives and contents in cariology for undergraduate dental students in Colombia. Eur J Dent Educ 2014;18:222–233.
44 Fontana M, Guzman-Armstrong S, Schenkel AB, Allen KL, Featherstone J, Goolsby S, Kanjirath P, Kolker J, Martignon S, Pitts N, Schulte A, Slayton RL, Young D, Wolff M: Development of a core curriculum framework in cariology for US dental schools. J Dent Educ 2016; 80:705–720.
45 Sbaraini A: What factors influence the provision of preventive care by general dental practitioners? Br Dent J 2012; 212:E18.
46 Elouafkaoui P, Bonetti D, Clarkson J, Stirling D, Young L, Cassie H: Is further intervention required to translate caries prevention and management recommendations into practice? Br Dent J 2015;218:E1.
47 van der Sanden WJ, Mettes DG, Plasschaert AJ, van't Hof MA, Grol RP, Verdonschot EH: Clinical practice guidelines in dentistry: opinions of dental practitioners on their contribution to the quality of dental care. Qual Saf Health Care 2003;12:107–111.
48 Davies KJ, Drage NA: Adherence to NICE guidelines on recall intervals and the FGDP(UK) selection criteria for dental radiography. Prim Dent J 2013;2: 50–56.
49 Witton RV, Moles DR: Barriers and facilitators that influence the delivery of prevention guidance in health service dental practice: a questionnaire study of practising dentists in Southwest England. Community Dent Health 2013;30: 71–76.
50 Brocklehurst P, Price J, Glenny AM, Tickle M, Birch S, Mertz E, Grytten J: The effect of different methods of remuneration on the behaviour of primary care dentists. Cochrane Database Syst Rev 2013;11:CD009853.
51 Suga US, Terada RS, Ubaldini AL, Fujimaki M, Pascotto RC, Batilana AP, Pietrobon R, Vissoci JR, Rodrigues CG: Factors that drive dentists towards or away from dental caries preventive measures: systematic review and metasummary. PLoS One 2014;9:e107831.
52 Monaghan N: Human nature and clinical freedom, barriers to evidence-based practice? Br Dent J 1999;186: 208–209.
53 Pitts N, Ismail AI, Martignon S, Ekstrand K, Douglas GV, Longbottom C: ICCMS™ guide for practitioners and educators. 2014. https://www.icdas.org/ (accessed December 2017).
54 Faggion CM Jr, Pachur T, Giannakopoulos NN: Patients' values in clinical decision-making. J Evid Based Dent Pract 2017;17:177–183.
55 Schwendicke F, Mostajaboldave R, Otto I, Dorfer CE, Burkert S: Patients' preferences for selective versus complete excavation: a mixed-methods study. J Dent 2016;46:47–53.
56 Mitchell ST, Funkhouser E, Gordan VV, Riley JL 3rd, Makhija SK, Litaker MS, Gilbert GH; National Dental PBRN Collaborative Group: Satisfaction with dental care among patients who receive invasive or non-invasive treatment for non-cavitated early dental caries: findings from one region of the National Dental PBRN. BMC Oral Health 2017; 17:70.
57 Cane J, O'Connor D, Michie S: Validation of the theoretical domains framework for use in behaviour change and implementation research. Implement Sci 2012;7:37.

58 Newlands R, Duncan EM, Prior M, Elouafkaoui P, Elders A, Young L, Clarkson JE, Ramsay CR; Translation Research in a Dental Setting (TriaDS) Research Methodology Group: Barriers and facilitators of evidence-based management of patients with bacterial infections among general dental practitioners: a theory-informed interview study. Implement Sci 2016;11:11.
59 Templeton AR, Young L, Bish A, Gnich W, Cassie H, Treweek S, Bonetti D, Stirling D, Macpherson L, McCann S, Clarkson J, Ramsay C; PMC Study Team: Patient-, organization-, and system-level barriers and facilitators to preventive oral health care: a convergent mixed-methods study in primary dental care. Implement Sci 2016;11:5.
60 Gnich W, Bonetti D, Sherriff A, Sharma S, Conway DI, Macpherson LM: Use of the theoretical domains framework to further understanding of what influences application of fluoride varnish to children's teeth: a national survey of general dental practitioners in Scotland. Community Dent Oral Epidemiol 2015;43: 272–281.
61 Bonetti DL, Clarkson JE, Elouafkaoui P, Stirling DA, Young L, Templeton AR: Managing patients on bisphosphonates: the practice of primary care dentists before and after the publication of national guidance. Br Dent J 2014; 217:E25.

Sophie Doméjean
UFR d'Odontologie
2, rue de Braga
FR-63100 Clermont-Ferrand (France)
E-Mail sophie.domejean@uca.fr

Schwendicke F, Frencken J, Innes N (eds): Caries Excavation: Evolution of Treating Cavitated Carious Lesions.
Monogr Oral Sci. Basel, Karger, 2018, vol 27, pp 146–154 (DOI: 10.1159/000487841)

The Problem: Relevance, Quality, and Homogeneity of Trial Designs, Outcomes, and Reporting

Gerd Göstemeyer[a] · Colin Levey[b]

[a] Department of Operative and Preventive Dentistry, Charité – Universitätsmedizin Berlin, Corporate Member of Freie Universität Berlin, Humboldt-Universität zu Berlin, and Berlin Institute of Health, Berlin, Germany; [b] Department of Restorative Dentistry, Dundee Dental Hospital and School, University of Dundee, Dundee, UK

Abstract

Clinical trials are the cornerstone of evidence-based medicine. By directly comparing different interventions they produce evidence on their relative efficacy and effectiveness. This, in turn, can inform secondary research and guideline development to facilitate evidence-based clinical decision making. However, the quality of evidence stemming from clinical trials is frequently poor. Here, the pathway of evidence from basic research to the generation of implementable clinical guidelines will be described. Relevant factors related to trial design and reporting, such as the choice of trial comparators, outcomes and outcome measures, will be described and their influence on evidence synthesis will be discussed. Finally, recommendations on how to improve trials in order to increase their usefulness for evidence generation will be given.

Pathway of Evidence to Practice

Medical research typically consists of formulating new approaches for interventions, which are first tested in laboratories and later, if proved to be safe and successful, within clinical trials. Data from clinical trials are then synthetised in systematic reviews, which are further used to inform clinical guideline development for clinical practice. This process is the ideal pathway of evidence into practice and should result in the clinical implementation of interventions based on the best available evidence [1].

At the beginning of this pathway, where new interventions are being formulated, it is crucial that these approaches are in accordance with patients' needs. Clinicians at universities are frequently involved in patient care and also in med-

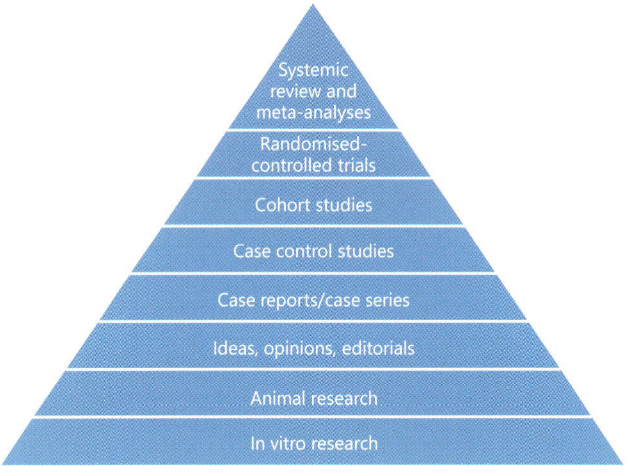
Systemic
review and
meta-analyses
Randomised-
controlled trials
Cohort studies
Case control studies
Case reports/case series
Ideas, opinions, editorials
Animal research
In vitro research

Fig. 1. The "evidence pyramid" illustrating the hierarchy of evidence stemming from different types of studies. The level of evidence increases from the bottom to the top.

ical research. Therefore, the development of novel interventions and the initiation of research has often been generated based on perceived patient needs based on clinical experience or from data of previously performed studies. However, with the emergence of new and more complex interventions and the development of more complex research methods there are growing barriers to communication between clinicians and scientists, as both roles are becoming increasingly specialised [2]. To overcome this, translational medicine has evolved as a new discipline in biomedical research. By building interdisciplinary collaborations, involving scientists, clinicians, and other relevant stakeholders, translational medicine aims at building a bridge between basic and applied research.

In primary research, unfiltered original data on the effect of an intervention is generated. Laboratory studies are usually the first step in the development of new interventions. They are used to assess the mechanisms of action, safety, and feasibility before the intervention can be tested in humans. Although laboratory studies are useful and necessary for preclinical testing, they do not allow conclusions to be drawn on the true clinical effect of an intervention.

To obtain such evidence, clinical trials are essential. By comparing 2 or more different interventions, evidence on their relative efficacy and effectiveness can be deduced. The quality of evidence of data from clinical trials is dependent on the type of study. Uncontrolled and observational studies such as case reports, case control or cohort studies are associated with a lower level of evidence (Fig. 1). Methodological aspects such as choice of patients, allocation to a treatment arm, and absence of blinding procedures may add a high degree of bias to the results of these studies and can limit confidence in their conclusions. Randomised-controlled trials (RCTs) are designed to minimise such bias in all steps of the study in order to provide the most reliable results [3]. Therefore, RCTs are considered to provide the highest level of evidence. However, there are still several factors that might influence the usefulness of an RCT on evidence synthesis, which will be described later.

Systematic reviews are the principal methodology for secondary research in medicine and dentistry. By using meta-analytic approaches, they combine and compare data stemming from different clinical trials on the same topic both qualitatively (assessing the data, its strengths and weakness) and quantitatively (deducing relative estimates of an intervention's efficacy or effectiveness). This minimises risk of bias and therefore increases the precision of effect size estimates. Systematic reviews and meta-analyses yield the highest level of evidence in the hierarchy of evidence-based medicine and provide the basis for the development of clinical practice guidelines. However, a key limitation of systematic reviews is that the validity of gained information is only as valid as the results of the primary studies the review relies on. If conducted rigorously, systematic reviews often report low-quality evidence that only allow for carefully drawn conclusions [4].

Clinical decision making in favour or against an intervention should not be based on a single study but on the totality of available evidence. Clinical guidelines aim to translate research findings from a systematic review of evidence (both from primary and secondary research) and translate them into recommendations for clinical care providers as well as to patients and policy makers. Guideline development follows a systematic approach to identify, select, assess, and summarise the available evidence. A consensus of a group of decision makers, also known as the guideline panel, must interpret the available evidence and develop recommendations considering the clinical context in which the recommendations will be applied [4]. Ideally, guidelines are produced using a rigorous and transparent process, where the shortcomings of contributing evidence are made clear [1]. This process should result in universally valid and robust recommendations for use in clinical everyday practice.

Even after evidence-based guidelines are produced with clear recommendations for practice, there is often a discrepancy between what they say and what is provided to patients [5]. Much work is being carried out investigating and understanding barriers and enablers of evidence-based practice [6]. What is clear is that guideline development is a link in the chain of evidence to practice, and not the endpoint.

Barriers to Evidence Synthesis

Evidence synthesis can be depleted or interrupted in quality and quantity at several stages, leading to waste of resources for research. The concept of research waste has recently been drawn to the attention of the life sciences and healthcare research community through a *The Lancet* series on research waste [7–11]. These papers highlight the fact that much of the research undertaken is of little additional value to the understanding of particular diseases and the benefits or harms of treatments or preventive measures. This is because they ask the wrong question, are not conducted to a high standard, are left unpublished, or are poorly reported. In fact, the authors suggest that the level of waste is USD 200 billion each year (85% of global life sciences research funding) [7]. There is no evidence to suggest that the caries literature is any different [12].

In some cases, research is undertaken which duplicates previously published work on a given intervention that already has sufficient evidence for or against it. Sometimes these studies are not carried out to a high enough quality standard to be of value either in their own right, or as part of evidence synthesis.

To prevent waste in the chain of evidence creation we must abide by the principles set out in the REWARD statement. These are:

- set the right research priorities;
- use robust research design, conduct, and analysis;
- regulation and management are proportionate to risks;
- information on research methods and findings are accessible;
- reports of research are complete and usable.

There have been attempts to improve caries research methodology in the past [13] and methodology is gradually improving, but in dentistry we are somewhat behind medical colleagues in the design of robust trial methods to improve the applicability or implementation of the results.

Table 1. Collaborative groups and organisations for improving the efficiency of clinical trials

Group	Aim
Trail FORGE (http://www.trialforge.org/)	Recommendations on evidence-based decision making for trial design, conduct, and analysis
Cochrane collaboration (http://www.cochrane.org/)	Recommendations that can be used to reduce risk of bias (e.g., due to allocation concealment or blinding) when designing an RCT
COMET (Core Outcome Measures in Effectiveness Trials) (http://www.comet-initiative.org/) COSMIN (Consensus-Based Standards for the Selection of Measurement Instruments) (http://www.cosmin.nl/)	Development of agreed standard outcomes for trials (COS) to facilitate trials that pursue relevant outcomes to clinicians, patients, and other stakeholders and to improve comparing results between different trials
CONSORT (Consolidated Standards of Reporting Trials) (http://www.consort-statement.org/) EQUATOR Network (Enhancing Quality and Transparency of Health Research) (http://www.equator-network.org/)	Aiding clinical researchers who conduct trials in accurate and complete outcome reporting
Clinical Trials (http://www.clinicaltrials.gov) AllTrials (http://www.alltrials.net/)	Registration and publication of study findings regardless of whether an intervention failed or not

Ask the Correct Questions

Many efforts have been made to improve the design and credibility of clinical studies in order to add valuable data to the evidence base (Table 1). However, even the most well-designed trial would generate results of low value if the comparisons of interventions that have been made are not relevant. The choice of trial comparators is a factor that can heavily impact the totality and robustness of available evidence stemming from trials in different ways: certain interventions might have been compared against each other more often, while other comparisons might have been avoided, leaving gaps in the evidence due to the associated segmentation of trials. Comparisons within the same intervention classes (e.g., on the same level of invasiveness) instead of across classes might be preferred, which weakens evidence about the relative effectiveness between different strategies. Furthermore, comparisons against weak comparators or against placebo can lead to the overestimation of effectiveness [14, 15].

Social network analysis (SNA) is an emerging methodology that can be used to analyse networks formed by comparators in trials. Through the use of SNA, a complete picture of comparisons that have been performed within trials in a certain medical field can be drawn and areas where evidence gaps exist can be identified. This method has recently been used to assess networks formed by comparators in caries prevention and management trials and found significant distortions within the assessed networks. A number of caries interventions that should have been compared have never been compared within clinical trials [15].

Outcomes as a Barrier to Synthesis

It is often said that "you cannot compare apples and oranges." That is to say, one cannot draw meaningful comparisons between 2 very different things or, in the case of trial design, outcomes. For example, imagine you want to compare the results of 2 trials comparing selective caries removal in a single stage and non-selective caries removal to hard dentine both followed by restoration with conventional composite resin. One of these trials selected "pulpal exposure" and the other "restoration failure" as the trial endpoint or outcome. Because these 2 outcomes are so different, it does not matter how they are measured, the data cannot be synthesised in a meta-analysis, which is a lost opportunity.

A systematic review of outcomes published in RCTs in caries management and prevention over the last 50 years has been undertaken [16]. The most common outcomes used are those focused on restoration performance and individual/population caries burden. Carious lesion activity, microbiological outcomes, and economic endpoints are growing in use, as are patient-centred outcomes. However, these remain at a low level.

Even in situations where the outcome domain is the same (e.g., restoration failure in the above example), differing outcome measurement tools can present difficulties in meta-analysis. Considering the previous example, some trials might assess restoration failure as survival of the restoration whilst others may have a scale where various degrees of failure are measured from marginal discolouration to complete loss. In this case, it may be possible to compare and combine the results at a given point (e.g., complete loss of the restoration) but not at points on the path to complete failure. Careful statistical handling of these scales is required to prevent distortion of the overall result. Differences in outcome measurement tools such as this are a barrier to evidence synthesis.

Outcome reporting bias occurs when a range of outcomes are measured at the end of a clinical trial but only those showing statistically significant differences make it into the final report. There is evidence that statistically significant results are more likely to be published: this is publication bias [17]. The result is that the published literature will tend to overestimate the benefit of a given intervention and underreport harm to patients. This is of obvious concern. Outcome reporting bias is acknowledged as a serious problem in medicine [18] but has not been assessed in dentistry.

Incomplete information in the trial report can lead to problems during evidence synthesis. Even when the trial has been undertaken to a high standard, lack of relevant information in the trial report can lead to inappropriate exclusion from the synthesis, reducing the statistical power and therefore strength of results and recommendations. Failure to provide adequate details can affect all aspects of the trial from details of the population under study to the intervention itself and the outcome assessment.

Limitations to the External Validity of RCTs

Due to their rigorous design aiming at minimising systematic error and bias, RCTs are considered to provide the highest level of evidence in clinical research. However, conducting clinical studies under such idealised conditions may limit their generalisability (or external validity) for general practice [19].

RCTs are conducted under very controlled settings, often in secondary or tertiary care, where interventions are provided under ideal conditions. This type of study design often has narrow inclusion criteria for participants resulting in interventions being delivered in a highly selected patient group which does not necessarily represent a cross-section of the whole population [20]. Even if trialists consider a perfectly representative sample when planning a randomised trial, it cannot be assured that all patients agree to participate and agree to be allocated to an intervention arm at random. Clinical decision making takes patients preferences into account in order to obtain informed consent for treatment choice. Such patient preferences might not always match with interventions offered within clinical trials. However, ethics do not allow the clinician or researcher to force an intervention onto a patient, even if it is thought to be beneficial.

For clinical trials on dental materials, reduction of some sources of bias is challenging or even impossible: practitioners have to follow a certain treatment protocol dependent on the material used. In case the operator has a favoured material, this might induce performance bias [20]. If the clinical appearance of tested dental materials is considerably different (e.g., for resin composites and glass-ionomers), blinding of the examiner or even the patient is also not possible, resulting in detection bias. In fact, a high number of RCTs on restorative materials are prone to performance and detection bias [21].

In RCTs, the entry of a patient into the trial and allocation to a certain treatment arm should be independent from the clinical decision making. This is achieved by true random sequence generation for the allocation of patients to different treatment arms and by concealing this allocation from the researchers responsible for recruiting patients to the trial [20]. Although random allocation to treatment arms reduces selection bias, it can increase the probability of failures as the choice of treatment is no longer based on personal clinical evidence which takes into account the nuances of clinical care.

Improving the Pathway to Practice

Different collaboration groups and organisations have developed tools in order to guide researchers in conducting trials, systematic reviews, and guideline development (Table 1). These involve guidance in design, conduct, analysis, and reporting. By using all these tools, losses in evidence quality and quantity at each step of the pathway to practice are reduced.

Marginal Gains Add Up

The success of the British cycling team at the 2012 London Olympics was attributed to the application of the principle of marginal gains in which improvements of 1% were sought at each stage. Added together, these small changes produced a dominant performance. If we apply the same principle to clinical research, we could generate more robust and relevant results in a more efficient way (Fig. 2).

If we begin by ensuring that research funding is only released to projects targeted where knowledge or evidence gaps exist, then we will reduce waste and channel resources into fruitful projects which answer pertinent questions. We must formulate questions based on need rather than on happenstance or the interest of the researcher [1]. Systematic reviews or guideline developers may help identify these gaps [15] which feedback to primary trial design.

It is helpful to begin by constructing our research question using the PICO (population, intervention, comparison, and outcome) formula. Once we have a question that addresses a knowledge gap we can break the question back down again and look for gains in each component. After trial design and conduct, we can then look at marginal gains in reporting methods. Let's first consider the PICO question.

Ask the Correct Questions

Relevant Population

When we consider our research question, we need to be sure that our sample population will be relevant to the population who will receive the intervention in a "real world" scenario. This relates not only to the age, gender, or socioeconomic characteristics, but also to the setting in which the intervention is delivered. This means that our sample should not simply be who happens to show up to our clinic in secondary or specialist care, but should be actively discussed, planned, and selected at an early stage in trial design. The population enrolled should not be accidental or incidental. Common variances should be con-

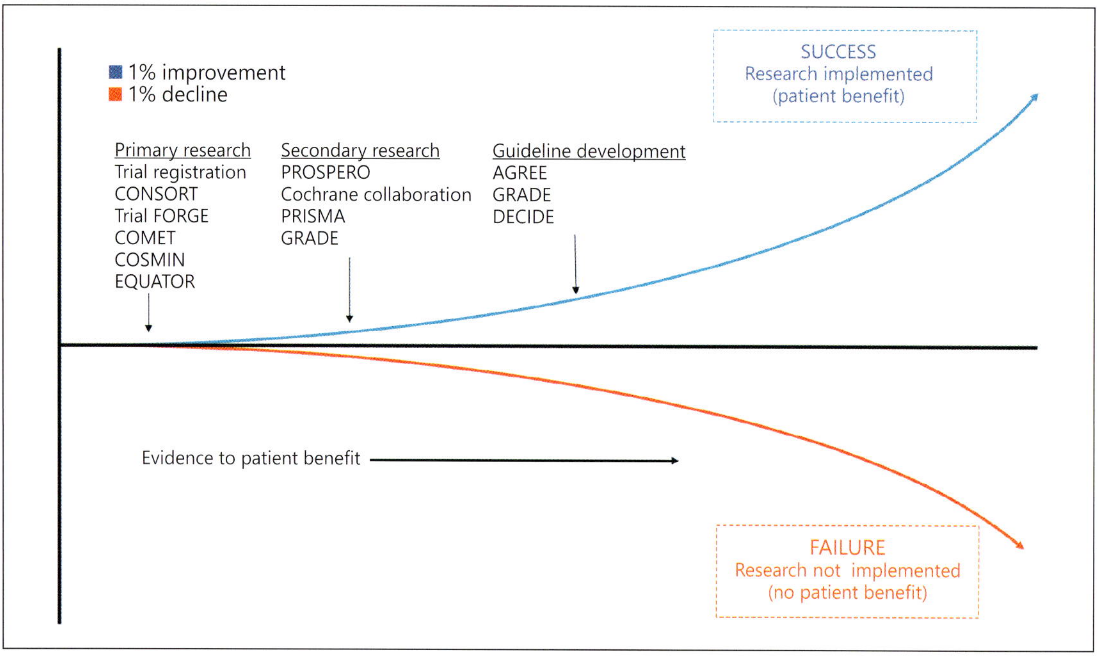

Fig. 2. Aggregation of marginal gains in evidence synthesis (from Innes et al. [1]). Small improvements at the different stages of evidence generation along the pathway of evidence from primary research to guideline development will considerably prevent loss of integrity and improve the quality of the final product.

trolled and the trial conducted within a setting that is relevant. In the UK, this will often mean that trials should be undertaken in a general practice setting, where most treatment is provided.

Make Relevant Comparisons

Trialists should be able to assess where evidence gaps exist. For this purpose, all trials should report their results, regardless of whether they yield a publication in a scientific journal or not. This will help to avoid unnecessary reproduction of trials by informing trialists where there might be evidence of an absence of effect rather than lack of evidence. To ensure this, all clinical trials should be registered before they are conducted and all results should be properly reported. Clinical Trials (http://www.clinicaltrials.gov) and AllTrials (http://www.alltrials.net/) are organisations where clinical trials can be registered to ensure the publication of all study results (Table 1).

Measure Important Outcomes

The outcomes chosen in a trial should be relevant for clinical or policy decisions [22]. That is, they should reflect questions that a patient, clinician, or funder would ask. For example, a patient might ask "if I have this treatment, how long will the filling last?" In this case, the outcome would be restoration survival. Another question might be: "will the procedure result in improved function?" In this situation, the outcome might relate to tooth loss or quality of life. Healthcare providers such as the NHS or medical insurance providers will also want to know about the economic costs of treatment relative to the effect size.

What is of importance to clinicians and patients with respect to outcome choice is not yet known. To address this problem, core outcome sets (COS) have been developed with input from patients and clinicians. A COS is a set of outcomes which should be measured in every trial of interventions for the prevention or treatment of a given condition. They are not intended to restrict the outcomes measured in a trial as researchers may measure others of interest or relevance in addition to the COS. If every trial comparing interventions for the management of dental caries used the same outcomes (a COS), it would simplify meta-analysis and systematic review. If adopted by publishers as a reporting standard, it would increase the relevance of clinical research and reduce outcome reporting bias. Work is currently being undertaken to generate a COS for caries management trials [23].

Align Research Questions to Clinical Questions
Translational research aims at improving the efficacy of research from the development of novel interventions in laboratory research to application in patients. This ideally results in a dynamic process where clinical questions drive scientific inquiry resulting in an increased understanding of biologic mechanisms of a disease and thus promoting development of new clinical interventions. By evaluating these interventions clinically, new clinical questions arise that drive the scientific process again [2]. To do so, multidisciplinary research teams have to be formed involving laboratory scientists, preclinical and clinical scientists, epidemiologists, and other stakeholders involved in oral health science [24].

Practice-based research networks (PBRN) are another way to connect science with everyday practice. PBRNs are designed to bring together a community of physicians or dentists in order to conduct studies of interest and relevance for patients in a practice setting. The infrastructure of a PBRN is built on a collaboration between academic health science centres and community practitioners [25].

Improve Reporting
After a trial has been concluded, partial reporting in the subsequent manuscript produces difficulties appraising the quality of the trial and extracting relevant outcome data to produce a meta-analysis. To improve reporting, there have been a range of initiatives aimed at standardising trial reports. These differ depending on the type of research being undertaken but can be found on the EQUATOR network website (http://www.equator-network.org/) [26]. For RCTs, the reporting tool of choice is CONSORT (http://www.consort-statement.org/; Table 1) [22]. The CONSORT statement is yet to be endorsed by the majority of dental journals and compliance is thought to be suboptimal in oral health compared with other healthcare areas [27]. Journals that have subscribed to the CONSORT statement should reject papers which do not fully report as per the guidelines. The pressure on authors to provide comprehensive data in the trial report means that these guidelines are considered at the planning stage. This ensures that decisions are made a priori and incorporated into the research protocol at the design stage, improving the quality of the investigation.

References

1 Innes NP, Schwendicke F, Lamont T: How do we create, and improve, the evidence base? Br Dent J 2016;220:651–655.
2 Hart TC, Pihlstrom BL, Tabak LA: Oral health research at the crossroads: translate we must! J Endod 2004;30:684–688.
3 Fabbro MD, Corbella S, Taschieri S: Principles of evidence-based decision-making; in Rosen E, Nemcovsky CE, Tsesis I (eds): Evidence-Based Decision Making in Dentistry. Cham, Springer, 2015, pp 7–18.
4 Carrasco-Labra A, Brignardello-Petersen R, Glick M, Guyatt GH, Azarpazhooh A: A practical approach to evidence-based dentistry: VI: how to use a systematic review. J Am Dent Assoc 2015;146:255–265.e1.

5 Clarkson JE, Turner S, Grimshaw JM, Ramsay CR, Johnston M, Scott A, Bonetti D, Tilley CJ, Maclennan G, Ibbetson R, Macpherson LM, Pitts NB: Changing clinicians' behavior: a randomized controlled trial of fees and education. J Dent Res 2008;87:640–644.
6 Clarkson JE, Ramsay CR, Eccles MP, Eldridge S, Grimshaw JM, Johnston M, Michie S, Treweek S, Walker A, Young L, Black I, Bonetti D, Cassie H, Francis J, Mackenzie G, Macpherson L, McKee L, Pitts N, Rennie J, Stirling D, Tilley C, Torgerson C, Vale L: The translation research in a dental setting (TRIADS) programme protocol. Implement Sci 2010;5:57.
7 Chalmers I, Bracken MB, Djulbegovic B, Garattini S, Grant J, Gulmezoglu AM, Howells DW, Ioannidis JP, Oliver S: How to increase value and reduce waste when research priorities are set. Lancet 2014;383:156–165.
8 Chan AW, Song F, Vickers A, Jefferson T, Dickersin K, Gotzsche PC, Krumholz HM, Ghersi D, van der Worp HB: Increasing value and reducing waste: addressing inaccessible research. Lancet 2014;383:257–266.
9 Glasziou P, Altman DG, Bossuyt P, Boutron I, Clarke M, Julious S, Michie S, Moher D, Wager E: Reducing waste from incomplete or unusable reports of biomedical research. Lancet 2014;383: 267–276.
10 Ioannidis JP, Greenland S, Hlatky MA, Khoury MJ, Macleod MR, Moher D, Schulz KF, Tibshirani R: Increasing value and reducing waste in research design, conduct, and analysis. Lancet 2014; 383:166–175.
11 Al-Shahi Salman R, Beller E, Kagan J, Hemminki E, Phillips RS, Savulescu J, Macleod M, Wisely J, Chalmers I: Increasing value and reducing waste in biomedical research regulation and management. Lancet 2014;383:176–185.
12 Lamont T, Schwendicke F, Innes N: Why we need a core outcome set for trials of interventions for prevention and management of caries. Evid Based Dent 2015;16:66–68.
13 Pitts NB, Stamm JW: International consensus workshop on caries clinical trials (ICW-CCT) – final consensus statements: agreeing where the evidence leads. J Dent Res 2004;83:125–128.
14 Schwendicke F, Blunck U, Paris S, Gostemeyer G: Choice of comparator in restorative trials: a network analysis. Dent Mater 2015;31:1502–1509.
15 Schwendicke F, Innes N, Levey C, Lamont T, Gostemeyer G: Comparator choice in cariology trials limits conclusions on the comparative effectiveness of caries interventions. J Clin Epidemiol 2017;89:209–217.
16 Levey C, Innes N, Schwendicke F, Lamont T, Gostemeyer G: Outcomes in randomised controlled trials in prevention and management of carious lesions: a systematic review. Trials 2017;18:515.
17 Easterbrook PJ, Gopalan R, Berlin JA, Matthews DR: Publication bias in clinical research. Lancet 1991;337:867–872.
18 Ioannidis JPA, Caplan AL, Dal-Ré R: Outcome reporting bias in clinical trials: why monitoring matters. BMJ 2017; 356:j408.
19 Rothwell PM: External validity of randomised controlled trials: "to whom do the results of this trial apply?" Lancet 2005;365:82–93.
20 Schwendicke F, Opdam N: Clinical studies in restorative dentistry: design, conduct, analysis. Dent Mater 2018;34:29–39.
21 Gostemeyer G, Blunck U, Paris S, Schwendicke F: Design and validity of randomized controlled dental restorative trials. Materials (Basel) 2016; 9:E372.
22 Moher D, Hopewell S, Schulz KF, Montori V, Gotzsche PC, Devereaux PJ, Elbourne D, Egger M, Altman DG: Consort 2010 Explanation and elaboration: updated guidelines for reporting parallel group randomised trials. BMJ 2010; 340:c869.
23 Schwendicke F, Lamont T, Innes N: Outcomes in trials for management of caries lesions (OUTMAC): protocol. Trials 2015;16:397.
24 Giannobile WV, Joskow RW: Clinical and translational oral health research: prospects for the future. J Dent Res 2012;91:633–636.
25 Curro FA, Vena D, Naftolin F, Terracio L, Thompson VP: The PBRN initiative: transforming new technologies to improve patient care. J Dent Res 2012;91: 12S–20S.
26 Dos Santos VE Jr, Filho AV, Ribeiro Targino AG, Pelagio Flores MA, Galembeck A, Caldas AF Jr, Rosenblatt A: A new "silver-bullet" to treat caries in children – nano silver fluoride: a randomised clinical trial. J Dent 2014;42: 945–951.
27 Sarkis-Onofre R, Poletto-Neto V, Cenci MS, Pereira-Cenci T, Moher D: Impact of the consort statement endorsement in the completeness of reporting of randomized clinical trials in restorative dentistry. J Dent 2017;58:54–59.

Gerd Göstemeyer
Charité Centre for Dental Medicine, Department for Operative and Preventive Dentistry
Assmannshauser Strasse 4-6
DE–14197 Berlin (Germany)
E-Mail gerd.goestemeyer@charite.de

Schwendicke F, Frencken J, Innes N (eds): Caries Excavation: Evolution of Treating Cavitated Carious Lesions.
Monogr Oral Sci. Basel, Karger, 2018, vol 27, pp 155–161 (DOI: 10.1159/000487842)

An Agreed Terminology for Carious Tissue Removal

Nicola Innes[a] · Falk Schwendicke[b] · Jo Frencken[c]

[a]School of Dentistry, University of Dundee, Dundee, UK; [b]Operative and Preventive Dentistry, Charité – Universitätsmedizin Berlin, Corporate Member of Freie Universität Berlin, Humboldt-Universität zu Berlin, and Berlin Institute of Health, Berlin, Germany; [c]Department of Oral Function and Prosthetic Dentistry, College of Dental Sciences, Radboud University Medical Center, Nijmegen, The Netherlands

Abstract

Understanding the carious process as a biofilm disease rather than an infectious disease has changed lesion management focus towards less invasive options. This has led to new and ongoing changes in recommendations for practitioners. However, the lack of clarity over what to do, and when, is complicated by different teaching, research, and policy documents containing different terms and definitions for carious lesions and management strategies. Lack of clear messages and communication over recommendations hampers moving evidence into practice. The International Caries Consensus Collaboration (ICCC) recommendations on terminology are one part of improving communication for discussing the diagnosis and management of dental caries and dental carious lesions. The term dental caries is the name of the disease, its use being limited to situations involving control of the disease using preventive and non-invasive measures at the patient level. Carious lesion management should be used where management is directly related to disease symptoms at the tooth level. As terminology cannot be used to directly relate the visual appearance of the carious lesion to the histopathology, the terms have been based around the clinical consequences of the disease: soft, leathery, firm and hard dentine. The 3 main carious tissue removal options are described as: (1) selective removal of carious tissue (to both soft and firm dentine), (2) stepwise removal, and (3) non-selective removal to hard dentine (previously known as complete removal and no longer recommended). Use of these terms across clinicians, researchers, dental educators, and even with patients, will help improve understanding and communication.

Background to Standardisation in Terminology

Understanding the carious process as a biofilm disease [1] rather than an infectious disease has changed the focus for managing carious lesions towards less invasive and more "sealing in" of lesions. This has led to new and changing recommendations for practitioners to follow when treating patients (and carious lesions) [2]. The recommendations have been developed, and are supported by evidence synthesised from clinical studies [3–5]. However, their implementation is complicated by the use of different terms describing the lesions and the same management strategies.

Making the shift from producing evidence to actually getting it used in practice is known to be difficult, as is discussed in detail in the chapter by Doméjean and Grosgogeat [this vol., pp. 137–145]. This process of translating knowledge to action is complicated by inconsistencies in clinical guidelines across dentistry, both among professional groups and dental educationalists. The guidelines often rely on outdated concepts, national healthcare policies, and are known to be influenced by local remuneration systems [6]. In addition, different terms for carious lesions, their presentation, and management strategies are used across teaching, research, and policy documents. Lack of consistent, clear messages and effective communication over recommendations hampers moving evidence into practice.

The International Caries Consensus Collaboration (ICCC) consensus process developed recommendations on terminology for carious tissue removal and managing cavitated carious lesions [7]. Standardising this terminology is one part of improving communication within the profession for discussing the diagnosis and management of dental caries and dental carious lesions.

Updating the Existing Terminology

In a systematic search for terminology describing carious tissue removal techniques, 23 different terms were found and a further 19 unique terms noted to being used by researchers, giving a total of 42 unique terms to describe 4 different carious lesion removal/management strategies (Innes terminology document). The ICCC group gathered and, through consensus [8], came up with definitions for dental caries/carious lesions where there was some confusion identified in the literature, terms for the stages of carious tissue removal, and terms for describing different carious management/removal strategies [9, 10].

Dental Caries Management and Carious Lesion Management

The term dental caries has historically been used synonymously as the name of the disease and the specific pathology seen at the tooth level. This meant that the patient would be described as suffering from dental caries and the tooth would also be described as having dental caries. However, the ICCC recommended that use of the term dental caries is limited to situations involving control of the disease using preventive and non-invasive measures at the patient level. The more accurate term, carious lesion, should be used where the management is directly related to the disease manifestation/symptoms at the tooth level, i.e., this should be referred to as managing the carious lesion.

Terminology for Descriptions of States of Carious Dentine

As terminology cannot be used to directly relate the visual appearance of the carious lesion to the histopathology, the terms have been based around the clinical consequences of the disease. Hard dentine requires a pushing force "with a hard instrument to engage the dentine, and only a sharp cutting edge or a burr will lift it. A scratchy sound or 'cri dentinaire' can be heard when a straight probe is taken across the dentine." Firm dentine is physically resistant to hand excavation, and "some pressure needs to be exerted through an instrument to lift it." Leathery dentine "does not deform when an instrument is pressed onto it but can still be easily lifted without much force being required. There may be little difference between leathery and firm dentine, with leathery being a transition on the spectrum between soft and firm dentine." Soft dentine will deform when a hard instrument is "pressed onto it and can be easily scooped up (e.g., with a sharp hand excavator) with little force being required." The definitions of these different clinical presentations of dentine affected by carious lesions are taken from the original ICCC terminology document [7].

Carious Tissue Removal Terminology

The 3 main carious tissue removal options are described as: (1) selective removal of carious tissue (to both soft and firm dentine), (2) stepwise removal, and (3) non-selective removal to hard dentine (previously known as complete removal and no longer recommended) with "soft," "firm," and "hard" as described above. However, we can make a comprehensive list of types of tissue removal by expanding this and group them under the following headings: atraumatic restorative treatment; no removal (which includes fissure sealants, the Hall Technique, and non-restorative cavity control; NRCC); selective removal to soft dentine; selective removal to firm dentine, and stepwise removal and non-selective removal. Table 1 (reproduced from the ICCC terminology document) details their previous names and provides descriptions of them and the indications for each technique to be used where there are non-cleansable dentine carious lesions.

Atraumatic Restorative Treatment

Atraumatic Restorative Treatment (ART) is a specific technique for carious lesion management using hand instruments only. Pulpally, excavation is carried out by removing demineralised enamel and soft dentine until firm dentine is felt in shallow/medium-sized lesions (or to the depth that will allow enough bulk of glass-ionomer to be placed) and until soft dentine is felt in deeper lesions. The cavity is restored usually with a high-viscosity glass-ionomer cement or other adhesive material and exposed pits and fissures are sealed. For lesions that reach the inner half of dentine (radiographically) soft carious tissue should be left on the pulpal wall to avoid pulp exposure. The decision between carrying out selective removal to firm dentine or to soft dentine depends on the extent of the lesion, the resulting cavity depth, and the possibility of pulp exposure. ART is suitable for primary and permanent teeth and has a large evidence base around it [see the chapter by Leal et al.; this vol., pp. 92–102].

No Removal (No Dentinal Carious Tissue Removal)

There are a variety of procedures where no dentinal carious tissue removal is carried out. Sealing includes: (1) fissure sealants (therapeutic), (2) the Hall Technique, and (3) NRCC. Despite being a diverse group of procedures, they have the same aim – to control the carious lesion without removing any diseased dentinal tissue.

Resin or glass-ionomer sealants (usually high viscosity) can be used to seal over pit and fissure enamel and dentine carious lesions. However, as described in the chapter by Fontana and Innes [this vol., pp. 103–112], care has to be taken in deciding when to place them and when it may be more appropriate to carry out a selective removal procedure. Although there is evidence to support placing sealants over carious lesions, there is a lack of evidence around how deep a lesion can be sealed and still be assured of success, especially for deeper lesions. The materials have limited abilities to resist forces occlusally. They are suitable for primary and permanent teeth with shallow and moderate carious lesions that appear

Table 1. Overview of carious tissue removal terminology and groupings (reproduced from the ADR Terminology Group) . From Innes et al. [7]. Reprinted by Permission of SAGE Publications, Inc.

Type of carious tissue removal	Previous names/ further details	Short description	Indications for non-cleansable dentinal carious lesions
Atraumatic restorative treatment (ART)	A specific technique for carious lesion management using hand instruments only	Carious tissue removal using hand instruments only Pulpally: excavate to firm dentine in shallow lesions and to soft dentine in deep lesions Restore cavity and seal available pits and fissures with adhesive dental material, usually a high-viscosity glass-ionomer cement	**Primary and permanent teeth** Shallow and moderate[1] dentine carious lesions to allow adequate depth for a durable restoration
No removal		No dentine carious tissue removal	
Fissure sealant including "ART sealants" (therapeutic)		Fissure sealants: place sealants (resins) or glass-ionomer cement over clinically intact enamel or enamel with signs of early breakdown; this can also be suitable where there is a microcavitation but the material is considered to have adequate mechanical properties to bridge any enamel breaches	**Primary and permanent teeth** Shallow and moderate[1] carious lesions that appear non-cavitated clinically, radiographically they might extend into dentine
Hall Technique		Preformed (stainless-steel) crown is cemented over the primary molar tooth to seal dentinal carious lesions	**Primary teeth** Moderate[1] and deep[2] non-cavitated and cavitated aproximal carious lesions **Permanent teeth** Not indicated
Non-restorative cavity control (NRCC)	Non-restorative caries treatment, non-operative caries treatment and prevention, slicing technique	Cavitated dentinal carious lesions are transformed to cleansable forms that can be cleaned by the patient or parent/carer with a toothbrush May or may not be supported by regular fluoride varnish application or placement of glass-ionomer-based material	**Primary and permanent teeth** Cavitated dentine carious lesions that can be made cleansable; might not be restorable (for permanent teeth, might also be suitable for root surface carious lesions)
Selective removal to soft dentine	Partial, incomplete, minimally invasive, or ultraconservative caries removal	Pulpally: remove carious tissue until soft dentine is reached Enough tissue is removed to place a durable restoration avoiding pulp exposure Periphery of cavity: clean to hard dentine (similar to sound dentine)	**Primary and permanent teeth** Deep carious lesions[2]
Selective removal to firm dentine	Partial caries removal, minimally invasive or incomplete caries removal	Pulpally: remove carious tissue until leathery or firm dentine (resistant to hand excavator) is reached Periphery of cavity: clean to hard dentine (similar to sound dentine)	**Primary and permanent teeth** Shallow and moderate dentinal carious lesions[1] to allow adequate depth for a durable restoration

Table 1. Continued

Type of carious tissue removal	Previous names/ further details	Short description	Indications for non-cleansable dentinal carious lesions
Stepwise removal	Stepwise caries removal, stepwise excavation, 2-step caries removal	Pulpally: selective removal to soft dentine during 1st step – remove carious tissue until soft dentine is reached Enough tissue is removed to place a durable restoration avoiding pulp exposure Periphery of cavity: clean until hard dentine is reached (similar to sound dentine) *Subsequently (6–12 months)* Pulpally: selective removal to firm dentine and place a long-term restoration	**Primary teeth** Not indicated – use selective removal to soft dentine **Permanent teeth** Deep carious lesions[2]
Non-selective to hard dentine (not advocated)	Complete caries removal	Pulpally and cavity periphery: carious tissue removal aims to remove all demineralised dentine to reach hard dentine, leaving no softened dentine Considered overtreatment	**Primary and permanent teeth** Not advocated

[1] Shallow and moderate lesions involving the outer pulpal two thirds or three quarters of dentine radiographically, or where there is no risk of pulp exposure.
[2] Deep lesions are those defined as radiographically involving the inner pulpal third or quarter of dentine, or with clinically assessed risk of pulpal exposure.

non-cavitated clinically, and radiographically are not too extensive in dentine either in depth or volume of lesion.

The Hall Technique [as described in the chapter by Santamaria and Innes, this vol., pp. 113–122] is a specific procedure suitable only for primary molars, where a preformed metal (stainless-steel) crown is used to seal dentinal carious lesions by cementing the crown using glass-ionomer cement onto the tooth with no tooth preparation or carious lesion removal. The crown is used to seal the dentinal carious lesion and slow down or prevent its progression to the dental pulp. This allows a carious primary molar to exfoliate without pain or infection. The Hall Technique is usually indicated for approximal lesions where there is still a radiographically visible band of dentine between the carious lesion and the dental pulp.

NRCC used to be known as non-operative caries treatment and prevention (NOCTP), non-restorative caries treatment (NRCT), and slicing preparations. These make up a group of techniques that aim to arrest carious lesions using a package of care involving caries management at the level of the patient. By creating a cleanable cavity (sometimes this involves altering the shape of the cavity through operative although not restorative intervention) and putting a successful preventive regimen in place, they aim to prevent further loss of tooth tissue through carious lesion progression. The regimen includes plaque removal through toothbrushing with a fluoridated toothpaste and/or application of fluoride varnish. NRCC is most commonly used for primary teeth but also has a role in the management of root surface carious lesions.

Selective Removal

Selective removal of carious dentine used to be known as partial, incomplete, minimally invasive, or ultraconservative carious tissue removal. However, these terms all focus on the end result of the carious tissue removal process. The new terms, selective removal to soft, leathery, or firm dentine, shift the focus to what is being carried out rather than the aim of the procedure. Selective removal uses different excavation criteria for the cavity walls (periphery of the cavity) where the aim is to have "sound" enamel to allow the best adhesive seal, using an adhesive material, to be achieved. The peripheral dentine should also be hard and should give the feel of hard dentine – a scratching noise if a sharp hand excavator is dragged across it. For deep lesions (extending beyond the inner, pulpal, third or quarter of the dentine radiographically), carious tissue removal should be selective removal to soft dentine (the main aim is to avoid exposure and irritation of the dental pulp), provided that there are no clinical symptoms of pulp inflammation present. Soft dentine will deform when an instrument is pressed onto it and little force would be required to lift it.

For less deep lesions, selective removal should take place to leathery or firm dentine pulpally (physically resistant to a hand excavator) in the pulpal aspect of the cavity. This is likely to be necessary to allow adequate depth for the restorative material bulk.

Although somewhat subjective, the tactile sense of dentine softness and hardness is probably the best guide that can be given as there is a lack of easily available or reliable diagnostic tools for this purpose.

Stepwise Removal (Stepwise Carious Lesion Removal)

Stepwise removal, or stepwise carious lesion removal, was agreed by the ICCC group to be a well-known and accepted term with less variability in its definition and understanding. As such, it was considered better to accept this as standard with just a clear and unambiguous explanation of the definition behind it. Stepwise removal involves "selective removal to soft dentine" at stage 1, followed 6–12 months later by "selective removal to firm dentine" for stage 2. This technique was previously also known as "2-step excavation." It is no longer recommended for primary teeth as selective removal to soft dentine would normally be carried out and a permanent restoration placed. The teeth have a limited lifespan and there is no demonstrable advantage to using a stepwise approach. Stepwise removal is indicated for deep carious lesions.

Non-Selective Removal

Non-selective removal to hard dentine was previously known as "complete excavation" or "complete removal." It is the approach to carious tissue removal that was accepted in the past and is now considered overtreatment. It is no longer recommended and is only mentioned here for completeness. The aim was to remove soft carious tissue to reach hard dentine resembling healthy dentine in all parts of the cavity, including pulpally.

Conclusion

It is difficult to change custom and habit as terms around dentistry, dental caries, and managing carious lesions have been in place for many decades and even a century in some cases. However, by standardising the use of these terms across the profession, clinicians, researchers, and dental educators will help improve understanding and communication. This, in turn, should help reduce some of the barriers we face in improving the standard of care for our patients by putting new evidence and effective practices into day-to-day clinical use.

References

1 Marsh PD: Dental plaque as a biofilm and a microbial community – implications for health and disease. BMC Oral Health 2006;6(suppl 1):S14.
2 Schwendicke F, Frencken JE, Bjørndal L, Maltz M, Manton DJ, Ricketts D, van Landuyt K, Banerjee A, Campus G, Domejean S, Fontana M, Leal S, Machiulskiene V, Schulte A, Splieth C, Zandona A, Innes NP: Managing carious lesions: consensus recommendations on carious tissue removal. Adv Dent Res 2016;28:58–67.
3 Ricketts D, Lamont T, Innes NP, Kidd E, Clarkson JE: Operative caries management in adults and children. Cochrane Database Syst Rev 2013:CD003808.
4 Schwendicke F, Meyer-Lueckel H, Dorfer C, Paris S: Failure of incompletely excavated teeth – a systematic review. J Dent 2013;41:569–580.
5 Schwendicke F, Dorfer CE, Paris S: Incomplete caries removal: a systematic review and meta-analysis. J Dent Res 2013;92:306–314.
6 Banerjee A: 'MI'opia or 20/20 vision? Br Dent J 2013;214:101–105.
7 Innes NP, Frencken JE, Bjorndal L, Maltz M, Manton DJ, Ricketts D, van Landuyt K, Banerjee A, Campus G, Domejean S, Fontana M, Leal S, Machiulskiene V, Schulte A, Splieth C, Zandona A, Schwendicke F: Managing carious lesions: consensus recommendations on terminology. Adv Dent Res 2016;28:49–57.
8 Frencken JE, Innes NP, Schwendicke F: Managing carious lesions: why do we need consensus on terminology and clinical recommendations on carious tissue removal? Adv Dent Res 2016;28:46–48.
9 Banerjee A, Kidd EA, Watson TF: In vitro evaluation of five alternative methods of carious dentine excavation. Caries Res 2000;34:144–150.
10 de Almeida Neves A, Coutinho E, Cardoso MV, Lambrechts P, van Meerbeek B: Current concepts and techniques for caries excavation and adhesion to residual dentin. J Adhes Dent 2011;13:7–22.

Nicola Innes
School of Dentistry, University of Dundee
2 Park Place
Dundee DD1 4HR (UK)
E-Mail n.p.innes@dundee.ac.uk

Schwendicke F, Frencken J, Innes N (eds): Caries Excavation: Evolution of Treating Cavitated Carious Lesions.
Monogr Oral Sci. Basel, Karger, 2018, vol 27, pp 162–166 (DOI: 10.1159/000487843)

Clinical Recommendations on Carious Tissue Removal in Cavitated Lesions

Falk Schwendicke[a] • Jo Frencken[b] • Nicola Innes[c]

[a]Department of Operative and Preventive Dentistry, Charité – Universitätsmedizin Berlin, Corporate Member of Freie Universität Berlin, Humboldt-Universität zu Berlin, and Berlin Institute of Health, Berlin, Germany; [b]Department of Oral Function and Prosthetic Dentistry, College of Dental Sciences, Radboud University Medical Center, Nijmegen, The Netherlands; [c]School of Dentistry, University of Dundee, Dundee, UK

Abstract

Non-cleansable carious lesions where sealing is no longer an option should be restored in the vast majority of cases. Prior to restoring the cavity, carious tissue removal is performed, mainly to increase the longevity of the restoration. Such removal, however, should not be conducted in a way that the vital pulp is harmed. This means that in teeth with shallow or moderately deep lesions, selective removal to firm dentine is recommended, while in deep lesions (radiographically extending into the pulpal third or quarter of the dentine) selective removal to soft dentine should be performed. In permanent teeth, stepwise removal is a possible alternative, while in primary teeth the Hall Technique can be considered, too. To assess carious tissue removal, the hardness of the dentine should be the primary criterion. Moisture, colour, and additional parameters (like fluorescence of bacterial porphyrins, etc.) might be used, but should be critically evaluated towards their validity and patients' benefit. There is insufficient evidence to recommend a specific single carious tissue removal method. However, hand or chemomechanical excavation seem useful, as they reduce pain and discomfort during treatment. Current evidence also does not support any specific restoration material or (bonding) strategy for restoring cavities resulting from different carious tissue removal strategies. Prior to restoring the cavity, cavity disinfection is not recommended any longer.

As previously discussed, a changing understanding of dental caries has led to new therapeutic approaches. Dental caries results from an ecologic shift within the dental biofilm, with acidogenic, aciduric, and cariogenic bacteria being highly competitive and eventually dominating the biofilm where there is a frequent supply of fermentable dietary carbohydrates; creating conditions that allow them to flourish. This also leads to a shift in the biofilm activity, with long-lasting periods of acidity and net mineral loss from the dental hard tissues, the result being a carious lesion.

The traditional view of caries being an infectious disease where the treatment approach required removal of all bacteria and affected tissue from the cavity therefore no longer applies. Alternative therapies, involving controlling caries-causing factors (carbohydrate restriction, biofilm removal) or re-establishing the balance between re- and demineralisation (fluorides and other remineralisation strategies, or placing sealants) are thus the cornerstone of "caries management," as they allow the "inactivation/control of the disease process, preservation of dental hard tissue, avoidance of initiating the cycle of re-restorations, and preservation of the tooth for as long as possible" [1].

However, once the lesion becomes cavitated it is usually no longer cleansable and so prevention is no longer effective in controlling and arresting the lesion. However, if the lesion is cleansable or made cleansable, there is some evidence that in primary teeth the carious process can be halted. The success percentages reported for these approaches vary widely, ranging from 89 [2] to 71 [3], 50 [4] and 45% [5] after 2–3.5 years.

For non-cleansable cavities, restorative approaches, reproducing the surface integrity, are usually needed. The same might apply to occlusal lesions that do not show frank cavitation, but show radiographic evidence of lesion extension into dentine. These lesions are sometimes known as "microcavitated," although the exact definition of this term is contested. Some have used a small excavator or a CPITN probe for measuring the orifice of the cavity, others consider a "microcavitated" lesion as not visually detectable but where there is evidence on a radiograph of a carious lesion extending into dentine, while others call a lesion without frank cavitation microcavitated. There is some evidence of success for sealing these small dentinal lesions in occlusal pits and fissures as another option for controlling the caries process [6–8].

Whilst the background pathophysiological evidence would show clearly that sealing can slow/stop the progression of lesions, the clinical evidence shows mixed success. This seems to depend on the particular lesions sealed (how large the cavitation is or perhaps how extensive the dentine lesion has become) although it may be to do with the quality of the bond and the lack of mechanical strength and limited fracture resistance of unfilled or low-filled resin sealant materials used. Fissure sealant materials wear and fracture and need to be replaced and "topped up," thus needing continual observation to maintain the seal. Further investigations are needed to pinpoint the exact factors that predict success/failure. There is no evidence on which to base recommendations on the size of lesion that can be sealed or the best sealant material.

Before placing restorations, dentists have conventionally removed all carious tissue from the cavity. As previously discussed, the historical reasons for this step (creating undercuts for macro-retentive materials, removal of bacteria, and removal of demineralised dentine) no longer provide a justification for complete removal of all carious tissue. The main factor that dictates the amount of carious tooth tissue to be removed is the depth of cavity required for the restorative material to have bulk to last or an adequate bonding area.

Based on the available evidence, the International Caries Consensus Cooperation (ICCC) has agreed on a number of guiding principles for carious tissue removal [1]:

- "preserve non-demineralised and remineralisable tissue;
- achieve an adequate seal by placing the peripheral restoration onto sound dentine and/or enamel, thus controlling the lesion and inactivating remaining bacteria;
- avoid discomfort/pain and dental anxiety as both impact significantly on treatment/care planning and outcomes – methods that are less likely to lead to dental anxiety are preferable;
- maintain pulpal health by preserving residual dentine (avoiding unnecessary pulpal irritation/insult) and preventing pulp exposure, i.e.,

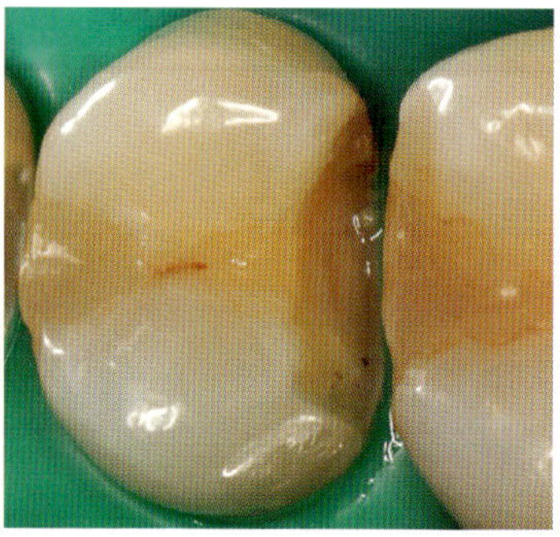

Fig. 1. Non-selective removal to hard dentine.

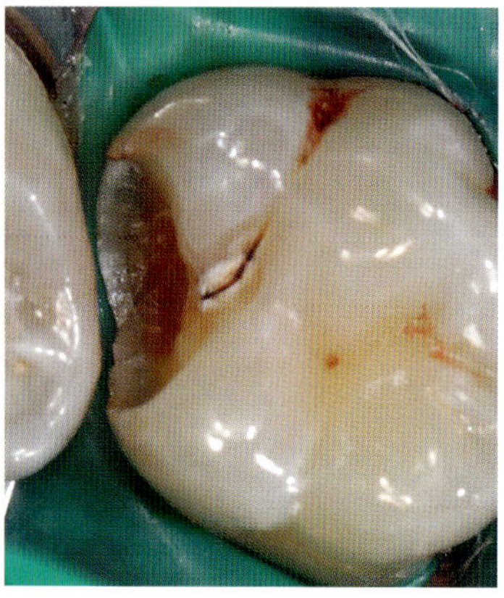

Fig. 2. Selective removal to firm dentine.

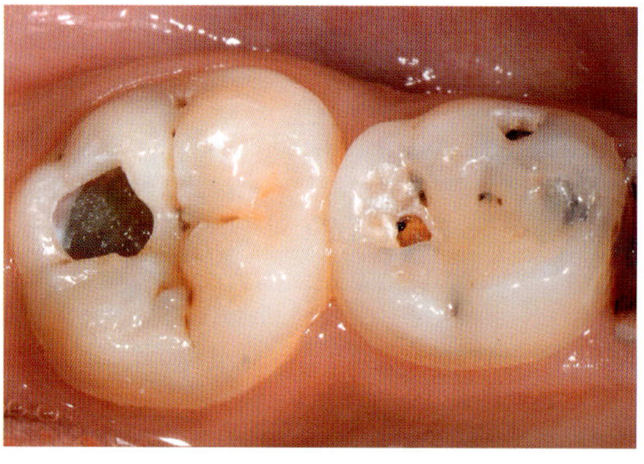

Fig. 3. Selective removal to soft dentine in both molars. With permission from the copyright holder, Prof. S. Leal, Brasília.

leave soft dentine in proximity to the pulp if required;

- maximise the longevity of the restoration by removing enough soft dentine to place a durable restoration of sufficient bulk and resilience."

There is conflict between the last 2 aims – maintaining pulpal health and maximising restoration longevity – but they carry different levels of importance for different lesions. In deep lesions in teeth with vital pulps, pulpal health is the priority, while in shallow or moderately deep lesions restoration survival becomes more important. Based on this, dentists can now choose between different carious tissue removal strategies:

- Non-selective removal to hard dentine removes all carious dentine from the cavity until the dentine is hard everywhere (Fig. 1). This is no longer recommended.
- Selective removal to firm dentine removes until firm dentine is felt. This gives a feeling of resistance to a hand excavator, centrally. The cavity margins are cleaned until hard (scratchy; Fig. 2). This is recommended for shallow or moderately deep cavitated lesions in both dentitions.
- Selective removal to soft dentine leaves soft dentine in proximity to the pulp, avoiding exposure, while hard dentine is left peripherally (Fig. 3). This is recommended in deep cavitated lesions.
- Stepwise removal is carious tissue removal in 2 stages (visits), with soft carious tissue being left over the pulp in the first step. This is then sealed using a provisional restoration which should be durable enough to last at least 1 year given that patients might not come back earlier. In a second step, the restoration is removed and carious tissue removal continued until "leathery" dentine remains over the pulp. This technique is an alternative to selective removal to soft dentine in permanent teeth, but given the additional treatment needs is not recommended for primary teeth any longer.

To assess carious tissue removal, hardness of the dentine should be the primary criterion. Moisture, colour, and additional parameters (like fluorescence of bacterial porphyrins, etc.) might be used, but should be critically evaluated towards their validity and patients' benefit.

With regards to how to remove carious tissue, there is insufficient evidence to recommend any single method. Hand or chemomechanical excavation seem possibly useful, as they reduce pain and discomfort during treatment, which is beneficial especially in children and anxious adults.

The resulting cavity can then be restored using conventional means. Current evidence does not support any specific material or (bonding) strategy for restoring cavities resulting from different carious tissue removal strategies. Prior to restoring the cavity, cavity disinfection is no longer recommended and treatments for inactivating dentine matrix metalloproteinase or to remineralise the dentine have so far no evidence of clinical effectiveness.

The recommendations presented here are in line with those from a recent international consensus meeting. These are summarised in the Appendix.

Appendix

Recommendations, taken from the consensus document of the ICCC 2015 [1]:

"1 Preventing carious lesions from occurring means managing the disease dental caries. For existing carious lesions, dentists should work with the patient to manage the disease and as a consequence to control the lesion activity, i.e., aiming for lesion arrest/inactivation, to preserve dental hard tissues, avoid initiation of the restorative cycle [9, 10], and retain the tooth for as long as possible (strong recommendation).

2 When carious lesions are non-cleansable and sealing is no longer an option, restorative interventions are indicated (strong recommendation).

3 Restorative treatments are carried out to aid biofilm control, protect the pulp-dentine complex, and restore the function, form, and aesthetics of the tooth, whilst causing no unnecessary harm. The carious tissue removal stage aims to create conditions for a long-lasting restoration, preserve healthy and remineralisable tissue, achieve a sufficient seal, maintain pulpal health, and maximise success of the restoration. However, this does not necessarily mean that close to the pulp all bacterially contaminated or demineralised tissues need to be removed (strong recommendation).

4 In deeper lesions in teeth with still sensible (vital) pulps, preserving pulpal health should be prioritised over restoration success, whilst in shallow or moderately deep lesions, restoration longevity might be the more important factor (strong recommendation).

5 For teeth with shallow or moderately deep lesions, selective removal to firm dentine should be carried out (weak recommendation).

6 In deep lesions (radiographically extending into the pulpal third or quarter of the dentine) in primary and permanent teeth, selective removal to soft dentine should be performed (strong recommendation).

7 In permanent teeth, stepwise removal might also be an option for deep lesions (strong recommendation).

8 Hardness (e.g., soft, leathery, firm or scratchy, or hard) dentine should be the primary criterion for assessing, describing, and reporting on carious tissue and their removal (weak recommendation).

9 Moisture (wet, moist, dry), colour (pale/yellow, dark brown/black), and additional optical characteristics of dentine or measures of different bacterial metabolic products might be useful as additional indicators (weak recommendation).

10 There is insufficient evidence to recommend any single method for carious tissue removal. Hand or chemomechanical excavation might reduce pain and discomfort during treatment and could thus positively impact on dental anxiety, especially when treating children (weak recommendation).

11 Cavity disinfection procedures currently have no evidence of patient benefit to support their use (weak recommendation).

12 Placement of cavity lining materials are not necessary to control the sealed lesion, but might be beneficial in impeding monomer penetration and avoidance of fracture of the remaining dentine when resin composite is the restorative material (weak recommendation).

13 The choice of materials for restoring cavities should be guided by the location and extent of the lesion, the caries risk, carious lesion activity, and the specific patient conditions and setting. There is no definitive evidence to support particular materials as more suitable than others for restoring teeth after selective carious tissue removal to soft or firm dentine (weak recommendation).

14 Retreatment of restorations should aim to repair by resealing, refurbishing, or repolishing where possible and replacement should be a last resort (strong recommendation)."

References

1 Schwendicke F, Frencken JE, Bjorndal L, Maltz M, Manton DJ, Ricketts D, van Landuyt K, Banerjee A, Campus G, Domejean S, Fontana, Leal S, Lo E, Machiulskiene V, Schulte A, Splieth C, Zandona AF, Innes NP: Managing carious lesions: consensus recommendations on carious tissue removal. Adv Dent Res 2016;28:58–67.

2 Mijan M, de Amorim RG, Leal SC, Mulder J, Oliveira L, Creugers NHJ, Frencken JE: The 3.5-year survival rates of primary molars treated according to three treatment protocols: a controlled clinical trial. Clin Oral Investig 2014;18:1061–1069.

3 Santamaría RM, Innes NPT, Machiulskiene V, Schmoeckel J, Alkilzy M, Splieth CH: Alternative caries management options for primary molars: 2.5-year outcomes of a randomised clinical trial. Caries Res 2017;51:605–614.

4 Hansen NV, Nyvad B: Non-operative control of cavitated approximal caries lesions in primary molars: a prospective evaluation of cases. J Oral Rehabil 2017; 44:537–544.

5 Lo EC, Schwarz E, Wong MC: Arresting dentine caries in Chinese preschool children. Int J Paediatr Dent 1998;8:253–260.

6 Griffin SO, Oong E, Kohn W, Vidakovic B, Gooch BF: The effectiveness of sealants in managing caries lesions. J Dent Res 2008;87:169–174.

7 Bakhshandeh A, Qvist V, Ekstrand KR: Sealing occlusal caries lesions in adults referred for restorative treatment: 2–3 years of follow-up. Clin Oral Investig 2012;16:521–529.

8 Hesse D, Bonifácio CC, Mendes FM, Braga MM, Imparato JC, Raggio DP: Sealing versus partial caries removal in primary molars: a randomized clinical trial. BMC Oral Health 2014;28;14:58.

9 Elderton RJ: Overtreatment with restorative dentistry: when to intervene? Int Dent J 1993;43:17–24.

10 Qvist V: Longevity of restorations: the "death spiral"; in Fejerskov O, Kidd EAM (eds): Dental Caries: The Disease and Its Clinical Management. Oxford, Blackwell Munksgaard, 2008, pp 444–455.

Falk Schwendicke
Operative and Preventive Dentistry, Charité – Universitätsmedizin Berlin
Corporate Member of Freie Universität Berlin
Humboldt-Universität zu Berlin, and Berlin Institute of Health
Assmannshauser Strasse 4-6
DE–14197 Berlin (Germany)
E-Mail falk.schwendicke@charite.de

Schwendicke F, Frencken J, Innes N (eds): Caries Excavation: Evolution of Treating Cavitated Carious Lesions.
Monogr Oral Sci. Basel, Karger, 2018, vol 27, pp 167–171 (DOI: 10.1159/000487844)

Caries Excavation: Evidence Gaps

Nicola Innes[a] · Mark Robertson[a] · Falk Schwendicke[b]

[a]School of Dentistry, University of Dundee, Dundee, UK; [b]Operative and Preventive Dentistry, Charité – Universitätsmedizin Berlin, Corporate Member of Freie Universität Berlin, Humboldt-Universität zu Berlin, and Berlin Institute of Health, Berlin, Germany

Abstract

Dental caries, the most common chronic disease in the world, affects over 3 billion people globally. Its management comprises a large proportion of dental care providers' clinical responsibility, yet despite the extensive evidence base for the management of cavitated carious lesions, gaps in the evidence persist. This promotes uncertainty and debate among providers. This chapter reiterates the 3 key components of evidence-based practice (EBP): clinical expertise, an awareness and appreciation of patient values, and use of best available evidence. Secondly, we give a brief summary of current best evidence pertaining to some key areas of caries excavation in the context of lesion management, and highlight respective gaps in the evidence. Consideration is given to the state of the evidence for: how carious-lesion excavation is best achieved, the extent to which excavation should occur, contemporaneous practice, the timing of dental intervention in relation to the extent of the disease, and some areas of contention. Finally, there is discussion around how dental care providers might proceed when high-quality evidence does not exist to inform that part of the EBP collective.

Currently, the best available evidence supports selective removal of carious tissue being superior to traditional, complete removal techniques, although the respective benefits of 1- and 2-stage removal remains contested. Furthermore, there are evidence gaps around dentistry for the ageing population and why clinicians display continued reluctance to adopt minimally interventive approaches to carious-lesion management. This chapter identifies the areas where the focus of future studies should be targeted to further inform the evidence base.

Evidence-Based Practice

This book has tried to take a research-based, hence evidence-focused, approach to discussing carious-lesion excavation and the evolution of treating cavitated carious lesions. Understanding the rationale behind approaches to carious-lesion excavation, and the evidence to support different strategies in different cases, should lead to consistent implementation of evidence-based practice (EBP). However, it is worth remembering that EBP, by definition [1], not only comprises the evidence to inform it but encompasses 3 areas:

- best available evidence;
- patient values/preferences; and
- clinical expertise (which also includes the wider clinical environment).

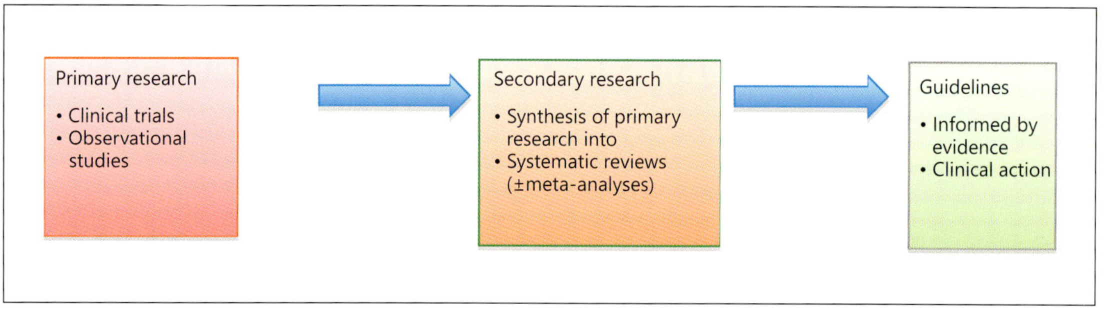

Fig. 1. The flow of evidence.

It is only when these 3 areas of practice are brought together successfully that we can claim we are practicing in an evidence-led way. It is worth noting that the areas of patient values/preferences and clinical expertise are often forgotten [2] or attributed less weight in undergraduate and postgraduate teaching, with the emphasis being on the best available evidence.

For the areas of carious-lesion removal, we need to look at where we have high-quality evidence and make recommendations based on this. To remind ourselves of the process that leads from evidence production to clinical recommendations that we follow in practice, see Figure 1.

Recommendations are ideally formed from evidence presented in high-quality systematic reviews, several of which exist and address caries excavation and sealing in carious lesions. Considering these together gives a picture of the information available for making clinical recommendations around carious lesion excavation and sealing, as well as showing up where the gaps in knowledge are.

How Much Caries Should We Excavate and How Should We Do It?

In their 2013 Cochrane review, Ricketts et al. [3] concluded that, for symptomless primary and permanent teeth, selective caries removal methods (including a stepwise approach) reduce the incidence of pulp exposure and are clinically advantageous over non-selective removal. There was no difference in signs or symptoms of dental pain and/or infection for stepwise removal compared with non-selective removal to hard dentine.

Gaps in the evidence include:

- Differences in success rates between partial and complete caries removal.
- Whether there was a difference in restoration failure for permanent teeth for partial compared with complete caries removal. Although there was less restoration failure for primary teeth, this was likely due to the use of crowns with the Hall Technique in one arm compared to plastic restorative materials in the other arm and preformed crowns consistently outperform plastic restorations in primary teeth for longevity. So there is also likely a gap in the knowledge for primary teeth where plastic restorations are concerned.
- Patient-centred outcomes should be investigated. These were only included in one of the contributing studies on primary teeth in children.
- Short-term follow-up times and high risk of bias were found overall, indicating that further trials need to have longer follow-up periods and be of a high quality.

It should be noted that this is quite an old review and more trials have been published since, although the review is in the process of being updated.

What Do Dentists Do Now?

There is a systematic review [4] and a further study that looks at dentists' behaviour around the management of deep carious lesions [5].

With regard to implementation of the evidence, a systematic review of dentists' behaviour towards adopting selective removal strategies, as reported by Schwendicke and Gostemeyer [4], showed that there are a number of barriers. Only around half of dentists accept the evidence base concerning caries removal.

Gaps in the evidence include:

- Information on what dental practitioners actually do, does not exist.
- Research to give better information on how to overcome the barriers to adoption is needed. This is further discussed in the chapter by Domejéan and Grosgogeat [this vol., pp. 137–145].

A questionnaire-based study by Schwendicke et al. [5] assessed the behaviour and attitudes of dentists in France, Germany, and Norway around the management of deep carious lesions and concluded that less invasive strategies, such as those discussed in this book, have not entered common clinical practice for dentists in general services. There is more information on this in the chapter by Domejéan and Grosgogeat [this vol., pp. 137–145].

Gaps in the evidence include:

- How to disseminate dentists and educate them in carrying out less invasive strategies.

When Do Clinicians Decide to Intervene?

A systematic review of observational studies by Innes and Schwendicke [6] looked at how deep a carious lesion had to be before dentists and dental therapists chose to intervene operatively. The studies included measured what dentists reported they would do in particular clinical situations rather than what they actually did. Despite recommendations that operative intervention should be mainly restricted to lesions that have reached a stage where they cannot be sealed or where a restorative option is required to restore function, aesthetics, or structural integrity, for proximal enamel lesions 21% of dentists/therapists would intervene operatively. For occlusal lesions with enamel discolouration/cavitation but no clinical/radiographic dentinal involvement, 12% stated they would would initiate operative treatment.

Gaps in the evidence include:

- There was a high degree of variability between countries and further understanding of this would help to explain decision making.
- How to implement interventions that translate research evidence into clinical practice.

Other Contentious Areas

There are 2 good examples within the realms of carious-lesion excavation where the wider barriers to adoption of new ideas and techniques can be clearly seen. There has been much debate over the last 20 years for Atraumatic Restorative Treatment (ART) [7, 8] and over the last 10 years for the Hall Technique [9], with both methods for handling carious tooth tissues seemingly polarising views. For ART, there have been a number of changes that have shifted the context within which the evidence is read. There have been improvements in materials and refinement of the technique and a wide evidence base leading to evidence, and therefore treatment recommendations, to support this as a management option that selectively removes carious tissue and is applicable to general dentistry settings for all patients. The evidence to support its use has been set in numerous different environments, from practice to field settings and with clinicians of different skill levels providing that evidence. The chapter on ART by Leal et al. [this vol., pp. 92–102] provides the evidence that shows that ART restorations provide no significantly different results in cavities for which ART is applicable than amalgam and resin composite restorations. Including ART sealants, evidence now runs to around 150 trials/ studies in the Chinese, English, Portuguese, and Spanish languages and has led the AAPD to endorse its use [10], following the World Health Organisation in 1994 and the World Dental Organization (FDI) in 2002. However, there is still opposition by many dental practitioners, and one can ask the questions [11]: do they not know about this evidence, do they know it but cannot change their practice, or simply do not want to change?

Viewpoints on the Hall Technique [described by Santamaria and Innes, this vol., pp. 113–122] are highly polarised among clinicians and the evidence base, now encompassing 4 randomised control trials with consistently high results and a number of observational trials (showing similarly high outcomes) [9], has had to grow to a level where the positive clinical results cannot be refuted, before it has begun to be accepted. In a recent meeting of the AAPD and Irish Paediatric Dental Association (December 2016), there was a debate held to showcase both sides of the argument for and against the Hall Technique. However, the paediatric dentist asked to argue against declined to do so, and stated it that he could not present a cogent argument that would stand up to scrutiny. The Hall Technique has now been included within the AAPD guidelines [10].

It is prudent and in patients' best interests to ensure we do not adopt new techniques, treatments, materials, or diagnostic tools without adequate checks. However, how do we know that there is enough evidence in an area for a new technology to be adopted? This is a very difficult question to answer because evidence, as we have seen in the cases of the Hall Technique and ART, can be produced in different clinical settings and under the delivery of different types and grades of clinicians. On top of this, the material science scene is a changing landscape, with different materials being produced and current ones being updated. The answer to how much evidence is enough has to depend on the question being asked. However, it is important to remember that we should be aware of "waste" within evidence. Waste can either be by not using it when it has been created and by overcreating it unnecessarily after a treatment has been verified as appropriate for use.

What Can We Do When Evidence Is Lacking to Inform Clinical Decision Making and Practice?

- Firstly, whether high-quality evidence is available to support practice or not, the other 2 areas of patient values and preferences and clinical expertise should play a part in determining the ideal course of treatment. However, where there is a lack of evidence to support treatment decisions, these 2 areas should perhaps have a bigger role and more than ever, clinicians must be prepared to have a full discussion with their patients on what the evidence does tell us and where uncertainty lies.
- There is also an opportunity for creating an internal database of evidence within the individual clinician's practice or the practice setting for a group of practitioners. Audit of outcomes within a practice can help to show where outcomes match those expected or where there is a deficit, perhaps related to materials or procedure.
- Clinicians need to keep up to date as evidence changes and be rewarded for following best practice.
- It is also important that primary care and other practitioners are prepared to contribute to building that evidence base by considering taking part in randomised trials.

Conclusion

Overall, it seems that there is strong, consistent evidence that less interventive methods are superior to previous, non-selective to hard tissue carious lesion removal approaches. However, it is still not possible to tell whether 1- or 2-stage carious tissue removal techniques give better outcomes.

There are gaps in the evidence around adults, especially older adults and older teeth, as most studies are carried out on primary teeth or adolescents/young adults. This is likely to be a research- or investigation-induced bias because it is easier to capture data on a population of children and ensure a good follow-up rate by virtue of them being in a school for certain parts of the year and less mobile than adult populations. Another major gap in the evidence is around clinicians' reluctance to adopt minimally invasive approaches to managing carious lesions. In many parts of the world, this approach is contra to the traditional dental school taught approach and, once decision-making paradigms are established, clinicians seem to find it difficult to adapt to new approaches simply through knowledge alone. In common with many other healthcare settings, there is a significant lack of understanding around clinical decision making and the barriers to translating research findings for less invasive options for caries management into clinical practice.

It is considered best practice to adhere to recommendations based on the highest available, contemporaneous evidence. EBP relies on not only the best available evidence, but also successful incorporation of the clinician's expertise and each individual patient's values and preferences into the clinical setting.

References

1 Sackett DL, Rosenberg WM, Gray JA, et al: Evidence based medicine: what it is and what it isn't. 1996. Clin Orthop Relat Res 2007;455:3–5.

2 Tsichlaki A, O'Brien K: Do orthodontic research outcomes reflect patient values? A systematic review of randomized controlled trials involving children. Am J Orthod Dentofacial Orthop 2014;146: 279–285.

3 Ricketts D, Lamont T, Innes NP, et al: Operative caries management in adults and children. Cochrane Database Syst Rev 2013;3:CD003808.

4 Schwendicke F, Gostemeyer G: Understanding dentists' management of deep carious lesions in permanent teeth: a systematic review and meta-analysis. Implement Sci 2016;11:142.

5 Schwendicke F, Stangvaltaite L, Holmgren C, et al: Dentists' attitudes and behaviour regarding deep carious lesion management: a multi-national survey. Clin Oral Investig 2017;21:191–198.

6 Innes NPT, Schwendicke F: Restorative thresholds for carious lesions: systematic review and meta-analysis. J Dent Res 2017;96:501–508.

7 Frencken JE: The state-of-the-art of ART restorations. Dent Update 2014;41:218–220, 222–224.

8 Frencken JE: The state-of-the-art of ART sealants. Dent Update 2014;41:119–120, 122–124.

9 Innes NP, Evans DJ, Bonifacio CC, et al: The Hall technique 10 years on: questions and answers. Br Dent J 2017;222: 478–483.

10 AAPD: Guideline on restorative dentistry. 2016. http://www.aapd.org/media/policies_guidelines/g_restorative1.pdf.

11 Innes NPT, Frencken JE, Schwendicke F: Don't know, can't do, won't change: barriers to moving knowledge to action in managing the carious lesion. J Dent Res 2016;95:485–486.

Mark Robertson
School of Dentistry, University of Dundee
2 Park Place
Dundee DD1 4HR (UK)
E-Mail m.robertson@hotmail.co.uk

Author Index

Subject Index